Dementia Care Programming:
An Identity-Focused Approach

Dementia Care Programming: An Identity-Focused Approach

by Rosemary Dunne

Venture Publishing, Inc. • State College, Pennsylvania

Production Manager: Richard Yocum
Manuscript Editing: Valerie Paukovits, Michele L. Barbin
Additional Editing: Richard Yocum

Library of Congress Catalogue Card Number 2002107737
ISBN 1-892132-35-4

Dedicated to those who care enough to live in and celebrate each moment and each other.

When we hear about compassion, it naturally brings up working with others, caring for others. The reason we're often not there for others—whether for our child or our mother or someone who is insulting us or someone who frightens us—is that we're not there for ourselves. There are whole parts of ourselves that are so unwanted that whenever they begin to come up we run away.

Because we escape, we keep missing being right here, being right on the dot. We keep missing the moment we're in. Yet if we can experience the moment we're in, we discover that it is unique, precious, and completely fresh. It never happens twice. One can appreciate and celebrate each moment—there's nothing more sacred. There's nothing more vast or absolute. In fact, there's nothing more!

—Chödrön (1994, p. 4)

Acknowledgments

My heartfelt gratitude to those who have supported my writing, my passion, and my being, *and* endured my humor.

First, my thanks to Geoff Godbey of Venture Publishing for making the call on a hot August day to discuss the possibility of this work coming to life in a new and exciting format. Thanks to Richard and the Venture team for welcoming my work and bringing it to life as you so graciously have. Special thanks to Michele Barbin and Valerie Paukovits for their tireless editing efforts and queries, for keeping me on track, and for just being fun to work with! Thank you, as well, to Carol Hansen for your patience and input in the reworking of this exciting new text.

Passion is a word that gives me goose bumps. I love language and the power within. There are so many words that influence my life: humor, compassion, responsibility, respect, laughter, dignity, celebration, encouragement, magic, professionalism, passion, tears, laughter, love, patience, support, mentors, friendship and family…did I say laughter? Those people I wish to acknowledge are individuals who at one time or another have found their way into my life and inspired and influenced my being and passions in one way or another through these words and no doubt many others. For this I thank and cherish you.

Professionally, I thank Mary Lucero, Carol Mothersill, Dr. John Tooth, Carol Hansen and so many others whose professionalism, dedication to care from the heart, and thought-provoking dialogue have moved me to action and charged my passion. And to the late Dr. Tom Kitwood, whose path in life I genuinely wish I had crossed, I say thank you for echoing and sounding the battle charge in my heart!

Personally, I thank my friends whose encouragement, support and loyalty have nurtured my own journey into identity and celebration—Alberta and Erin McNamara, Jessica and Jason, the CanGO girls: Karen Schaefer and Shelley Purdon, Dianne Simpson, JoAnne Harrison and Darlene Murphy.

Finally, my family: Mum and Dad; Pat and Sande; Maureen, Gerald, Jack, and Leo; Terry and Abe; Mary Beth, Michael, Annabella, and Samuel. You have given me joy in your love and support. Your humor, reality checks, and individuality make our family a wonderfully colorful quilt with which to warm myself. I am proud to restitch seams and iron wrinkles with you as we grow and experience life's joys and sorrows both together and apart through the years.

May you always have someone to celebrate your unique self and may your life be filled with dignity, respect, and love.

In the spirit of the journey—Rosemary

Table of Contents

List of Figures and Tables xii

Foreword xiii

Preface xv

PART 1
Building a Foundation: The Attitude of Discovery ... 1

The Key to My Heart 3
Creating a Community 5
Rear Admiral Richard 10
Lesson Number One: Never Assume 13
Coping: Needs Response 16
Expressing Reality: Is It Theirs or Ours? 18
Piecing the Puzzle Together 20
In the Moment 23
Nurturing Permissiveness and Safety 26
Tempus Fugit? 29
Defenders of Dignity 31
The Awakening 33
Attitude of Discovery 35

PART 2
Making A Life-Enhancing Difference 37

Understanding and Valuing Individual Identity 39
Celebration of the Self 45
Common Understanding 51
Discovery Kits 56
Stimulating Success 58
Autobiography in a Box 61
Celebrating Life Creatively 62
Family Gold 64
Aggression: Siding with Anger 66
Just the Facts 71
The Bonus Round 75
Great Discovery Challenge: Creating Kits 76
Possibility Thinking: Educating for Action 80

PART 3
Promoting Success through Program Framework... 83

Breaking the Pattern 85
Trouble in Paradise 87
Coming Together: A Framework for Success 92
Repetition Is the Path to Achievement and Success........... 94
The Connection Continuum.. 98
Making Friends Out of FOAs 105
Social Meals Programs and Dining Solutions 108
Creative Problem Solving... 116
At the End of the Day 120
Silence Is Golden 124
A Little Soft Shoe Goes a Long Way 128
Wrap Your Mind Around It 130

PART 4
Sharing the Program Magic................................... 133

Care versus Control 135
Seasonal Scheduling 137
Off-Unit Program Criteria and General Programming Guidelines .. 143

PART 5
Meeting the Challenge 147

Real, Honest, and True 149
Daniel's Journey 150
The Visit 152
Rules of the Game.. 156
Discovering Humanness 158
Journey's End 160

PART 6
A to Z: Programs, Stories, and Content 161

Armchair Travel 163
Arts and Crafts 166
Baking 168
Ball Toss 171
Bean Bag Toss 174
Bowling 176
Bus Outings (GP) 178
Dancing 180
Discovery Kits 182
Entertainment (GP) 184
Exercises 186
Five-Card Bingo (GP) 188
Gardening 190
Group Talks (Spontaneous) 192
Happy Hour (GP) 194
Ice Cream Making 196
Intergenerational Program (GP) 198
Manicures (GP) 200
Pet Visitations 202
Putting (GP) 204
Puzzles 206
Reminiscing 208
Social Teas 210
Stamp Pad Club 212
Theme Parties 215
Walking 217
Word Games 219

References 223

Additional Resources 225

List of Figures and Tables

FIGURE 1
Community Development Cycle/Pyramid and
Maslow's Hierarchy of Needs 7
FIGURE 2
Basic Application of Needs Response: Responding to the
Individual and Unique Needs of the Person 16
FIGURE 3
Personal Fact Sheet 73–74
FIGURE 4
Discovery Kit Advertising Ideas 78–79
FIGURE 5
24-Hour Reverse Clock 80
FIGURE 6
Breaking the Pattern 86
FIGURE 7
Adaption based on the Leisure Ability Model as applied to
dementia care programming interventions 96
FIGURE 8
The Connection Continuum: A Cyclical Model of Approach 99
FIGURE 9
Creative Problem Solving in the Dementia Care Environment 118

TABLE 1
Community Environment versus Individual Environment 5
TABLE 2
Examples of Task Breakdown 30
TABLE 3
Caregiving Behavior: Positive Person Work 43
TABLE 4
Global Deterioration Scale (GDS) 52–53
TABLE 5
Sample Discovery Kits 60
TABLE 6
Categories of Stimuli 70–71
TABLE 7
Potential Programs and Activities 140
TABLE 8
Potential Programs and Activities—Domain Involvement 141

Foreword

Ever-increasing numbers of people with dementia are entering professional care settings and creating a sense of urgency among caregivers. What can we do to help them? How do we ensure that their lives continue to be filled with meaningful relationships, interaction, and activity? How do we get them to accept the care they need but so often refuse? In essence, what do they need from us?

In this book *Dementia Care Programming: An Identity-Focused Approach,* Rosemary Dunne helps us to recognize that there is no single right answer to how we meet the needs of persons with dementia in these professional care settings. Each facility cares for people in different stages of their dementing disease progression. These people come from different cultural, ethnic, and religious backgrounds and have had different life experiences. The common thread that binds these individuals, however, is that their dementia places them on a heart-wrenching, relentless journey—one often filled with frightening obstacles, frustration, and loneliness. This knowledge helps us to understand what our residents need from us. They need, as Ms. Dunne so compassionately points out, for us to join the dementia journey with them—entering their reality, viewing the world from their perspective. They need us to be their guides on this journey; to anticipate what will be required along the way; and to be comforters, encouragers, problem solvers, and validators of their experiences. They need us to help them maintain their connections to themselves, to others, and to the world around them.

How we accomplish this is what identity-focused dementia care programming is all about. It provides a foundation of identity-discovering, dignity-defending, and life-enhancing insights that set us up for success as caregivers. Before we embark on this journey, Ms. Dunne compels us to first examine how we view ourselves as caregivers to persons with dementia. Our perceptions, she points out, will make a tremendous difference in what approaches we use in problem solving to overcome or avoid obstacles; in building trusting, meaningful relationships with our residents; and in enabling our residents to have more joyful moments than fearful ones. They will also influence how we measure our experiences as caregivers and, equally important, how our residents experience our care.

Dementia Care Programming: An Identity-Focused Approach points out how dementia caregiving is filled with opportunities for adventure, nurturing, being nurtured, and creative problem solving—plenty of opportunities to meet difficult challenges. When we are able to meet our residents' needs at particularly trying times, we will also have opportunities to experience that magical "high" that comes from meeting a challenge head-on and succeeding.

Rosemary Dunne also gives us some gentle reminders to listen to our residents' responses to our care with our eyes, hearts, and minds. Perhaps one of the most powerful messages in this book is that when we strive to empathize with our residents' experiences of dementia, we move away from the power struggles that have caused much of their resistance to our care and become more creative and more successful caregivers.

I know that after reading this book you will be filled with excitement and an eagerness to get started testing your new skills. May your travels with your dementia residents enrich your life as well as their lives. Bon voyage!

Mary Lucero
President, Geriatric Resources, Inc.
Las Cruces, New Mexico, USA

Preface

Join their journey...

—Mary Lucero

With all the ups and downs I could link with my father's life, there is one consistent theme: his memorable optimism, generosity, and creativity—each of which formed his identity as seen by all those who loved and knew him. At the time of his death, he was fortunate—his dignity and identity were still intact. It was my father's heart that failed him, not his brain. I speak of my dad with affection and with the intent of creating a connection. All who read this will say "I know someone just like him." The feeling in the heart is light, the memories warm, and the sense of closeness is strong. However, this state of intactness or wellness is not the state lived by all. For some who read this they may say, "My dad *was* like yours but not anymore...he's gone, he has dementia." This may be so from a pathophysiological perspective, but the good news is that Dad, Mom, spouses, friends and family will always remain. It is simply his or her ability to express identity and life experience that has become impaired by loss of brain function.

There are those whose lives have been abundant with experiences of joy, sorrow, mystery, humor, happiness, and health like my father's was. For others, in times of "less than health," the challenge of a rediscovery becomes an even greater adventure. Undying love puts others in the challenging and sometimes painful role of caregiver. It is this role that enables the person living with the dementia to maintain their dignity and express their identity. We become the battery that powers the memories and experiences. As caregivers, we take on the responsibility to support the individual in maintaining dignity and expressing identity.

Dementia Care Programming: An Identity-Focused Approach proposes that disease or no disease each person has the right to be treated well and to be respected for whom they are and what they have accomplished. It gives the reader introductory models and approaches to apply the philosophy and theory, as well as examples supported by relevant research and data.

The goal of this book is to teach a respect and dignity focus based on recognition of individuality—whether there is a disease present or not. It offers practical philosophy supported by research, examples, and adoptable practice for the reader. It further offers a supportive and easy-to-read presentation from which both families and professionals can benefit. This is a practical teaching tool with simple models of caregiver approach and behavior that will result in the programs listed (and ADLs) being successfully implemented. It is a book of learning, celebration, and reassurance.

I firmly believe in our responsibility to seek out and provide creative tools to assist our residents, friends, and families in celebrating themselves and their lives when they can no longer do so without assistance. This publication ventures to suggest and to share with you philosophies and proven models of approach for use with persons with Alzheimer's disease and related dementias.

As a send off on this literary learning journey, I offer you the wisdom of Dr. Maya Angelou from her marvelous book of reflections *Wouldn't Take Nothing for My Journey Now*.

> Life is pure adventure, and the sooner we realize that, the quicker we will be able to treat life as art: to bring all our energies to each encounter, to remain flexible enough to notice and admit when what we expected to happen did not happen. We need to remember that we are created creative and can invent new scenarios as frequently as they are needed. (1994, p. 66)

PART 1

BUILDING A FOUNDATION:
THE ATTITUDE OF DISCOVERY

The Key to My Heart

Christmas 1996

He didn't recognize me when I approached. I asked if I might sit down beside him. He indicated there was no reason why I shouldn't. I waited a moment and then introduced myself again. I did this every time I visited. Why should I assume that I was so important in his hectic life amidst 40 other men struggling to coexist? "Hi Daniel, I am Jackie—your niece." BINGO! It is like putting a key in and turning it. Given a moment to make the connection, everything unlocks and opens up. He opens up and begins to outline everything that has gone wrong and everyone who is at fault. He's mad as hell and he ain't gonna take it any more! I don't blame him. He's a guy who has spent the years since the war running. Now he is in a cage with animals—or so he perceives. They are all out to complicate his life. He knows who is well and who is not. He can tell you who is able and who is not. He knows. He watches. He listens. He gets angry.

The nurse tries to tell him to get up so we can go out for lunch. He wants no part of her. I gesture "thanks" to her—we're okay on our own. Once alone the complaints begin again. In Daniel's eyes, these are terrible people always telling him what to do and how. And those other people (resident peers) are noisy and get in the way. Anyone who enjoys independence and personal space and privacy would empathize with him or any of these men. I immediately side with him, and ask if he would like to get away from it all. The idea is a hit and we gather his belongings (not an easy task). We are off on another wonderful journey together. The time spent is reflective and humorous. This is the uncle I loved growing up—funny, teasing, young at heart, and free in spirit.

As we were leaving the nurses said, "Good luck." I looked at them baffled. Inside I was hurt and angry for my uncle. We had a wonderful day together. He knew his limit and when asked he told me when it was time to go back. Upon our return they inquired of our outing with some strange combination of trepidation and "I told you so" mixed together: "How was he?"

I responded truthfully—"He was great once we got out of here." I felt let down. I have learned, however, these times do occur. But once the spontaneity of caring and compassion takes over, you share the deepest and most human of relationships with another human being.

Thoughtful Reflections

This journal entry and those in the latter part of this text are not fiction but absolutely true. You will read much about approaches, interactions, and the difference between success and failure in this book. As you open your heart to learning you will open your care experience to a greater experience of joy. The difference between joy of life and the experience of frustration and aggression is found in our

- approach
- respect of the uniqueness and ability of the individual (We do not know everything, not even ourselves…How can we claim to know others so well?)
- asking for input and making suggestions (instead of "telling" or just "doing")
- asking permission…set up the scene so the individual understands, agrees, and gives consent (It is generally *our* willingness and commitment, not theirs, which brings about success!)
- ability to explain how we feel

There is an emotional understanding that exists on many levels with the individual. We simply must be open enough and circumspect to trust the individual with our feelings at times. How do we do this? It is as simple as this story.

> One day I was riding the elevator with a woman from our
> special care unit. She was agitated and so was I. I was tired
> and bothered by something. I turned to her and said quietly,
> "Laura, I feel lousy today. I am tired and sad." Immediately
> her demeanor changed and she began to console me! She
> supported me with positives and care. She empathized with my
> experience and offered me care, expressing her concern…her
> own version of TLC. The tables had turned. Her demonstration
> of behavior familiar to all and needed by each of us gave us
> both strength to continue without incident. Not only did the
> situation improve and not only did I actually feel better, but
> also the situation was esteem enhancing for Laura. I learned
> a great lesson, one that we can all benefit from over and over
> again: We are none the wiser for our caregiver roles. Defer-
> ence to our residents or clients may be the healthiest and most
> empowering action we take in many scenarios.

Creating a Community

To understand the message of this text, one must first have a clear understanding of what I believe to be the foundation of dementia care success. We achieve success when a care team can establish a sense of community. The definition of community is simple: *Community* is found where a sense of normalcy has been achieved within the confines of dementia-related losses. Community acknowledges the potential for individuals, in spite of the disease process, to experience

- dignity
- safety and security
- sense of belonging
- familiarity
- humor
- trust
- companionship

The presence of a community environment suggests that an external focus is encouraged and exists for residents (see **Table 1**). Participants in a community maintain a degree of awareness of others coexisting in their environment. They are expressive or interactive in their own often nonverbal or confabulatory languages.

TABLE 1
Community Environment versus Individual Environment

Community	Individual
External	Internal
Explosive (Expressive)	Implosive
Connected	Disconnected

I will never forget the joy on the faces of two elderly women deep in conversation. Their faces were lit with brilliant smiles as they leaned in, attentive to one another's message...The uniqueness of this interaction was that both women had reverted to their first language. One woman spoke Ukrainian and the other woman spoke Cantonese. Everything is possible in the dementia care environment!

We must adjust the perception of "explosion" (as seen in Table 1) to a *positive* perspective. This is not a description of agitation or aggression but a description of *positive self-expression* among one's peers. Community presence generates the opportunity for a sense of belonging or connection with peers. It suggests external interaction of a positive nature.

Without community, we disconnect the individual and create an environment where the person is more at risk. The potential for agitation, aggression, and withdrawal increases. An internal focus decreases the individual's ability to relate to others and to cope with situations as they arise. This inevitably confirms withdrawal as the person's world narrows or implodes upon them. Communication diminishes. They lose touch. Contact or effort to interact and pursue a place within the community decreases.

Later in this book you'll meet the "turn-up man" (p. 171) who is a charming example of an established role within a well-established community. Not only is he connected through the other residents' recognition of his presence, but also he is included in their activity. We will explore the relationship of personhood and identity extensively throughout the book to elaborate on the importance of each individual in the context of the dementia care community, regardless of cognitive or physical ability. The definition of *personhood* by Dr. Tom Kitwood is

> the standing or status that is bestowed upon one human being, by others, in the context of relationship and social being. It implies recognition, respect and trust…the according of personhood, and the failure to do so, have consequences that are empirically testable. (1997, p. 8)

In this we recognize the value of nurturing a community and those who form it. Without recognition of individual roles, strengths, and needs, we fail to promote personhood and the community cannot unite to grow and to support one another. It simply functions aimlessly, seeking only to meet needs in a given moment from a survival standpoint rather than a mutually satisfying and success-oriented perspective. The difference is an empowered and esteem-enhanced community versus a self-absorbed, survivalist mode that minimally qualifies as a "community" by definition. This dichotomy is vast and the sacrifice of worthy individuals is too great. It is imperative that we promote the growth of our special dementia care communities.

We must first keep in mind that every community experiences cycles of growth and change, building and rebuilding based on

- admissions and discharges

- levels of wellness (e.g., flu seasons, untreated pain or other symptoms, levels of hydration and nourishment)

- fluctuations in resident functional levels
- insights and attitudes of caregivers

A typical cycle of community development includes the stages of admission/ transition, familiarity/role setting, acceptance/participation, belonging, and trust/companionship. Each stage the individual cycles through is a graduation from being the outsider to experiencing inclusion, satisfaction, and happiness. This is the Community Development Cycle or Pyramid. It may be compared to Maslow's Hierarchy of Needs for its essential construction of building on comfort, safety, acceptance, and belonging, and having at its highest level trust and companionship (see **Figure 1**). Within the experience of dementia this would equate to self-actualization.

Community Development Cycle/Pyramid	**Maslow's Hierarchy of Needs**
Trust/Companionship	Self-Actualization
Belonging	Esteem Needs
Acceptance/Partipation	Belongingness/Love Needs
Familiarity/Role Setting	Safety/Security Needs
Admission/Transition	Physiological Needs

FIGURE 1
Community Development Cycle/Pyramid and Maslow's Hierarchy of Needs

Admission/Transition

Admission is a high stress period for all involved with the new resident's arrival—from the new resident to the existing resident population to caregivers. This is where we begin the trust and relationship-building phase. At the same time, we seek to become familiar with the individual's identity and history.

Transition is a period of familiarizing routines, faces, and environment (from noise to location to lighting). This is an opportunity to observe coping and communication mechanisms used by the individual. It is a time to offer support while noting abilities and strengths as one looks ahead to the next phases.

Familiarity/Role Setting

If allowed and promoted, trust begins to develop at the familiarity stage. We must be aware of how we communicate. We must offer consistency in our approach and support choices made by the individual.

Consistency of approach is enabling in its own right. Familiar routine and approach lend clarity to the environment. These provide additional cueing for comfortable choices or actions by the resident. Choices on their own are often overwhelming for individuals with dementia. In this context, I propose that the term suggests a new interpretation of choices as *supportive* or *controlled choice*. Yes, I am proposing a form of benevolent manipulation. While being mindful of our ethical practice of "do no harm," we enable residents by suggesting the options available to them, rather than taking control of their lives and dignity. We provide choices that lead to the achievement of desired outcomes. We enable the individual to maintain a measure of control with a safety net of alternatives to benefit both caregiver and receiver. Some individuals will make a choice, others are not able and defer back to us. The point to take away from this example is that we are enablers (promoters of dignity) and deferring back to the individual is still as valuable a choice as the options we may have originally proposed or demonstrated.

Controlled Choice

Provide planned options (choices) to achieve successful outcomes by using gestures and/or careful wording. A nonthreatening manner that may take the approach of seeking help or assistance from the individual, and allowing them to own the situation. *Controlled choice* is using the power of suggestion to achieve an outcome for the benefit of the other person.

Having established a level of comfort and familiarity, the individual begins to express needs and behaviors that we can support. We carve out a role for this individual. Often a person becomes known for this activity or task, and identity begins to form within the community. For those who have difficulty relating to individuals with dementia, it becomes easier to understand and to respond to this person.

Acceptance/Participation

With understanding comes acceptance. This is the reality experienced by resident peers, family members of other residents, volunteers, and staff. We must find some way to relate to another person before we can feel safe and accept them. This is how we come to form a responsive community.

As a result of this acceptance, we find that individuals begin to partici-pate in the variety of programs available. Whether this is a meal or a ball toss, the individual has developed the basic feelings of safety and security as outlined by Maslow's Hierarchy of Needs.

Belonging

When an individual feels safe, feels secure, and has found someone with whom he or she can relate, the individual experiences a sense of belonging. This is essential to community development. Belonging requires reciprocal behavior. Therefore, more than one person must have reached this stage for the com-munity to form. This is often why we find residents congregating at nursing stations or making strong staff connections. It is essential that staff facilitate connections and belonging among residents. This is achieved successfully through programs like the social meals program (pp. 108–116).

Trust/Companionship

Like a row of dominoes toppling and touching one to the next, the commu-nity of residents passes on feelings and behaviors among themselves. The resulting connection formed through shared feelings and behaviors is a level of companionship unlike that which we experience. This simplifies the commu-nity development, or when positive and supportive behaviors are lacking, causes barriers to community.

Community Development

The ultimate goal is to be part of a functional special care community. This is not an easy or rapid process—for some it takes years. Having a foundation of trust, security, safety, and support promotes achievement of this outcome with greatest efficiency. At this point, regardless of ability, members of the community experience safety and comfort at such a level that their self-expression and self-esteem is worthy of celebration by both caregivers and receivers. This is an outstanding accomplishment for all involved.

Unfortunately, there will always be individuals whose dementia has advanced to such a degree that their behavior threatens the peace, and some-times cohesion, of the community. This is a reality of caring for those living with dementia. Nevertheless, care and attention to agitated residents and those whose comfort is threatened can reduce the impact of such dementia behavior. *Dementia behavior* is used because recognizing that given a choice the indi-vidual would not choose to behave this way is important. It is the dementia we are seeing as it surfaces—not the individual. We must remember that the individual is doing the very best to cope as he or she can based on the func-tion that remains in the brain. All the more reason to know and to recognize the person and not to take the behavior personally. This is how we build a community—through knowledge, love, respect, dignity, and support.

Programs and activities through a routine day vary according to season, time of day, and the goals we seek to achieve. Because of this reality, we must strive to promote each person's role and participation in our communities with flexibility, awareness, humor, acceptance, and love. These supportive behaviors, as demonstrated by caregivers, are what ultimately promote the success of our community. With this awareness and a desire to connect with our care receivers, we are truly on a wonderful journey! And so, the journey begins…

Rear Admiral Richard

Richard had been trying in vain to get his message out—no one understood.

A page went through the building: "Nurse call second floor—STAT!"

An errand happened to draw me to the second floor special care unit at the same time, so I looked around for the problem. Richard had been thrashing aggressively at the LPN who was trying with all her energy to encourage him to take his medication. But Richard had been trying in vain to get his message out—no one understood. In her best efforts the nurse advised everyone to leave him alone so he could calm down.

Unable to resist a challenge, I began a journey into Richard's adventure. I think he welcomed the help. I stood back observing, listening, and waiting for my cue.

"Get up!" he said as he moved through the dining room. "Everyone move down the ship!"

My first clue: the ship.

He approached me saying to someone I couldn't see, "Get to it sergeant."

I took the lead. "Sir, could you tell me your rank?" I asked (no response) "Is it Captain, sir?"

"Oh, higher than that," he said. And so the guessing continued as I asked several more times only to receive the response "Much higher than that."

"May I walk with you sir?" I asked.

"Yes, but move quickly, man," he said as we moved down the hall. He then began pushing open doors calling, "Is everything all right in here?"

Realizing his apparent distress aboard his ship I began responding to every statement with "Everything is clear, sir," or "Help is on the way, sir."

Each response seemed to appease his urgent concern. We continued up and down the hall as I took on the rank of someone junior to him. (I had no idea what or whom.) Respectfully I posed questions to my senior officer. "Sir, may I ask a question?"

"Yes," he would say patiently each time I asked.

"Sir, may I ask your rank or role here?"

"I am Chief Engineer," he responded. He then ordered me to start up the engines. I told him I was new to this and asked if he would be patient with me. "I'll be patient with you," he said kindly and then barked, "The key is in, now get going!"

"Aye, aye, sir," I said and was off to the balcony, out of his sight so he could not see I had absolutely no idea how to operate his ship! He moved in such a way so he could peer out and watch me. I invited him onto the balcony saying "Shall I call attention on deck, sir?"

"Yes, do," he said, and I did. He then barked the command "Speed it up will you!" I repeated his order to someone I could not see to which he responded, "Quit repeating everything I say!"

"Yes, sir!" I said, embarrassed by my lack of Navy prowess. We began our tour of the ship again, inspecting cabins, calling for help and asking questions all punctuated with "yes, sir," "no, sir," and other polite deferences to my senior officer. Each time his distress resurfaced we went through the motions and I discovered new ways to guide him to moments of peace—moments which he clearly needed more than any other resident or staff on *his* ship.

Shortly thereafter he observed one of the ladies entering her room. He called out, "Into your cabin, get in, get in!" I pushed her door open and guided her shoulders, talking her into her room, as his shouting frightened her. Although she spoke no English, I attempted to put her at ease with a calming voice and gestures, including gently rubbing her back. Just as I had closed her door, he pushed his way into her room, frightening her even more. It had crossed my mind—don't let him in—but he clearly needed to enter the room. Something was on his mind he needed to work through. So instead of stopping him, I turned my attention to comforting the other resident. Straight to her window he went with great urgency and concern.

"Is everything OK, sir?" I asked.

"Yes, it will be all right now." That was easy for him to say, I thought. Now how do I get him out of this terrified woman's room?

"Sir, you are needed on the other side of the ship." I blurted out with great imagination and hope. He turned on his heel and followed me out of the room without question. He clearly did not want the sailor to leave the cabin with us however. Sensing this, I turned to the woman and said calmly, "It's

OK now, sailor, stay in your room." She backed up and closed the door. We were off to the other side of the ship.

As we came around the corner, a group of ladies were wandering the opposite way. "Stupid CPOs," he muttered and shook his head as we passed them. (I later learned he was referring to Chief Petty Officers—senior enlisted personnel.)

Our next mission? To attempt the previously refused medication. First, although not preferred, we tried ice cream with a crushed pill. "Is it on the up and up?" he asked. Although I assured him (with a sense of guilt) it was, he tasted a half spoonful then flicked the rest away. I offered to relieve him of the empty spoon and he obliged. Medication in hand, I pondered my next strategy.

"Sir, I have just come from the telegraph room. The water is contaminated and we must all take our water pills to avoid sickness. I brought you yours, sir." He took it in thumb and forefinger, opened his mouth and popped it in. I then asked to be dismissed. My request was granted and my senior officer praised my work.

A short while later we crossed paths again. He had taken two chairs, tipped them over, and dragged them out on the balcony, creating somewhat of a hazard. Reporting back to him I asked, "Sir, may I assist you by moving these chairs?"

"Of course," he replied, "Salvage what you can." Picking up the first chair, I asserted that it was in fine shape and indicated I would go for the other if this were all right. He appeared agreeable, so I brought it in from the balcony. I asked if I may move them and he granted permission. With a polite request and numerous "sirs" I was granted the privilege of strolling back toward the dining room with him.

Upon arriving, I suggested Richard sit for refreshment. He requested whiskey or rye. He then asked my rank and again I was stumped. Using my imagination and knowing nothing of the Navy, I rationalized that a Chief Engineer would have a junior. I dubbed myself "Junior Engineer" and received a good laugh from the Chief. A subsequent laugh was achieved later when I suggested he meet the ship's dog. Richard's grin was beautiful and stretched ear to ear as he turned to observe the visiting pooch. Despite the grin, his manner remained that of an officer throughout.

Still perplexed and wanting to know his rank, I persisted with the polite curiosity of a junior seaman. "Sir, may I ask again, what is your rank, sir?"

"Rear Admiral," he stated with a dignity to which one could only respond with a high salute. I was dismissed.

Lesson Number One: Never Assume

We have a distinct responsibility to aid the individual to reexperience himself.

My new friend the Admiral taught me a great lesson in aggressive behavior: Never assume.

Admiral Richard appeared to be in the midst of a most distressing wartime flashback. He was giving out clues by his nonsensical gestures and statements. However, the question is: Nonsensical to whom? After all, this was his reality he was experiencing, not mine. In situations such as these we must validate the person and his or her situation by attempting every means of clue gathering, puzzle piecing, and pure improvisation.

To say that we are merely acting and to view this as making light of the individual is wrong. These efforts are in no way to be interpreted as "humoring" the individual. We respectfully support the person and guide them through their experience with the least amount of distress and conflict. We have a distinct responsibility to aid the individual in reexperiencing himself. Whether it is a tool such as a life book or kit, a story, or a familiar activity (especially if it is what we might call a flashback), our role is to recognize and be familiar with the person's history and the reality the person might be living at any given moment.

Life Kits and Life Books

Kept in a familiar case such as a box, briefcase or chest, a life kit is a personalized collection of recognizable items that may cue reminiscence visually. A life book is a two-dimensional version of a life kit. Both are used by family, staff, volunteers, or other visitors to verbally cue reminiscence with residents.

I have been asked the question: When is it lying or deception? I suggest that we let the individual guide us in our choice of responses. We must respond based on the information they give us. If the question merits a direct and truthful answer, give it. If it is clearly a displaced reality question (When does this train get in? Where is my mother?) using validation is the kindest and most acceptable choice of response. We use neither lies nor deceit in our interactions.

Q: I don't live here, do I?
A: Yes, you've lived here three years (soften by adding a positive) and we have so enjoyed getting to know you. You have a way of making everyone around you feel good.

A compassionate answer eases the distress of the individual and may improve the individual's mood so that he or she moves from a questioning frame of mind to a different focus.

Q: Is my mother/husband dead?
A: Yes, you've spoken fondly of ____ many times. He/she's been gone now for ____.

Further validation of feelings may be achieved through reminiscing. In these scenarios the person is asking a direct question, and any other response would be a deception. It is the time we take and how we cope with the reality of the answer that makes the difference.

In the case of a displaced question or comment, the use of the Feil (1993) method of validation and support seems the most appropriate means of providing a caring and satisfactory answer or diversion to meet the needs of the person. We do *not* deny this is the focus for the person. We *help them through* their remembrance.

Q: I have to get back to the farm. I don't know how I got here, but it's getting late. Where do I get the train?
A: Your farm was in Granum, is that right? Can you tell me about it? What was your role on the farm? I always felt at home on our family farm. I can understand your need to be there.

Validation

Respectful attitude of communication and empathy for use with older adults experiencing dementia. The caregiver listens and supports the individual's view of reality. (Feil, 1993, pp. 27–28)

Ask questions which redirect and assist the resident to deal with memories that have prompted him or her to seek out the farm. This may help the resident find calm or be put at ease. As we work through the issue or memory concerning the person, the resident usually recalls it as a present or current situation. Remember the "deception" issue? By using past tense: "Your farm *was* in Granum, is that right?" we are not deceiving the resident. We are validating his or her memory.

> **Q:**   Thank you for everything, I've had a lovely time but
> mother will be worried if I don't get home to help with din-
> ner. Where do I get out?
> **A:**   You are a very caring person, worrying about your
> mother this way. You must have very fond memories of her.
> Please tell me more about her.

Allowing the person to retrieve memories and feelings helps them to cope
with the situation at hand. Validation of the person rather than cutting down
with painful reality (not to mention that it is *our* reality and not *theirs*) is a
far more acceptable means to an end.

There will always be the repeaters: those who come time and again
with the same question. It is always a question or statement for which we
have no answer or comfortable response:

- I have to go now.
- Where do I get the bus?
- I have to pick up the boys.
- I have to cook supper for my children now.
- My family needs me now.

These are the "kid glove" questions and statements to which no one has the
absolute answer—the types of questions or statements which, if not handled
with great care, can lead to a variety of troubles. My feeling is to try every
approach (leaving reality out—potentially far too damaging—or use as a last
resort). "If at first you don't succeed try, try again" certainly applies here. The
quality of our intervention is at issue here. Ultimately, it is the *time we take*
or the *time we do not take* that makes the difference in the success or failure
of our interactions with residents.

We must remember, absolutely and without question, that our reality
is different from that of our residents. We must step outside ourselves and
join their journey. Every experience is truly an adventure.

Coping: Needs Response

Good care requires a very highly developed person—one who is open, flexible, creative, compassionate, responsive, and inwardly at ease.

—Kitwood (1997, p. 120)

Many wonderful outlets and opportunities exist for addressing the needs of individuals and small groups: planned reminiscence, spontaneous improvisational interactions, and discovery and life kits to name a few. Meeting the needs of our residents is a multifaceted challenge successfully addressed through Needs Response (see **Figure 2**). I chose the term Needs Response to simplify the understanding of what we do from moment to moment: We *respond* to the individual and to the unique *needs* of the person.

Discovery Kit

Three-dimensional, multifaceted, themed tool assembled for the pursuit of adventure through reminiscence and exploration, totally without expectations.

Our role with residents is to provide an environment in which they may live safely, happily, and comfortably within whatever reality they may experience at a given moment. Needs Response suggests that throughout a person's day they may be independent and appropriate to their level of functioning or totally dependent and experiencing distress. They may project distress through flashback experiences, agitation, acts of aggression, or emotional dependence. We must be aware of these factors, center ourselves, and depart our reality to join theirs. As Mitchell (1990) proposes, "I listen to and watch individuals as their speaking and moving changes to reflect what is important to them" (p. 173).

Needs Response calls on us to step out of our space—to listen and to be there for the resident. We must be prepared to shut down our own thoughts and needs and to genuinely listen and respond to the needs of others. We must be prepared to stop and let go of our current task to meet the needs of an individual as they are expressed in that moment. Kitwood explains this in his positive person work theory of effective caregiver behaviors. In this case the behavior is termed *relaxation*.

As a result of this respite, we can better understand and address the specific needs of the individual. Not only must we understand the needs,

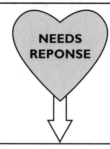

NEEDS REPONSE

SHUT DOWN SELF:
Focus on the other person

- Let go of personal worries
- Let go of the task at hand
- Check and adapt the environment
- Communicate actions with team

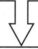

APPLY TOOLS:
Use interventions to facilitate positive outcomes

- Improvisation
- Validation
- Detective work
- Puzzle piecing

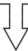

Achieve outcomes of positive support and identity-focused care:

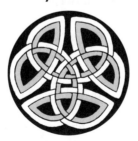

Acknowledge and support the person *and* his or her experience in that moment in time.

FIGURE 2
Basic Application of Needs Response:
Responding to the Individual and Unique Needs of the Person

> **Relaxation**
>
> The caregiver is free to stop active work for a while and even to stop planning. He or she positively identifies with the need that many people with dementia have: to slow down and allow both body and mind a respite. (Kitwood, 1997, p. 120)

but also we must apply this understanding with cognizance and skill. The essential element of this behavior is in being able to give ourselves permission to be available to the person for the duration of Needs Response.

We must develop skills to piece together the puzzles and to unravel the mysteries presented through their realities. On this journey, we enter a world where the language may have changed but there is plenty of room to translate. Detective work, improvisational responding, and caring from the heart are clear requirements for success in aiding the resident in need.

Needs Response may be spontaneous or planned (if we have been successful in establishing a pattern of behavior and a solid history for a specific individual). However, when we are responding to needs how can we be sure whose needs we are responding to? To establish this we must address and clarify the issues of reality—but whose reality?

Expressing Reality: Is It Theirs or Ours?

It is much more important to know what sort of patient has a disease than what sort of disease a patient has.
—Sir William Osler
Canadian Physician (1849–1919)

The first question many people ask is: What is the diagnosis? The first answer that crosses my mind is: Who cares?

Do we use a diagnosis for positive purposes beyond the medical treatment? If not, let us step back to a humanistic and holistic approach and leave the diagnosis to the treatment and prescriptive needs of the physician. When we apply a diagnosis, do we not also tend to apply a series of limitations and frequently inappropriate expectations?

What is essential in the context of diagnosis is the recognition of the strengths and limitations with which the individual is now coping. That is, diagnostic data is essential to the caregiver's success as it tells us what brain function is lost or remains. As effective caregivers, our responsibility is to know the range of brain functions and what the outcome is when the various parts of the brain deteriorate. This way we can continue to acknowledge *individual strengths and needs* as the disease progresses. A blanket diagnosis for all residents serves no one. Each person living with dementia is a unique person, as is their experience of the disease and its progression. Yes, patterns and stages have been distinguished; however, because each person is unique his or her coping skills and behaviors will reflect individual life experience as well as the ability to cope within the contexts of the environment.

Expectations based on diagnoses are rarely realistic, as our insight into the reality of the person with dementia is always incomplete. In fact, I suggest that the word "expectations" is failure oriented and should be dropped from the vocabulary of those who associate with people who have special care needs. After the initial treatment the diagnosis becomes irrelevant as we focus on the individual. The Needs Response approach

- decreases incidences of aggression or agitation
- serves as a backup for providing required medication or treatment, if necessary
- allows for safe expression of the reality experienced at the time

It is my belief and experience that if applied appropriately, with knowledge of the disease, Needs Response is the most respectful and positive caring approach one can take within the context and goals of providing supportive care.

Does the illusion of limited time deter use of this intervention? I would again suggest the time, concern, and risks involved in alternative approaches is far greater and much more stressful than the effort required in validating a person by joining in their journey. Some attempts may never get off the ground; others may soar joyfully. The issue is simple and clear: Their reality and their journey calls on us to try. We must lose our inhibitions and challenge our creative selves. Simply stated, *we must always try*. Nothing is embarrassing, shameful, or wrong in the resident's behavior—unusual as it may seem. This person is doing the best they can under the circumstances. We as caregivers have significant control over the circumstances outside of the disease itself. This person maintains the same needs, rights, and value as you and I. Therefore, he or she reserves the unspoken right to expect our actions to fulfill their needs and rights. In Kitwood's own work, he sought to view the application of personhood in dementia care based on four main criteria. Dementia care must

- reveal our moral obligations
- be valid in terms of a psychology that focuses on experience, action, and spirituality
- illuminate care practice
- be fully compatible with the well-supported findings of neuroscience (Kitwood, 1997, p. 55)

Again, we recognize and understand the brain and the resulting disease pathology, but we do this in such a manner that over and above the disease the person ultimately is acknowledged as the first priority. We create a genuine interpersonal relationship with this individual. Adapted to respond to the person based on strengths and limitations, this interpersonal relationship is both dignified and respectful. It is important that wrong or right; strange or intriguing; serious, sorrowful, or humorous—*this is their reality,* not ours. We must leave appearances, judgments and our past as we know it behind to once again join their journey.

Never will there be a dull moment if we adopt the approach of leaving our reality. Each "incident" becomes less of an incident and more of a "challenge."

Piecing the Puzzle Together

"I can't do this puzzle," said the child sadly.
"But think of how beautiful it will be when done,"
urged her mother.
The child listened, smiled, and with great hope she
went back to piecing the puzzle together.

Recently I suggested to a relative that the anatomy and physiology of aging and the comprehension of disease processes may be very important to total care. (Make no mistake, I do believe this.) Nevertheless, being able to maintain objectivity and an explorer's sense of adventure are equally important.

Have you ever watched the game shows *Wheel of Fortune* or *Jeopardy*? If you recall the shows, take the format back to your resident population. (If you are not familiar, do some exploring on your own.) *Who Wants To Be a Millionaire?* also challenges one's thinking and deductive reasoning. These and other popular shows challenge one's thinking on many levels, thus generating the unique and (often after questions are answered) obvious answers. We can apply the logic and puzzle piecing of game show challenges to our observations and practice in dementia care scenarios, from personal care challenges to reality challenges.

It might even be that the scenario playing out in the mind of the person we seek to support is a combination of life stages and events flashing back and forth. Such occurrences contribute to confusion for the interpreters. For example, "Rear Admiral Richard" was not a Rear Admiral, but a Chief Engineer. The Chief, as we knew him, did rank highly—he was second to the Captain of the ship and would take over in the event the captain could not lead. Richard was only briefly in the Navy. He actually served through the war in the Merchant Marines. His references to soldiers, the army, and other distressing situations are likely a combination of events he experienced. Although his ship was, by his family's account, never in distress, his was one of the most vulnerable sailing units during the war. His family account supports that he did carry troops and was a major player in the evacuation of Singapore. The puzzle pieces do link together!

I suggest to you that we will be more successful in the challenges presented to us if we include in our situational assessments the previous analogy and description. The person with dementia gives us clues to his or her reality. These clues may be fragmented like individual letters or in chunks like phrases or similes. With this in mind, you may find yourself looking more carefully for clues and asking yourself questions from different angles:

- He is referring to a ship—is this a clue?
- He appears to be a leader, giving direction, encouraging, and supporting—is he a high-ranking officer?
- He is anxious, calling for help—is his ship in trouble?

Listen carefully, consider the clues, and apply the logic of respect, response, inquiry, and redirect.

Respect

Demonstrate clear respect for the individual. Do not question or challenge actions, but respect them.

Response

Acknowledge the situation or reality the person is experiencing (i.e., their needs). Do not ignore the situation just because you may not understand it.

Inquiry

Ask! Probe for details or clues to unravel the mysteries being presented to you. You may just learn something.

Redirect

Offer suggestions in a nonthreatening and supportive manner ("May I make a suggestion?"). *Ask permission* to develop rapport and redirect the individual toward a positive and safe outcome. For example

"May I go with you, sir?"
"Everything here is under control, sir."
"You are needed on the other side of the ship, sir."
"May I be dismissed, sir?"

While the interaction may be unusual or out of the norm from our traditional training, the outcomes will provide sufficient justification for use of this approach.

∞   ∞   ∞   ∞   ∞

I encountered Frances as she hurriedly left the dining room abandoning her lunch. It seems she felt she had been deceived into coming and wanted to go home. I validated her feelings of anger and distress, and with her consent took up the walk at her side. We strolled around the unit twice while I learned of her concerns. Frances was originally from the Prairies, which is where we strolled that day, on a street of her hometown.

As we passed each resident's room, she remarked on the apartments. She asked me to take her to the bus stop so she could get back to her home. I told her I didn't know the bus routes involved but that I would happily walk with her. I began to make suggestions of eating lunch as she described her fatigue and worries. Our stroll took us close to the dining room for the second time. Having established we were on a city street, I said, "Oh, look at the restaurant there. They seem to be serving lunch."

She acknowledged my statement. I then suggested we go in and have a look at the menu. As she did not object, I directed her to a dining room seat and asked, "Waitress, is this seat taken?" For lack of a menu, I asked the waitress what today's special was. Having caught on, the care aide explained the chicken dish being served for lunch. Although my friend Frances was still concerned about getting home, for the moment she was settled and eating something to sustain her tiny, fragile frame.

∞   ∞   ∞   ∞   ∞

Perhaps it seems too simple, but the truth is we often complicate life. Simplify your thinking, evaluate the situation, know your resident's history, and respect wherever he or she may be. Overall, when you join their journey, this twist on your reality proves the range of joyful adventures we can experience in dementia care.

In the Moment

Cherish each thought, every experience, and always live in the moment.

I believe that if everyone truly lived in the moment we would have a genuinely different, and perhaps better, world. With this thought in mind, I suggest our experiences in dementia care would have a different flavor and feeling if we "lived in the moment" of the person with dementia. Again, this calls on us to step through the looking glass and into their reality. More than this, it calls on us to attend to and observe our residents very carefully. It calls on us to apply Needs Response. The person with dementia becomes the director; however, there is no script. We must decipher our role and responses. This is improv in its most challenging form.

The time we spend in a resident's reality is often fragmented. Their remembrances may be a complete story from their past or broken pieces of flashbacks disjointedly linked together through environmental triggers. In this reality, we coexist from moment to moment. The art of improvisation suggests the same approach: Without a script, each player writes as they go. In this case we follow the lead of the person with dementia.

The first piece of advice leaders in improv offer: *know your subject*. It is important to be thorough in our knowledge of the individual's social, career, marital, family, and leisure/recreation history. Being knowledgeable of the individual's era, including major historical events, is important. This includes knowledge of history, trends, fads, vehicles, and nuances of specific trades. It is natural, when we are unsure of specific details, that we refer to things current and familiar to ourselves. It is crucial to know the era of the person involved. Our frame of reference has no relevance to those who are reexperiencing their past. For example, modern pilots fly blind using instruments. In the early days of flight, pilots leaned out the cockpit window to look for a pasture in which to land. Know the specifics of their era, as they may not have a firm grasp of current technology.

Kitwood's breakdown of "that special resourcefulness that dementia care requires" from caregivers encourages us to be present for our residents in a more deeply personal way (1997, p. 119). He speaks of the twelve caregiver behaviors known as *positive person work*. He suggests twelve different ways through which we can better support our residents through modeling specific actions and behaviors. These twelve, to be expanded later, include creation, recognition, play, and facilitation.

Creation

The creative action initiated by the person with dementia is seen and acknowledged as such. The caregiver responds without taking control.

Recognition

The caregiver brings an open and unprejudiced attitude, free from tendencies to stereotype or pathologize, and recognizes the person with dementia as an individual.

Play

The caregiver is able to access a free, childlike, creative way of being.

Facilitation

Here a subtle and gentle imagination is called into play. There is a readiness to respond to the gesture that a person with dementia makes—not forcing meaning upon it, but sharing in the creation of meaning, and enabling action to occur (Kitwood, 1997, p. 20).

These elements of positive person work parallel the concepts of improvisational theater. The added touch is the deep sensitivity and respect for the dignity of the person with dementia. Improv instructor and author Delton Horn (1991) describes the "stop–start" form of improv as the "most fun." In this form we find actors proceeding through a scene until stopped, a new twist is added, and someone calls to begin again. What a treat then to have regular access to the most fun form of improv! Residents with dementia call stop and start with each new situation they present. The increased challenge is in the type of twist: Is it a change of story line, changed emotion, or even a reversal of roles? It is a challenge, but a fun one if we allow it to be so. Support, cooperation, and trust are key in the discussion of any relationship, including improvisation and dementia care.

Caregiver efforts to support residents must establish genuine trust within the relationship. We must be prepared to cooperate with the person with dementia through Recognition and Facilitation. (One cannot assume or expect that they will cooperate with us!) This can be accomplished by taking a soft spoken, quiet, passive, and agreeable approach. We must not argue or force our needs on them. Doing so could be compared to pulling a pin on a grenade—explosive!

If you are not successful in your attempts to support an individual or to accomplish a specific task

- leave well enough alone
- evaluate your approach (see The Connection Continuum on p. 98 for evaluative questions)
- try again later
- give the person some space and ask someone else to try
- be fair to yourself—everything is not always going to be effective

What works with one individual may *never* work with another. Then again, what works one day with one individual may not work the next. We are called on to be creative and innovative!

Everything seems to have rules. If we call these "guidelines" instead we can take the following suggestions and apply them to our own experiences. We will then become successful at building supportive, cooperative relationships with those for whom we provide care. The guidelines for ensemble improv are simple and act as a fair guide for interaction:

- Do not make excessive movements when the other person is talking.
- Keep in character, listen, react, and respond.

"Acting is reacting. Let your body listen and react as well as your brain," says the author of *Improve with Improv,* Brie Jones. In our supportive practice, I prefer the word "respond" to "react." However, I strongly believe this is good advice. According to Jones (1993), to achieve success ensemble actors use eye contact, personal space, open and closed body positions, and touching.

Ensemble actors, like us, do not distract or upstage the person opposite through Creation—they attempt a balance. Keeping a boat steady is easier than righting a capsized boat. It is amazing how well interaction and support in improvisation overlaps with caring for and responding to a person with Alzheimer's or related dementias.

The British director Keith Johnstone describes improvisation as "steering a car by looking through the rearview mirror. You don't know where you're going, you can only see where you have been." Clearly, this is often true for those who care for persons with dementia.

Take up the challenge. Find the supporter/nurturer in you and add improvisation to your list of talents. When we feel safe, when we feel we have permission to explore and be creative, we are successful. Share your understanding of improvisation with others and allow yourself to be free to explore, to improvise. Develop your skills in positive person work to bring satisfaction to your caring role and quality to the life of those for whom you provide care. Trust yourself first and residents will increase their trust in you.

Nurturing Permissiveness and Safety

It is not what can *I do, but what* will *I do.*

When I think back on my life, I chuckle at several things. I think (though some who know me may find it hard to believe) of how shy, in fact terrified, I was to speak my mind, to try new things, or to ask permission. It was easier to go about my business and do what I was told. While in the privacy of my own space I would be tackling the world with my imagination, leadership, and creativity—it was quite a little world.

Thanks to my experience, I find I have more patience for those who struggle to feel safe and ask permission. Whether it is permission to pursue a specific activity or permission to be themselves, I find it easier to empathize and to create a safe environment for them to ask permission based on my own experiences.

Today, I can freely motivate myself to different levels of creativity, leadership, and imagination that I am able to share with others. It is a joyful feeling and experience. How this personal freedom came about, I cannot question; I can only nurture it. One could ask: What can I do to nurture self-expression and an environment in which the residents can peacefully exist?

The answer isn't simple, but here are some points to ponder as one prepares to nurture those in one's care:

- Once the momentum is created it cannot be lost.
- Making mistakes is easy enough, but these are inherent to the adventure.
- Success will almost always follow.

If we as caregivers accept that the individual with Alzheimer's or a related disorder is living in a different reality and that this reality is ever changing, we begin to create momentum. We need an anchor for the pursuit of our beliefs and goals. Understanding the idea of a different reality existing for each individual anchors us. This stabilization of beliefs gives us a starting point for each situation. Now, with ease, we give residents permission to be themselves comfortably. We create a safe and nurturing environment. We begin to create community as we create momentum.

∞   ∞   ∞   ∞   ∞

A resident who repeatedly brought his daybook to the nurses' station and asked the nurse on duty to verify the appointments listed was apparently "driving the staff crazy." The book was intended to reduce his visits to the nurses' station by listing all his appointments so he would be able to see them and answer his own questions. They were close in their theory, but not right on.

He still needed confirmation. The staff termed this as harassment. The dictionary defines harassment as disturbing, repetitive behavior. Based on the potential areas of the brain that may be damaged, one could speculate that this individual was forgetful, lonely, or bored, yet unable to directly communicate the specific need. It was these needs he was expressing, not harassment.

∞   ∞   ∞   ∞   ∞

Again, we blame the resident for his needs! Shouldn't this behavior be described as self-validating rather than harassment?

With this in mind, consider the following coping routine. By reversing the approach and going to the resident to check his calendar the staff would validate his need for reassurance, interaction, attention, planning, organization, and socialization. Let us make a conscious effort to validate the person's reality. By creating a nurturing environment in which we give permission to safely be ourselves, we nurture the soul. A conscious point of emphasis is that this concept not only applies to the resident, but also to the family, volunteers, and staff. The question is not what *can* I do, but what *will* I do?

In this safe environment of special care, we provide permission to take risks. There are no guarantees in any approach we try, yet we must try just the same. Through support and shared understanding we acknowledge the permission and create feelings of safety to try new approaches. Yes, mistakes are part of the package, but they are part of the process of elimination. Mistakes are growth and part of the progress toward ideal care and support, which is unlimited in its potential.

The meditation on page 28 may help caregivers to center and focus themselves prior to beginning their interactions.

Permission: A Caregiver's Meditation

I am one who answered a unique call
to respond to the needs of people who
have experienced life just like me:

joys, sorrows, health, happiness, family,
careers, travel and a host of adventures.

Today I am called to discovery
to support them in celebrating themselves
as they can no longer do this on their own.

I am important to the success of this celebration.
I have a unique responsibility and I have permission
from my peers and supervisors, families, and most of all
permission from myself.

With this comes freedom to improvise and creatively
allow individuals to experience their reality.

I have support to take leave of my assignment and
to join their journey.
I am called to express the nurturer, detective,
improvisational actor, and "clown," the supporter in me.

I am called to adventure and discovery
to awaken to the needs of others...
I give myself permission to answer the call!

—Rosemary Dunne, June 1995

Tempus Fugit?

Stepping out of our reality and into theirs means accepting that our clock runs too fast.

Almost everyone who drives has had the experience of witnessing someone racing from lane to lane, tailgating and zooming down the road only to stop at the next light. At this point, all the cars this person has dangerously maneuvered around have safely found their way up to the very same stoplight. In our desire to get everything done, we have become obsessed with speed and time. These phrases come to mind as I think of our obsession with time:

- I simply don't have time.
- Time's up!
- We haven't the time.
- Take time to smell the roses.
- Time is of the essence.

When the staff told us that the residents couldn't set the tables in the dining room, the first thing that came to mind was the concept of *task breakdown*. We suggested they try giving simple, brief instructions and going step-by-step through the process of setting each table with the residents. We later observed that more often than not the staff quickly set the tables for the sake of time. In this great challenge of discovery and adventure, time cannot be the main issue.

Task Breakdown

Divide a specific activity into its smallest, most basic components. This enables the person with dementia to successfully, step by step, acheive the desired outcome of the activity as a whole. Assign tasks or steps based on the individual's skill level, interest, desire, and potential for success. Do not assign a task that will create a negative or unsuccessful outcome.

Dr. William Thomas, father of the Eden Alternative, speaks of the three plagues of nursing homes as loneliness, helplessness, and boredom (1996, p. 27). As he suggests, these "major barriers to growth" reflect our inability to apply common sense to the daily living experience of someone with dementia. While cognitive losses are scientifically evident and behaviorally demonstrated, spiritually the person is intact. This is where true nurturing and understanding are essential. We must protect and promote the dignity and spirit of the person. Using time, "management," or "my coworkers will get mad" as an excuse is inexcusable. True caregivers, *gift givers*, are leaders and role models to others. It is their primary directive to find ways to adapt the routine to manage time to the benefit of the resident. This can be done quite simply by breaking tasks down, incorporating resident participation, and achieving required tasks while boosting the morale, dignity, activity, and spirit of the individual. This initiative may take time for some to become both comfortable and adept.

The person with dementia gradually loses the skills and comprehension to complete simple, familiar tasks, such as the lifelong skill of setting a table. These losses lead to isolation, which leads to loneliness, helplessness, and boredom. Without total or partial breakdowns of the specific tasks and supplies used (see **Table 2**), we cannot create a successful and positive experience or outcome for the persons involved. As a result we cannot make a difference to eliminate Thomas' three plagues.

What might take you or me five minutes can take up to 25 minutes with a person whose ability is affected by dementia. (Using task breakdown with two residents, setting the tables took 20 minutes of quality, purposeful, esteem-building time.) Stepping out of our reality and into theirs means accepting that *our clock runs too fast* for their abilities and needs. We must not assert that the person cannot complete the task. We can only suggest that the person will complete the task in a longer period than would be considered normal. It may also be said that the person requires more assistance and direction to complete the task. We must begin to understand and to adapt our approach to

---

TABLE 2
Examples of Task Breakdown

Baking	Gardening	Setting the Table*	Washing Dishes
Read the recipe	Turn soil	Set placemats	Set plug
Crack, beat eggs	Plant	Place napkins	Run water
Measure	Water	Place silverware,	Add soap
Mix	Weed	one item at a time	Place dishes in sink
Grease sheet/pan		Set plates, one at	Wash
Pour/drop batter		a time	Rinse
		Set drinking glasses	Place in dryer rack
			Dry, stack dishes
			Place in cupboard

* Give only enough for table guests

include a breakdown of the task at hand. When we do so, we will create a sense of purposefulness, dignity, and worth for the person. This means taking the time to break activities down to subtasks, which will accomplish the goal in the space of time needed by the individual. The more skilled we become at breaking down tasks and simplifying instructions, the easier the job will be. Tasks will become increasingly successful for both staff, family and the individual involved. As a result, self-esteem and self-confidence rebound as well.

A final comment on this issue. The question may remain for some: "How do I meet the resident's needs and complete the other duties required of me during a given shift?" First, we must evaluate the model of care we are applying to ensure it not only focuses on meeting the needs of the residents but also considers the demands of a day's required routines. This requires explicit teamwork: uniting all levels of staffing, blending roles, and acknowledging the equal contribution of each member of the team.

Teamwork on a special care unit often means staff may not always accomplish all routine responsibilities. It suggests that staff share responsibilities. Team members working together pick up the tasks when others are addressing or responding to resident needs through the Needs Response approach. Being a member of a care team is a great responsibility and is not to be taken lightly. Team players must recognize when it is important to let a task go for the sake of a resident and when to relieve another team member so that the individual may resume their responsibilities. This is the essence of the meaning of community. When handled maturely—and filled with adventure, humor, flexibility, creativity, and compassion—the practice of Needs Response is a challenge worth striving toward.

Defenders of Dignity

We must create a secure environment where the individual
is safe from misunderstanding and misrepresentation.

If you haven't taken your role in special care seriously yet, I challenge you to consider the following word: Toys.

If your first cued response relates to children, you may guess my direction: age appropriateness. Toys, dolls, and stuffed animals are controversial subjects of discussion and argument. This is a true dignity and identity issue.

If an individual comes to you or your facility with a toy or animal with which they have had a longstanding "relationship" or for which they have sentimental feelings, this is their choice. I suggest that they established the connection made with the creature at a point or stage when the person had a greater awareness. The key word is *awareness*. This person made a choice and kept the toy for whatever personal reason. This, by choice, is part of his or her identity. Therefore, we must endeavor to support their choice. We have a responsibility to do just that.

On the other hand, a conscious choice made by staff to give toys to distract, soothe, or quiet a person must be made responsibly and with care. It is wrong if it replaces one-on-one caring interventions because it is convenient for the staff. Ask yourself this question: Do you know, *absolutely and without question*, that this individual would have chosen to handle and interact with a toy if dementia had not invaded their world?

I suggest that unless we are family, a friend, or a significant other we have no way of knowing. Now, what if a stuffed animal is sitting on a shelf and a person seeks it out? I do not suggest that we take it away. Despite the dementia, the individual has still made a choice. We must always respect the choices of our residents unless that choice will cause harm to themselves or another individual.

The reality of the issue is this: We are defenders of dignity. We may have some insight, or possess a perceived understanding of the resident's interaction with a toy. However, if a stranger arrives on the unit lacking the familiarity and insight we possess, they will likely pass incorrect judgment on the animal-hugging individual. Because individuals may be unable to speak for themselves, they are perceived as childish and therefore infantilized. This is where our responsibility is greatest. We must defend their dignity. We must create and protect a normal, stimulating, comfortable, and soothing, age-appropriate environment. We must create a secure environment where the individual is safe from misunderstanding and misrepresentation.

Our interventions and approaches must

- be age appropriate
- enhance image and identity
- preserve dignity

These concepts are part of the mission to which we are entrusted as caregivers. Understanding and promoting the image of our residents based on age-appropriate interventions must be the foremost goal when we address their care needs. We go to great lengths to collect appropriate and accurate social histories. Why should we contradict our information by introducing a potentially inappropriate intervention such as a toy? There are those who argue in favor of "doll therapy" and other such concepts. However, it is my opinion that our responsibility is much too great to resort to what could be described as the easy way out.

Nurses Isabel Milton and Judith MacPhail, in a limited sample investigation, found that residents they interviewed used dolls and toys for several reasons: to reminisce, to express anger, or to stimulate the senses. Most family and staff supported the use of dolls and toys and felt there were distinct benefits to residents. Some families placed appropriate restrictions on the use of the toys in an apparent effort to preserve the individual's dignity. They describe the use of toys as a "sensitive, fundamental issue which causes nurses much discomfort and disagreement" (1995). Milton and MacPhail suggest

> This may be because we find the use of these objects a silent but visible accusation related to the health care system's failure to meet certain basic human needs of people entrusted to our care. (1995)

Perhaps there is no true right or wrong, and as with most approaches to special care, we must individualize the selected approach. The reality is that we are charged with the care and preservation of dignity in addition to the personal and leisure care aspects of special care. Therefore, we must demonstrate empathy for the position of the person with dementia. Unable to assert himself or herself, we must not assume he or she would benefit from dolls or toys. Based on the knowledge at hand and the role with which we have been entrusted, we must assert ourselves as *defenders of dignity.*

The Awakening

It is not they who should cooperate with us,
but we who should cooperate with them.

It is *simplicity* to which we are called: slowing down, taking time to be a backbone of support and direction, listening, allowing the person to communicate clues to what is on his or her mind. We respond to the individual's needs quietly and reassuringly. The concepts of slowing, listening, and responding are too simple to apply in a complex world. Bear in mind that once we convert to slowing, listening, and responding we become much improved at cooperating with the person with dementia. We begin to recognize that the person is not *misbehaving* as some would describe, but *coping* as best he or she can with the cognitive resources remaining in the brain. As a result, fighting for power or control on the part of the caregiver ceases. The stress we cause our-selves and our residents, or family members, ceases. Incidences of agitation and aggression decrease, and enjoyment of our roles as caregivers increases.

"We need to manage the residents better." Language has a major impact on our application of care. When words such as *manage* are used in the con-text of completing tasks of *care* we miss the point. Manage suggests control on the part of the caregiver over the care receiver. A preferred word would be *support*. Dr. William Thomas suggests that "we place too much emphasis on treatment and too little on helping residents to grow" (1996, p. 27). In our own growth process as caregivers we must recognize that by awakening to the individual, the humanity, and uniqueness of our residents we enhance care. My goal is to have all caregivers genuinely personalize the care expe-rience—*to apply aspects of care and the language of care to our own lives*. As we seek to grow what do we place our focus on? Do we manage our rela-tionships or do we seek to nurture (promote growth) in our relationships? In healthy, growth-oriented relationships we slow down, listen, and respond. We do not "treat" our partners or family. We love and care for them. When we can awaken to our own experiences we can better awaken to the experi-ence and needs of others.

This proactive behavior of awakening is simply the action of taking time to listen and respond. As she reflects on a change of nursing practice, Mitchell identifies her new, supportive behavior:

> The way I am with individuals is different now…My focus is not on diagnosing people from my perspective but on listening to the individual and his or her perspective of what is occurring. I no longer tell people what I think they need, rather I ask them what they want and where they want to go. I ask indi-viduals what is important for them, rather than trying to get them to do what is important for me. (1990, p. 176)

As a result of such proactive changes in thinking and approach, we reduce the time spent in a reactive mode cleaning up from and documenting unnecessary disasters. By taking the time to implement Needs Response we can truly make a difference in the life of a person living with Alzheimer's or related dementia. Making a difference may be a challenge, but the satisfaction is rewarding.

Attitude of Discovery

Attitude:
The more I live the more I understand that life is not a
50/50 proposition, but rather life is 10% what happens
to me and 90% how I react to it.

—Anonymous

Attitude forms the basis, either positive or negative, of our adventures. If we believe, it will be. If we do not, it will also be. Stories abound of achievement and success surmounting what was seen as impossible or foolish. In the case of those with disabilities or struggling with disease, we may be blinded by the clinical and not see the potential.

Attitude is a foundation on which to build. It is the essential ingredient to a successful outcome. A hint of doubt or negative thinking can prevent successful caregiver action. This is where the "attitude of discovery" comes into play.

Attitude

An *attitude* is a set of learned predispositions to respond either favorably or unfavorably in an evaluative manner toward someone or something. Through the example of others and our own experiences we learn to respond to situations or stimuli either positively or negatively. These form beliefs from which an attitude is developed. We are then predisposed to respond in a specific manner. These predispositions are bricks that form the foundation of our attitude.

Attitude is such a powerful element of our being. Maintaining a sense of objectivity, especially with the person with dementia, is a serious challenge for the most determined care adventurer.

One family said "We wish you had known Mother five years ago. She is not the same person today." While this is true from a communication, skill, and behavioral perspective, it is at the same time false. Mother is still there and even the staff see glimpses of her. For example, when Mrs. Orr was in the final stages of life with Alzheimer's she still communicated her "hot-headed French Canadian side," as the family describes. "If she was angry or in pain we knew it, her eyes would come ablaze, a look we knew well not to cross throughout our lives!" This gave the family and the care team a means of maintaining a focused perspective of her needs. Part of her identity as each member of the family knew her still shone through. The attitude that was adopted was one of seeking to communicate best with limited resources. The approach was an acceptance of a lifelong behavior and applying it to the current situation. It is how we choose to remember as well as what we look for that counts.

To say "this is not our mother" is to speak of the disease process. Attend to her finer, individual points: humor, caring, nurturing, leadership, sadness, and even anger. This is to seek out and find the mother you knew five years ago. There remains a wonderful person to celebrate in spite of the thievery of the disease process. We must adopt a belief system, an attitude of discovery, which says in spite of the illness and change affecting the individual, there remains someone just like us—someone with an identity worth searching out and celebrating. That someone has a rich history of experience, joys, and sorrows from which we can learn, if we so choose.

This is the attitude of discovery!

PART 2

MAKING A LIFE-ENHANCING DIFFERENCE

Understanding and Valuing Individual Identity

Who I am and how I got here is no secret—if you care enough to listen and hear what I may not be saying.

Once we have diagnosed and prescribed treatment, the true challenge and magic of the caring relationship begins. Often I hear that people want very concrete tasks or things to do with people. The idea here is that we will resolve and address every need of an individual by slotting them into a program or activity or putting them in front of the television. People want a succinct recipe for success. In truth it is not, nor will it ever be this simple. While this book will later offer a broad selection of programs and interventions, the best care lies in listening to and being present for residents. We can all be this caring person—a meaning maker. A *meaning maker* is someone whose life and experience has an impact on others by virtue of being here. If we can recognize that each person (including ourselves) in his or her own right and experience (in this case, dementia) is, was, and will always be a meaning maker, we then recognize that to support another person is to simply be with them. In care, supportive interventions are intuitive interventions.

Successful caregivers know four secrets about caregiving:

1. To walk a mile in another's shoes, and only then, is to understand what that person needs or wants.

2. Listening and sharing information builds relationships.

3. Trust is the heart and soul of any relationship regardless of physical or cognitive ability or impairment.

4. We receive what we give.

How we *provide support* and *promote individual identity* is central to this discussion. How you choose to use this information will impact your success as a caregiver and a supporter. Your increased awareness will directly influence the quality of your clients' lives and your own.

You are there to provide care and support because *within the limitations they are living* these people are doing the best they can with the brain function that remains. We tend to see people as ourselves: with normal healthy brains. We must remember the deficits and losses created by the dementia destruction. Like a war zone, dementia destroys the brain and steals one's independence and ability to express oneself. People living with dementia and other sensory or physical deficits need us to remain sensitive to their basic human needs.

Therefore, it is paramount that we recognize the role we play as caregivers and the potential we have to give back to the person for whom we provide care.

In essence, we are gift givers. Ours is an awesome role, a challenging role, an exciting role. We seek to celebrate the unique self of those who can no longer initiate the celebrations on their own. This is truly a magical gift. These gifts are borne of the four secrets of caregiving.

Secret #1

To walk a mile in another's shoes, and only then, is to understand what that person needs or wants.

This secret acknowledges the importance of identity. It suggests that recognizing the person and their life experience results in a greater presence of dignity in the caring relationship. *We are nothing without our story.* Further, when dementia steals one's ability to express the story and the self, and thus to continue to experience life, individuals are in danger of becoming a more raw form of nothing. It is a raw form because this is what we as caregivers contribute to by stripping away or denying the person's story. When the brain becomes irreversibly damaged, the individual remains. *This is a disease of the brain, not the spirit.*

There is no research that can prove that the spirit, the story, or the self has been destroyed by this disease. As the ability to communicate, express, share, and participate becomes impaired by the dementing process, the person still remains. This person continues to do the very best he or she can do as the odds stack against him or her. *This is an admirable quality of survival.*

In his outstanding identity-focused research, Dr. Tom Kitwood's concept of personhood acknowledges the status "bestowed upon one human being, by others, in the context of relationship and social being." We as caregivers are in a powerful position, as we are in the position of according or denying another's personhood or identity. Kitwood describes the uniqueness of people in the following way:

> At a common-sensical level it is obvious that each person is profoundly different from all others. It is easy to list some of the dimensions of that difference: culture, gender, temperament, social class, lifestyle, outlook, beliefs, values, commitments, tastes, interests, and so on. Added to this is the matter of personal history. Each person has come to be who they are by a route that is uniquely their own: every stage of the journey has left its mark. (1997, pp. 15–16)

The beauty of Kitwood's description is its obvious and simple *matter-of-factness* or as he puts it, common sense. The simplicity of personalized dementia care is the basic common sense approach. Imagine—in the midst of the clinical, diagnostic part of care one can create successful interventions and outcomes with pure common sense. (But it is a rare quality!)

Nurtured with an astute insight into the history and identity of the person, care is simplified even further. It is essential to have a knowledge base comprised of understanding the disease process and resulting effects on the different areas of the brain/behavior. It is also essential to back this up with an in-depth and concrete awareness of the individual that we are trying to support. It is a balancing act.

Secret #2

Listening and sharing information builds relationships.

Through listening to residents and sharing ourselves we become more adept at providing successful and natural Needs Response. We are able to continue building our understanding and the care relationship effortlessly.

We build our understanding of other's identity through information gathered about the *story and the self.* The Greek root of *communication* is *common understanding.* Have you established a common understanding with your residents? Or have you *assumed* a common understanding, which therefore negates its existence. By understanding the importance of identity and acknowledging the uniqueness of each person in spite of the disease, we verge on providing care in the truest form. This is what true care is all about. Ask yourself: am I a "people janitor" or a "caregiver?" People janitors are those in an intended supportive role who in the midst of the interactive process deny the person and focus only on the task. Their mission is purely to accomplish the task. There is no intention of making contact with the person within. If you are actively working to become a stronger caregiver, a gift giver—returning the gift of life and identity to those from whom it is being stolen by a ravenous disease—then you will want to know what comes next.

How can we, as caregivers, prevent the *nothingness* of a stripped identity from happening and from overtaking this marvelous individual's life? This is what I call sharing the magic.

Secret #3

Trust is the heart and soul of any relationship regardless of physical or cognitive ability or impairment.

Trust is the most essential element of the dementia caregiver–receiver relationship. It makes perfect sense that in a world where one may lose the ability to communicate (aphasia), the ability to identify things (anomia), and the ability to interpret stimuli (agnosia), the relationship with caregivers becomes essential for stress-reduced survival. We become the eyes, ears, and defense system for our residents. Our success in the care relationship is enhanced by familiarity and trust as the person knows we will protect and guide their journey.

In Kitwood's research he reflects on the person-to-person relationship and how it impacts care. He suggests twelve actions of positive person work (see **Table 3**), some of which have been referenced already in this text. These twelve caregiving behaviors or supportive actions promote trust and a nurturing, healthy, caregiving relationship.

The most significant and aspect of this list is in the final two descriptions. You will notice that the first ten actions originate from the caregiver. The final two are initiated by the care receiver. The success of this initiation is based first and foremost on trust. This trust would not be well-established were it not for the caregiver's ability to practice the other elements of positive person work. Trust is formed as a direct result of our actions, behaviors, skills, and awareness. Secret #3 demands that we put into action Kitwood's methodology with the generous outcome of a trusting relationship that will benefit both caregiver and receiver. Secret #4 further validates the practice of positive person work and reflects how our approach can be mutually beneficial.

Secret #4

We receive what we give.

In my heart there is little explanation required for this valuable secret. However, some lives have become so closed and isolated, even with daily interpersonal contact, that it may be a distant concept. For many caregivers stressed lifestyles, unresolved personal conflicts, lack of personal awareness, and desensitization to one's own needs frequently restricts one's ability to create a balanced interpersonal caring relationship. We must work toward a "balanced existence, with a proper place for recreation, social life and personal renewal" (Kitwood, 1997, p. 125) to understand and promote the well-being of residents. It is our responsibility to care first for ourselves so we may genuinely care for others. This means stringent self-evaluation toward the celebration of the self on a journey of self-healing and self-care. In doing so we develop greater clarity of what would make a difference to the quality of our own lives so that we may make a difference in the lives of those for whom we provide care.

I suggest to you that the familiar words "do unto others as you would have done to you" must form the basis of our practice, regardless of our caregiving role. We truly do receive what we give. In building and maintaining a successful relationship, our accomplishment empowers those whom brain disease disempowers. It is very easy to do everything for someone, especially

TABLE 3
Caregiving Behavior: Positive Person Work (adapted from Kitwood, 1997)

Recognition
The caregiver brings an open and unprejudiced attitude, free from tendencies to stereotype or pathologize, and recognizes the person with dementia as an individual.

Negotiation
The caregiver sets aside all assumptions about what is to be done, and dares to ask, consult, and listen.

Collaboration
There is a deliberate abstinence from the use of power, and hence from all forms of imposition and coercion. Space is created for the person with dementia to contribute as fully as possible to the action.

Play
The caregiver is able to access a free, childlike, creative way of being.

Timalation
The person with dementia receives pleasure through the direct avenue of the senses. The caregiver is at ease with his or her own sensuality—untroubled by guilt or anxious inhibition. This neologism is from the Greek *timao* (I honor, hence I do not violate personal and moral boundaries), and *stimulation*. This interaction provides contact, reassurance and pleasure with very few demands on those involved. Timalation is particularly valuable when cognitive impairment is severe.

Celebration
Beyond the burdens and immediate demands of work, the caregiver is open to joy and thankful for the gift of life.

Relaxation
The caregiver is free to stop active work for a while and even to stop planning. He or she positively identifies with the need that many people with dementia have: to slow down and allow both body and mind a respite.

Validation
The caregiver goes beyond his or her own frame of reference, with its many concerns and preoccupations, to have an empathic understanding of the other person. Cognitions are tuned down and sensitivity to feeling and emotion is heightened.

Holding
Whatever distress the person with dementia undergoes, the caregiver remains fully present—steady, assured, responsive, and able to tolerate the resonances of all disturbing emotions with in his or her own being.

Facilitation
Here a subtle and gentle imagination is called into play. There is a readiness to respond to the gesture that a person with dementia makes—not forcing meaning upon it, but sharing in the creation of meaning and enabling action to occur.

Creation
The creative action initiated by the person with dementia is seen and acknowledged as such. The caregiver responds without taking control.

Giving
The caregiver is humble enough to accept whatever gift of kindness or support a person with dementia bestows, and honest enough to recognize his or her own need. Ideas of being a benefactor or an old-time dispenser of charity have no place.

when there is difficulty communicating and acting on messages exchanged. A hidden truth in this caregiving–receiving relationship is that when things become difficult the spirit of the person (giver or receiver) rises above the challenge if given the freedom to do so. If we let go of our pride, express our own feelings in an appropriate way, and give permission (and time) for the other to respond, we will be pleasantly surprised and blessed by the response. This is the art of letting others help us rather than always doing for them and taking away their expression of empathy (in positive person work terms, giving). This is the ultimate dignity-enhancing gesture.

In living these four secrets of caregiving

- Every person who is being cared for will have his or her identity and dignity gloriously restored.
- The "us" versus "them" roles will blur between caregivers and receivers, making the relationship happier and more mutually satisfying and successful.
- As caregivers you will develop a greater sense of confidence and self-esteem or pride in your work.

Because of your success in these efforts you will smile more, laugh more, relax easier, and make the lives of many living with dementia and the associated losses more comfortable. As a result your clients will also smile more, laugh more, relax more, and respond to your caring efforts with greater ease and understanding. For having cared and for having shared these secrets, you will contribute to many people breathing easier in this world. Perhaps my favorite words from Kitwood's writing will best conclude this chapter and guide us further into the valuable journey of celebration. He proposes that

> the best dementia care is, paradoxically, a paradigm for human life. The excellent caregiver is, so to speak, a moral artist, and sets an example to all of us as we search for the right and the good. (1998, p. 34)

Celebration of the Self

*My grandmother was an amazing woman in every way...
Artist, seamstress, extraordinary hostess, a devoted wife
and mother, athlete, actress, business woman, teacher,
multitalented, interior and fashion/design wise—she was
all of these and more. Then and now, years after her
death, she remains a woman celebrated.*

To acknowledge another's worthiness means to view or to treat him or her with respect, honor, greatness, stateliness, or importance. Ask yourself: Is this what the care I provide is founded in? To respect someone is to acknowledge them in their entirety—to treat him or her with special consideration or high regard. Is this how I interact with residents, families, and peers? A living application of dignity and respect is an understanding and conscious application of the four secrets of caregiving. It is a journey of conscious awareness of ourselves and others.

To succeed in our journey we must be prepared to explore, to learn, to grow, and then to celebrate the outcomes. A celebration is not to be a forced gesture. It is one initiated and pursued with excitement, energy, and effortlessness.

I remember thinking one day that the primary benefit of the discovery and life kits was significant, more significant than originally perceived. Each of these is a venture in self-expression, an expression of identity. Each can be profoundly esteem enhancing while at the same time a celebration. For every individual experiencing and benefiting from one of these tools, it becomes a celebration of the self. But that is too easy, too simple.

It's true there is more to the celebration of the self. This is not just an occasion for the individual living with dementia. It is an experience or celebration for each of us every day. How, who, when, and why we celebrate is the bottom line in determining what matters.

Let's start with the easy one: **When?** If we understand our personal value and that of those around us, we will celebrate every day at every turn.

Who? Him, her, them, us...you and me. We celebrate others best when we can freely celebrate ourselves. When we are healthy (spiritually, emotionally, intellectually, and physically) and we are taking the best care of ourselves, we are then able to take the best care of others. (Thus aiding in the implementation of Secret #4—*We receive what we give.*) This is true of the celebration of the self: First understanding myself helps me to understand you.

How? Well, that is up to each individual. Certainly in the case of the person with dementia he or she is relying on the caregiver to promote and maintain the celebration, acknowledgment, or expression of that person's identity. The method of celebration may be as simple as a smile, a hug, or a gentle touch. It may be as complex as listening to the individual with dementia as she muddles through a jumbled message of great personal importance. Valuing the individual's right and need to communicate a message despite loss of language skills (aphasia) is a challenging way to celebrate that individual. It involves time, respect, patience, focused listening, reflecting, and observational skills—a true challenge.

I am reminded of a resident whose life career was as a woodworking instructor (industrial education teacher) at a secondary school. He was very focused in his career, highly respected by his students, and clearly a man of great patience and no doubt wisdom. It is through his patient, quiet, and gentle manner some of these inferences have been formed. Periodically he strolls the unit as if he were at school. Perhaps he is on his way to class. He will stop passersby—interestingly enough he always chooses staff and not other residents for his tête-a-têtes—and politely asks for a moment to "discuss" something. He is "such a gentleman," as described by staff, that he is difficult to turn down. Yet like a spider's web, once into the conversation you can never get out, or so it seems. His message is so tangled inside his mind that despite his efforts he only circles around and around. Sometimes strong reflective statements and paraphrasing guide his message and satisfy his communication needs: "Yes, will you take care of it then?" he will say. (Perhaps implying: "Yes, that was what I was trying to say.") Other times, no effort can decipher his cryptic communications. These are the times when all he needs is a patient, unrushed listener. Often these are the times for which he is most grateful. Often these are the greatest moments of celebration.

One day the recreation worker on the unit realized it had been some time since she had spent some true quality time with George the industrial education teacher. She reintroduced herself to him, as is her practice, and asked if she might visit with him for a while. At his gracious bidding, the two found a comfortable, semiquiet place to connect. The visit went on for some time. From a distance they appeared engaged in a fascinating exchange of ideas and opinions. Upon reflection following this valuable interaction, the recreation worker stated:

> I am exhausted. He doesn't always make sense and it is difficult to understand him at times. But, you know, when it came time for me to say good-bye he thanked me so sincerely for taking time to listen to him I was overwhelmed. It was all he wanted—someone to take the time to listen to him.

Listening to someone who has difficulty communicating is a very demanding experience…or it is a very beautiful celebration of the self. The gift of celebration is not only free but also a very easy one to satisfy.

So you still are not sure what the gist of the "celebration of the self" is or *why* it might have great value? Well then, let's explore the concept further. If you ask someone "Who are you?" the answer is often a name or a career description, maybe an address, or in some places rank and serial number. Simply put, who we are is the experiences, ideas, and beliefs as well as the more unique elements of our personality that together form our identity. It is our identity that we take the time to celebrate. In the formation of discovery and life kits and personal fact sheets, a reflection of strengths, interests, experiences, and associations come together to represent our unique being. For example, I am a recreation therapist, love to write, cherish my niece and nephews, love cats, dolphins, water, Mickey Mouse, theater, mystery novels, classic films, impressionist art, comedy (especially Lucille Ball, Carol Burnett, and Ellen DeGeneres), big band music, and old radio plays. This is only a part of my identity; I have only scratched the surface. There are my family, friends, travel interests, hobbies, dreams, passions, values, spirituality, ethics, and beliefs. What about losses—my Dad and eldest brother—and other painful experiences or memories? These hold great value.

One's identity is *never* entirely full of the good stuff. What makes a whole person is a balance of all that life has offered, gifted, and challenged each individual and how that individual has responded to the experience. A compilation of good and bad experiences contributes to the formation of one's identity.

The celebration of the self is truly a lifetime adventure. Our identity is formed over the course of years. For those who can no longer initiate remembrances and celebrations, we as caregivers take on that challenging and exciting role. It matters not whether we are a professional, family member, volunteer, or friend of the celebrant—the joyful potential of a celebration is unbounded. It is up to us to cue the magic. I love to view the experience like opening a treasure chest or Christmas gifts or birthday gifts. As the observer we never know what will be inside but we can be sure we will observe and uncover much to celebrate.

How we succeed in this is simple. The first thing I will ask of you is to completely shed your preexisting perceptions and beliefs about an individual. I want to ask you for an "attitude change." It is easy to prejudge another by appearance, shape, color, mannerism, or behavior. I invite you to a new attitude. Attitudes influence all our interactions and outcomes. Attitudes affect the beliefs that define our choices, actions, and behaviors. In turn these influence our perceptions and their resulting positive or negative outcomes. A bad attitude can be a dangerous thing. Through a shift of beliefs our attitude may be revised to see beyond the illness or influence causing a specific behavior or negative outcome. The shift invites us to see the potential cause and to look for the person beyond the problem. In the case of the person with dementia, this shift invites us to acknowledge that the individual, before the illness, would not have chosen this path of behavior. For that matter, we acknowledge that the individual has not chosen this path at all—this is the disease process we are seeing in action, not the person.

Once we accept and believe this, we begin our search for the true identity. Understanding our own identity and the value we place on ourselves gives us the insight and awareness to seek out the same in the other person. And so we begin the quest for potential (past, present, or future) in the individual. We seek, as Kitwood defined, to establish the personhood of the individual. This is achieved through observation and interaction, personal, family and other forms of interview and assessment. On this quest we look for

- **History:** Every piece of the person's puzzle must be gathered to give us insight.
- **Identity:** As seen by others, what can we find out from family or friends?
- **Strengths:** What made this person stand out to others in the community, family, workplace, and to himself or herself as he or she might identify for you?
- **Humor:** Humor can be the ultimate saving grace for so many of us. What role has humor played in this individual's life? What is its use and value?
- **Talents:** Everyone has talents. Find out what unique gifts or special skills the individual has developed throughout life and celebrate these as well.
- **Experience:** What is the good, the bad, and the ugly in this person's past? How has it influenced his or her life attitudes, outcomes, and celebrations?

Once we have gathered the information the challenge grows. We have a responsibility as caregivers to promote lifelong learning and to expand the parameters of knowledge. We must devour details about carpentry, gardening, and other areas of interest that may be relevant to residents. In doing so, we show both respect and skills to competently cue, validate, and support the person. We must get inside the information—see it, feel it, and experience the positives and negatives surrounding it. This is why it is so invaluable to prepare ourselves through deep self-awareness and ongoing skill/knowledge acquisition. To be truly successful at supporting another individual's celebration of the self we must have experienced it first ourselves. If we have seen, felt, and experienced—and understand our own life and developing identity—we are then qualified to assist others to do the same.

Oh sure, anyone can do it. "Hey, you were a great carpenter. Way to go!" But in this cursory acknowledgment, what do they understand about this identity and why? It is not simply the acknowledgment of another's experience. It is the *celebration* of what we know of the other person's experience. Appreciation, reflection, and learning from our knowledge give depth and value to the celebration of the self when initiated for another individual.

A veteran 15-year extended care unit nurses' aide recently summed up the place from which we should all start in our minds as caregivers. Maria McGinley practices what she believes and it is from the heart. She says, "We are the young people delivering care and it's only a matter of time before we are the care receivers." Her message can be summed up as *protect what we seek*. As simple, once again, as "Do unto others as you would have done to you." Maria also points out

> Sometimes I am standing at the bedside of someone who is dying. Her husband, friends, and children may be gone. I, as a nurses' aide, am often the one who holds the hand. We don't know what fears may be there. We do know the person. All there is here now is me. My message must be "somebody cares." This is how important it is to know the person. (personal communication)

Her message is simple and an eloquent acknowledgment of the value of the celebration of the self at all stages of life—even at death.

To truly experience a celebration is to take all that you have learned so far and bring it together. In this journey of celebration we acknowledge the individual by recognizing that we are, in fact, entering another's journey. It is their reality, not ours. Recognition and acceptance of this fact makes the celebration happen. We utilize the tools of reflective listening and paraphrasing where appropriate. We empathize. We use the tools of validation and improvisation as they call upon us to respond. Sometimes, as Maria McGinley indicated, we are simply present for the person. Educator Carol Hansen reminded me that silence is misunderstood. "It is an action. To be still allows for a real movement of exchange. I am not reacting, defending, or planning. I am receptive to what is in this moment." Our silence honors and respects the person's identity and dignity. More often, we observe and

Celebration of the Self

Rising with the sun,
new day challenges
face more than one.

Lost lives,
not found in mirrors
reflect brilliantly in
celebration of the self
through others' caring.

As disease consumes,
thievery abounds.
Silent witness to the losses,
trembling heart fears all.
Memory succumbs to the thief.
Answers not found...

Illumination through celebration!
Thieves run and hide
but those who care solicit knowledge
—themselves they share.

Magic spells not found here,
Simply—
patience, attention, time,
a listening ear.

The answer's clear
through celebration of
others' sphere.
Identity lost is identity found
Mere time together
brings stolen pasts near

The question is simple:
who are we?
But ones responsible
to set others free.

—Rosemary Dunne, 1996

respond, drawing from the information we have gathered. Each situation, if we are prepared, is yet another adventure in our mutual journey. A journey in which it is a privilege to participate.

Celebration of the self is captured in the words of a genuine pioneer woman of the late 1800s as she was fictionalized by Janice Woods-Windle in her book *True Women* (1993). Reflecting back on their full lives, the character Euphemia addresses her older sister Sarah:

> I don't feel a bit old, Sarah. I believe there's something in us, I
> am sure, a kind of flame that does not change through time. It is
> as alive when we're old as when our eyes first see the world.

These words give us ample reason to acknowledge and promote the celebration of the self at all stages of life. They confirm the heat of the flame inside us all and the desire to keep the flame of our identities burning. For those whose spirit is weak, or those from whom disease has appeared to steal their identity, we as caregivers accept the awesome responsibility of keeping the individuals' brilliant and colorful flames alive.

Whether we are chronologically young or young at heart, every day we add to our treasure chest of reasons to celebrate ourselves. It is a joyful moment when we acknowledge our potential for personal celebration at any age. This is the bottom line: The celebration of the self is an exciting journey into discovering and preserving our cherished identities and those of the individuals for whom we provide care. It is the foundation on which we build all our caregiving tools and interventions.

Common Understanding

The Greek root of communication is *communus*, which means *common understanding*. Though difficult, this is what we strive to achieve among caregivers and within the caregiver–receiver relationship. The disease itself often stands in the way, or at minimum creates barriers to a common understanding between caregivers and residents.

There are ways, however, to enable both caregiver and receiver. It is possible to bring about optimal outcomes and enhance a common understanding of needs and desires. Many tools have been designed to assess and treat those who require care and assistance. One tool is the *Global Deterioration Scale* (GDS; Reisberg, Ferris, de Leon & Crook, 1982; see **Table 4**, pp. 52–53) Effective use of the GDS to establish a functional baseline will

TABLE 4
Global Deterioration Scale (GDS)

Choose the most appropriate global stage based upon cognition and function.

1. **No subjective complaints of memory deficit. No memory deficit evident on clinical review. [*normal aging*]**

2. **Subjective complaints of memory deficit, most frequently in the following areas: [*normal aging*]**
   (a) forgetting where one has placed familiar objects.
   (b) forgetting names one formerly knew well.

   No objective evidence of memory deficit on clinical interview.
   No objective deficit in employment or social situations.
   Appropriate concern with respect to symptomatology.

3. **Earliest clear-cut deficits. [*border stage between normal and PDD, such as Alzheimer's disease*]**
   Manifestations in more than one of the following areas:
   (a) patient may have gotten lost when traveling to an unfamiliar location.
   (b) coworkers become aware of patient's relatively poor performance.
   (c) word and/or name-finding deficit become evident to intimates.
   (d) patient may read a passage or book and retain relatively little material.
   (e) patient may demonstrate decreased facility remembering names upon introduction to new people.
   (f) patient may have lost or misplaced an object of value.
   (g) concentration deficit may be evident on clinical testing.

   Objective evidence of memory deficit obtained only with an intensive interview. Decreased performance in demanding employment and social settings. Denial begins to become manifest in patient. Mild to moderate anxiety frequently accompanies symptoms.

4. **Clear-cut deficit on careful clinical interview. [*evidence of mild AD*]**
   Deficit manifest in following areas:
   (a) decreased knowledge of current and recent events.
   (b) may exhibit some deficit in memory or one's personal history
   (c) concentration deficit elicited on serial subtractions.
   (d) decreased ability to travel, handle finances, etc.

   Frequently *no deficit* in following areas:
   (a) orientation to time and place.
   (b) recognition of familiar persons and faces.
   (c) ability to travel to familiar locations.

   Inability to perform complex tasks. Denial is dominant defense mechanism. Flattening of affect and withdrawal from challenging situations.

5. **Patient can no longer survive without some assistance. [*moderate dementia*]**
   Patient is unable during interview to recall a major relevant aspect of their current life—for example,

TABLE 4 (continued)
Global Deterioration Scale (GDS)

(a) their address or telephone number of many years.
(b) the names of close members of their family (e.g., grandchildren).
(c) the name of the high school or college from which they graduated.

Frequently some disorientation to time (e.g., date, day of the week, season) or to place. An educated person may have difficulty counting back from 40 by 4s or 20 by 2s. Persons at this stage retain knowledge of many major facts regarding themselves and others. They invariably know their own names and generally know their spouse's and children's names. They require no assistance with toileting or eating, but may have difficulty choosing the proper clothing to wear.

6. **May occasionally forget the name of the spouse upon whom they are entirely dependent for survival.** [*moderate to severe dementia*]
Will be largely unaware of all recent events and experiences in their lives. Retain some knowledge of their surroundings, the year, the season, etc. May have difficulty counting by 1s from 10, both backward and sometimes forward. Will *require some assistance with activities of daily living:*
(a) may become incontinent.
(b) will require travel assistance but occasionally will be able to travel to familiar locations.

Diurnal rhythm frequently disturbed. Almost always recall their own name. Frequently continue to be able to distinguish familiar from unfamiliar persons in their environment. Personality and emotional changes occur. These are quite variable and include
(a) delusional behavior (e.g., patients may accuse their spouse of being an imposter; may talk to imaginary figures in the environment, or to their own reflection in the mirror).
(b) obsessive symptoms (e.g., person may continually repeat simple cleaning activities).
(c) anxiety symptoms, agitation, and even previously nonexistent violent behavior may occur.
(d) cognitive abulia (e.g., loss of willpower because an individual cannot carry a thought long enough to determine a purposeful course of action).

7. **All verbal abilities are lost over the course of this stage.** [*severe dementia*]
Early in this stage words and phrases are spoken but speech is very circumscribed. Later there is no speech at all—only grunting.
Incontinent; requires assistance toileting and feeding.
Basic psychomotor skills (e.g., ability to walk) are lost with the progression of this stage.
The brain appears to no longer be able to tell the body what to do.
Generalized and cortical neurologic signs and symptoms are frequently present.

Reisberg, B., Ferris, S. H., de Leon, M. J., and Crook, T. (1982). The Global Deterioration Scale for assessment of primary degenerative dementia. *American Journal of Psychiatry, 139,* 1136–1139. Reprinted with permission.

aid caregivers in understanding and interpreting needs as they are presented. Through appropriate assessment using relevant instruments such as the *Brief Cognitive Rating Scale* (BCRS) and *Functional Assessment Staging Test* (FAST), we may determine functional levels of residents. We may monitor changes through annual reassessment, as significant changes occur or as pharmacological intervention may be required. These tools are not discipline specific—they reflect on the function or loss of function in the brain. Therefore, the tools may be used by any discipline, giving a consistent and clear picture for everyone on a team.

The *Brief Cognitive Rating Scale*, like Folstein's *Mental Status Exam* (MSE), assesses cognitive and functional decline to a certain level. The BCRS covers five axes: concentration, recent memory, past memory, orientation and functioning, and self-care. Each of these axes is further classified or scored 1–7 (parallel to the GDS) from "no subjective/objective evidence of decline" to "severe change." This, like the MSE (or mini-MSE, a shorter format which evaluates only cognition), is a procedure that can be done quickly and easily (20 to 40 minutes). The measurement allows the scorer to determine age-associated memory impairment (AAMI), primary degenerative dementia (PDD), and the extent to which it is present.

The FAST scale is a valid, relevant tool for those who rate very low on other testing or are untestable. This is most helpful, for example, in the case of those individuals who would otherwise score zero in the mini-MSE for lack of cognitive or communication skills to respond to the assessor. The scale is broken into detailed stages based on the BCRS and the GDS, thus enabling the scorer to obtain more telltale data.

It cannot be emphasized enough that without appropriate assessment we cannot meet the needs of those for whom we care. Without a functional understanding, we cannot unite in a common understanding of needs we seek to fulfill together with this resident. Remember, in spite of the demands and losses presented by the dementia, we are coming together to serve the individual. He or she is not present for our convenience and survival. The disease was not devised to create jobs for caregivers. Rather, caregivers were sought to support the individual needs of people struck by dementia so they may live with dignity.

On that note, the Global Deterioration Scale acts as a guide to help us to understand, to support, and to enable people knowledgeably and consistently:

> The Global Deterioration Scale (GDS) is a seven-point rating instrument for the staging of the magnitude of cognitive and functional capacity in normal aging, age-associated memory impairment (AAMI), and primary degenerative dementia

(PDD). The GDS is one of the most widely used instruments for the clinical assessment of the overall magnitude of severity of AAMI and PDD, particularly PDD of the Alzheimer's type. (Reisberg, Ferris, de Leon & Crook, 1988, p. 661)

As we as caregivers come to know with what strengths and losses a person lives, we become more creative in our supportive interventions and efforts. When we identify what is involved in a task or activity, we can match this to what we know of the individual's strengths based on the GDS ratings. As we become familiar with the scale, our ability to recognize strengths and needs becomes more fine tuned. The grand reward is simple: greater quality of life for the receiver of care, less stress for caregivers, and increased successful outcomes.

To further clarify the rating scale we can describe the seven levels as follows. Stages one and two may be described as "normal aging." Stage three is subtle in presentation and a border stage between normal and Alzheimer's onset. In stage four we begin to see evidence of mild Alzheimer's disease. At stage five the individual is no longer able to survive in the community without assistance; they are functioning with moderate dementia. Moderate to severe dementia is present at stage six. Stage seven is one of progressive loss and referred to as severe dementia. This continuum of ongoing loss, due to unpredictable damage to various areas of the brain, is nothing less than tragic. The challenge presented to caregivers is one of recognizing individuality and promoting the use of remaining strengths.

The Global Deterioration Scale is used here with the goal of focusing caregiver energy on skill awareness and promotion through purposeful and enjoyable activity. As you continue to read this book, take time to see the possibilities as you recognize strengths in your own resident population. Everything is adaptable and anything is possible.

You may find that the rating assigned to a specific program (e.g., one of the programs in Part 6) does not seem to match your own experience. Based on the flexibility and adaptability of programs and their implementation, this may be true. You are encouraged to review the rating scale from all angles to find the skill match. Tasks may need to be broken down further. Volunteer roles may change. Many variables play on the success of a program. Let us not forget the all important question: Is this the right program for this population at this time? The GDS is a valuable tool to assist you in better recognizing your role and your resident's needs.

The Global Deterioration Scale has been presented here with two goals in mind: (a) to introduce you to a concrete and recognizable measure which assists us in identifying and meeting needs, and (b) to lend some insight into abilities retained as well as those required for the programs found later in this text.

The important consideration to emphasize at this point is that we can all identify familiar behaviors as they are listed here. Assessment gives us a guideline on which to base our actions. The tendency to disenable our residents comes from incorrect assumptions and skill judgments without qualifying or conclusive evidence. Using consistent measures is invaluable as we seek to implement relevant goals and approaches with those for whom we provide support and care. Personal biases and individual judgments are inappropriate and unsuitable. If there is a question of functional ability, reassess to establish the team's baseline. We provide support based on individual strengths and needs. We establish strengths and needs through appropriate assessment and reassessment of the individual.

Discovery Kits

When a person loses the ability to draw from his or her
own personal vault of adventure experience, he or she
relies on us as caregivers to stimulate them to adventure.

There is joy in individuality. Each of us has a unique perception of what is or is not, of reality and fantasy. These perceptions are what contribute to the adventure of experiential prop kits or *discovery kits*.

Discovery Kit
Three-dimensional, multifaceted, themed tool assembled for the pursuit of adventure through reminiscence and exploration, totally without expectations.

Reminiscence is a powerful tool. It can be used by almost anyone. Reminiscence requires skill in the areas of establishing, directing, and maintaining a discussion. It also requires skill in asking open-ended questions (questions which do not result with a "yes" or "no" response and usually begin with who, what, where, or when). *Discovery* is equally unique because it may require knowledge of specific subjects and confidence in pursuing and celebrating the reminiscences shared. There are immediate advantages offered through the use of specifically themed, three-dimensional discovery kits. Using props increases the participant's success because it provides them with something concrete and recognizable. Response is cued even though their language comprehension and expression have been affected. We are also able to observe and assess their level of comprehension and ability to cope with the theme of the chosen kit by their cued response and appropriate demonstration or use of the specific props. For example, a fisherman who can show the group how to cast with a fishing rod or the best way to bait a hook displays his or her comprehension. (*Note*: Use barbless hooks or remove barbs for safety before use.) A homemaker able to demonstrate the use of a traditional meat grinder accomplishes the same goal.

Through the creation and use of discovery kits, elements of familiarity, recognition, sharing, demonstration, and enjoyment add to the concept of one-dimensional verbal reminiscence. In exploring and understanding discovery kits we must first try to understand the individuals who would benefit from their use.

Adult reference to *adventure* draws from our education, memories, life and work experiences, courage, and imaginations. When a person loses the ability to draw from his or her personal vault of adventure experience, he or she relies on us as caregivers to stimulate them to adventure. We take on the responsibility of cueing and guiding them. This is achieved through assessment or information gathering.

We must develop strong social and experiential histories. We must make full use of our interviewing and observational skills to listen and to look for pieces of their puzzles and clues to their realities. At times the answers may be nonsense to us, but they are pieces to the individual's unique puzzle. Having gathered our information, which may reflect one person or the demographics of the unit as a whole, we begin to create our kits. Discovery kits have limitless possibilities. They may be based on

- specific careers (e.g., railway, clerical, airline pilot, military)
- seasonal or cultural celebrations (e.g., Valentine's, Day, St. Patrick's Day)
- rites of passage (e.g., Sweet 16, courting, marriage)
- hobbies or favorite pastimes (e.g., trains, stamps, woodworking)
- domestic activities or chores (e.g., cooking, sewing)

Through the use of the themed kit, a person with Alzheimer's or a related disorder now receives an opportunity to restore or experience adventure. The individual is offered the chance to take a road less traveled.

Stimulating Success

Once staff found the courage and figured it out, it was
amazing how fun and exciting our job became!

Successful interactions and self-expression for people with Alzheimer's can
have an impact on more than just the individual with dementia. Celebrating
ourselves can take place through the successful expression of our knowledge,
experience, and personality with others. With the onset of dementia this expression can be an even greater challenge. The benefits offered by discovery
kits can turn this challenge around. With the successful creation and use of
the kits, everyone involved blossoms. There are many benefits to encouraging
the development and use of discovery kits, including social, intellectual,
identity, sensory, functional, and self-esteem advantages. Kits that encourage
the discussion and exploration of common experiences result in social interactions that might not otherwise take place. Interpersonal relationships begin
developing through increased familiarity. Because we are social beings, we
naturally seek out the company of others. Small groups or one-on-one interactions allow for a direct social, learning, and sharing experience. As individuals express themselves, bonds develop and the potential for isolation is
reduced. Interaction promoted through small groups or initiated by the residents themselves strongly supports the "thirst" for social interaction that exists
long into the onset of dementia. Even when some individuals seem to have
withdrawn, they may still return to a higher social interaction level given the
right supportive environment. In her book *Activities and Approaches for
Alzheimer's* Sally Freeman further clarifies and supports the value of encouraging and stimulating such interactions:

> Activities should be used to encourage conversation and friend-
> ship. Socialization provides a way in which an activity can be
> approached at an adult level and at a level at which the patient
> can succeed. A person may prefer to watch passively or con-
> verse rather than actively participate. If a sense of accomplish-
> ment can come from conversing about an activity, rather than
> participating in the activity, it should be considered a success.
> (1990, p. 35)

We have seen residents who have gradually reintegrated back into the
social network. Their initial involvement is often extremely superficial (e.g.,
merely being present in a room). Yet they can gradually increase to observing

a group, supporting a group, and participating in a group. This is another example of constructing a community.

> *One day most of the residents were off unit for a special event in the auditorium. Returning to the unit to address the needs of the remaining residents, the recreation worker encountered one individual who fit the progression of a resident reintegrating into the social and program environment. This resident had been a busy wanderer, routinely strolling the wandering path. She lacked interest in events, and perhaps in part due to a hearing impairment, remained mostly in her room when not wandering. Gradually her wandering decreased. She began spending more time sitting in the lounge and observing, sometimes clapping or laughing at the particular activity in progress. On this day she smiled and observed the quiet lack of activity. She asked the recreation worker, "Where are the people you amuse?" This resident had progressively developed an interest and social awareness of those around her—including the valuable role of the recreation worker.*

It may take several months, but a noninvasive and supportive approach using open communication can restore a person's curiosity so that they seek out more interaction. Discovery kits offer a specific, noninvasive, and supportive focus. Proper use of a kit promotes open communication and sharing as a great means to an even greater end. **Table 5** (p. 60) presents a sample listing of kit possibilities.

Specific discovery kits are carefully assembled based on the history, geography, and demographics of the area and population. This includes generational considerations that can increase familiarity for the specific population or group involved. For example, *prairie life* reflects farming, ranching, small town life, the schoolhouse, and trips into town. *Coastal life* reflects seaside cottages, city life, boating, office work, college, and the port industry.

Although overlap exists with each focus area, it is easy to see that there also will be differences. We find the same differences in the residents or families for whom we develop our themed kits. We must recognize that kits are as disposable as they are priceless. A change in population will make a kit temporarily useless as the familiarity or appeal is lost. Our awareness of changes in the population is what maintains effective use of discovery kits. Start small and grow. Interchange parts of kits to build and develop functional effective tools. As Mary Lucero indicates, some success may come by accident. She elaborates on her own experience, successes and failures:

TABLE 5
Sample Discovery Kits

Photography	Fishing	Jewelry
old-fashioned camera	tackle box	earrings
old/famous photos	weights	brooches
camera equipment	fishing hat	bracelets
book on photography	fake/live bait	table mirror
Life magazine	bobs, other gadgets	jewelry box
Construction/Tools	**Silver Polishing**	**Motoring**
large PVC pieces, joints	empty Silvo bottle	models of cars
large nuts, bolts, screws	polishing cloth	books about cars
wood blocks	old silver	driving music
sand paper/sanding block	silver chest	hat, scarf
tool box		driving gloves
Military	**Business**	**Sewing**
medals	briefcase	sewing basket
photographs, albums	alarm clock	buttons, zippers
letters	ruler	bows
uniform elements	pen	fabric/fabric book*
canteen, mess kit	clipboard, paper	thimbles
ration books	book	spools of thread
music of the war years	abacus/calculator	patterns
Seaside		
sea shells	* *Fabric book:* A mixture of 6x12-inch swatches	
sponges	of brightly colored, multitextured material	
crab shell	sewn together down the short edge (like a	
driftwood	book) with a button, snap, or Velcro so it can	
bathing suit	be folded over and tucked away or "fiddled"	
picnic basket	with by the user.	

The first ones I developed focused on the props our residents used in their occupations. I found that these kits were successful not only in engaging residents, but also their development alone created excitement and enthusiasm in family members and the staff. I believe these occupation kits also had a powerful psychological impact on the way staff and family members perceived residents. Given things that were familiar and meaningful, residents astounded everyone by doing very "normal" things and using many props very competently. (personal communication)

Lucero further elaborates on their success by explaining the advantage and adventure that failure experiences present:

> We had more failures in the beginning than successes, but eventually we realized that the successful ones related directly to our unique group of residents' individual and collective past life experiences. Most of our failures were because we tried ideas that were more related to our interests and/or backgrounds. That experience was pivotal in helping me realize how important it was for every facility to learn about the unique demographics of their dementia residents so that commonalities could be identified, and programming and props developed specifically around those commonalities. (personal communication)

Mary Lucero's experiences and successes, not to mention failures, advocate for adventure in the pursuit of discovery kits as well as suitable program development. Her insight and experience can help to motivate us to continue the quest for props that will benefit everyone whose needs we endeavor to address, including staff, volunteers, family, and residents.

Autobiography in a Box

Life kits open us to the uniqueness of a person long after the individual is able to open up to us.

It didn't take long to realize the value of individualizing the concept of discovery kits to create the life kit. It may not be a universally useful proposal, but who says everyone must use everything in special care? The individual exists beyond the losses experienced through dementia, and life kits keep this promise. The joy in the development of the life kit is the opportunity provided for families to maintain relationships through the familiar history of the person. It acts to cheat the disease process despite the brain's attempt to abandon the individual, and serves as a mini personal archive or museum that promotes the celebration of the person. Not only do families benefit from enhanced interaction, but also volunteers and staff receive the opportunity for more purposeful and satisfying interactions. Development of individual life kits offers families positives to focus on in what can often be a bleak process of debilitating loss. What do we give Mom for Christmas or Dad for Father's Day? The answer is easy: the gift of themselves.

Special occasions or day to day, we can add to quality of life. This also serves to augment our coping resources by creatively challenging us to seek out items to add variety and familiarity to the kits we develop. We can suggest these positive options to families as they clamor for ideas and options to maintain hope and energy. Caregiver batteries do drain—life kits can offer a recharging. The Orr Family found a recharging in their pursuit of a life kit.

Celebrating Life Creatively

Today they describe her with respect for the strong woman she once was.

The Orr family struggled with the understanding and management of the needs of their mother (Vera) whose battle with changes due to Alzheimer's appeared at age 82. Like other families, they attempted to learn about the disease process, what to do to cope, and how best to support their mother and their father. After the initial and ongoing grief processes began to lessen, time took their mother through the many stages of the disease. They traveled with her, valiantly coping along the way.

Today, they describe her with respect for the strong woman she once was. She is sometimes unrecognizable—although her physical health remains, her mind has wasted away. Their undying love and admiration for the woman who made them who they are today takes them regularly to spend time with her. They visit out of love and make sure she has all the comforts she needs, but this is a struggle. When each visit became more difficult with little response and even less recognition, it became harder to go to her. How many times could they water a plant, straighten her clothes, or read the newspaper—with no response?

Help came in the form of a personal life kit. Together, we explored memories of the woman they love. It was a thought-provoking, sensory exploration of their recollections as they reminisced about: the shampoo she always bought, her love of seamstressing, her loyalty to family, and her generosity to friends. Her talents in the kitchen were undeniable. They viewed her French Canadian spirit as her strength. Her faith a devout Roman Catholic came to fore. Her general strength of character provided us with the means to piece together possibilities to create a valuable tool for both Mrs. Orr and her devoted family. In a large plastic box we gathered

- religious reading material
- oversized rosary (one-inch, round beads)
- scented hand lotion (her shampoo was no longer available)
- mini photo album with photos labeled for descriptive reading and reminiscing, including people in the photo, their relationship to Vera, location, and year
- various sensory stimulation props of different textures to call her attention (e.g., cosmetic puffs, compact puffs, feather duster)
- a soft, multicolored ball for stimulating small hand movements
- a bowl to soak her hands, and lotion with which to massage her hands
- recycled film canisters now filled with her favorite spices (Aromatherapy oils on cotton balls work well and may be changed or replenished from time to time.)
- a fabric book of brightly colored and various textures of material sewn together for her to handle

This kit is quite basic in its approach. Although it primarily focuses on sensory stimulation, it is assembled based on her personal history. While she benefits from the interaction and stimulation secondary benefits must be acknowledged.

The Orr family now experiments with different approaches. By using their creativity, they find their visits less stressful and more satisfying. Family members read the newspaper aloud to her (she is soothed by a familiar voice), massage her hands (soothed by a familiar touch), pray the rosary (placing the large beads in her hands, they include her by moving each bead through the sequence of prayers). They even find pleasure in watching her with the fabric book as she instinctively folds half-inch pleats in the individual pages.

By creating a multidimensional kit as a source of props to enhance interactions, this family turned a devastating situation around making it as pleasurable and filled with warm memories as possible. Families can continue to refresh the kit over time to maintain interest. By changing items we continue to open up bits of information about the individual to others. This is a great way to rally the family together when one is unsure how to recognize or celebrate a loved one during those special days of the year (e.g., Christmas, Mother's Day, birthdays).

Family Gold

They traveled with her, valiantly coping along the way...

After a lifetime of family sharing and memories, it is heartbreaking to witness a loved one experience the gradual onset of dementia. The changes, losses, confusion, and grief experienced are many and varied. Caregivers search for resources to help their loved ones and themselves in coping with the changes. Professional caregivers search for tools to facilitate the best possible care on behalf of the individual and his or her family.

By personalizing the approach of discovery and creating an individualized kit, we provide a specific and accurate means of interacting with the individual. A personal life kit reflects the identity, experiences, and memories of the individual. It is an effective tool that provides

- families with familiar props to enhance time spent together
- professional caregivers with props that may be used to become more familiar with the individual, and used to stimulate discussion
- valuable insight into the individual's history and possible realities

The example of a life kit information sheet (opposite) is a special summary provided to families and friends. It adds clarity to the purpose of kits and shares how to create a personal life kit. Feel free to use and adapt this format.

Now for a cautionary note: One of the most important elements to emphasize in promoting life kits is the labeling of personal items. I mean this in two specific senses. The first is that people are not the only wandering elements in special care. Possessions wander in such a way that they may never be seen again. This is a reality for family and staff. Equipment can disappear as easily as your favorite or most cherished family photos, clothing, or souvenir. Preadmission information often includes this caveat. Unfortunately many families take action only after a cherished item disappears. There are two solutions to this. Either leave items of value at home or keep an inventory and offer to help with the occasional search of the unit to recover items and restore a touch of order. Certainly everyone involved in the unit will appreciate this. Sadly, many people don't look for items until they are clearing out a relative's room after they have passed on. This is a difficult enough time as is—to discover a further loss only serves to salt the painful wound of grief. Be proactive.

You Can Make a Meaningful Life Kit

Let me share my life with you so you can bring my life to me...

The losses experienced with the onset of dementia can be discouraging. Still, there are ways to stay connected with those we love and care for while sharing, remembering, and relaxing together. Life kits are effective tools which enhance interaction with your family member.

Families with a relative experiencing the consequences of later stage dementia describe the distress, guilt, and frustration felt when visiting. The life kit is a valuable tool that may move us from frustration to fulfillment of quality interactions. Although some individuals in later stages may not be able to respond in an observable manner, the comfort offered visitors by the life kit makes spending time together more positive and gratifying.

Stored in a familiar case such as a box, briefcase, or chest, life kits contain recognizable items that may cue reminiscence visually. For those unable to respond to visual stimulus, the contents of the kit may provide direction for the family, staff, volunteer, or other visitors to verbally cue reminiscence, thus creating a mutual atmosphere of comfort. Life kits may comprise any or all of the following ideas:

- career-related props
- family/personal memorabilia
- photo album (remember to label photos)
- items relating to life periods (e.g., childhood, marriage)
- familiar knickknacks, souvenirs
- samples of or photos of hobbies or achievements

Don't limit yourself, however: Be creative and put *life into your kit.* Think of the uniqueness of the person you celebrate. Be sure to include descriptive cards and labels to enhance effectiveness for all users.

The second and perhaps more important reason for labeling items is to share knowledge toward promoting the celebration of the individual. As caregivers we become the memory. A labeled photo does two things. First it tells us a little more about the person, thus enhancing our appreciation of his or her identity. This helps to form the feeling of having something in common with another. For example, after working with a volunteer for more than five years I learned she worked as a nurse for 23 years. I have a greater appreciation of her identity now plus an understanding of where she is "coming from." Second, the label is a tool that helps us help the resident. A clear label will tell us, for example, who is in a photo. It may describe the location and relationship of others in the picture to the resident and give a date to orient us to the memory, thus assisting the resident to enjoy the memory. In *Aggression: Siding with Anger* you will read about this benefits of labeling and how to use it to the advantage of both yourself and the resident.

Aggression: Siding with Anger

> *Ninety percent of catastrophic behaviors are inadvert-*
> *ently provoked by caregiver behavior or a [perceived]*
> *unsafe environment.*
>   *Knowing the strengths and limitations of our resi-*
> *dents is the first crucial step in providing the most sup-*
> *portive and respectful quality of care.*

It is imperative to keep an open mind with reference to our props and kits. Their uses cannot be limited to planned one-to-one visits. They can be elemental to offsetting potentially disastrous situations. The more applications we find for our props and kits, the greater their value becomes. Laura's life book made all the difference when she needed to depart a painful experience in her reality.

∞   ∞   ∞   ∞   ∞

We had just finished an energetic exercise class and were cheerfully strolling through the hall on our way to stop in for manicures. It was quiet as usual when we came upon the hair salon. Laura's eyes were ablaze and her hands gripped the arms of her wheelchair. She stood and faced the hairdresser, who held the handgrips at the back of the chair in an attempt to steady it. Laura's anger had brought a rush of adrenaline which gave her the strength to lift the chair several inches off the ground and repeatedly slam it back down. She shouted angrily at the hairdresser, "Leave me alone! Just get away! Get away or I'll kill you! Someone get me out of here!"

    Standing in the gap between the seat and the footrests, Laura was in danger of being tripped by her own chair and falling to the ground. She shook, her dress torn down the front, and glanced terrified at the number of onlookers who had come to the aid of the hairdresser.

    Fearing a fall, I stepped closer and looked at Laura, smiling. "Hello Laura, it's Rosemary," I said slowly and gently. She broke her gaze from the hairdresser and looked at me—no recognition. I stopped a few feet from her, lowered my voice again, and asked what I could do for her.

    "I can't stand it here. Get them away!" she said.

I came a bit closer and asked her gently "What exactly can I do for you, Laura?"

Still shaking, she shouted "Tell her to go away!"

At this point, it was crucial to show my support and gain her trust. Standing protectively between the two, I matched her energy, and with the same anger, I turned to the hairdresser and shouted "Go away, Sheila!" (I must admit I had little concern for the hairdresser's feelings at that point—because there was no time for explanation—although she seemed to catch on.)

Sheila backed off the chair and moved out of sight into a small supply room. I looked directly at Laura and said. "There, she's gone. Now Laura, I am very worried about you." She was completely agitated and disoriented at this point and totally without awareness of her wheelchair and the potential danger she was in. I explained I would like her to sit down and rest. She shook the chair, confused by the apparatus, and apparently unable to release her grip. I explained she was holding the armrests of an unusual chair.

Looking down, she let go, we then held on to each other and slowly she turned to sit. Together we left the salon. I promised to take her to her apartment so we could make her more comfortable and change her torn dress.

Once at her suite we sat quietly for a minute. (I refer to resident rooms as apartments or suites, as they are their rental homes. It tends to reduce the confusion regarding going home somewhat. Although, I often must elaborate to explain the luxury aspects of housekeeping, personal care, and dining facilities as being all-inclusive with their rent.)

I had initiated a reminiscing-focused discussion on the elevator ride up. In her suite, I reached for her life book—a loving gift created by her devoted daughter. Laura had no recollection or familiarity with the book, her family, or her long-term memories as we began—her level of distress and anxiety was still too high. As we began going through the book, I would read ahead the descriptions, but relate the information as if I knew the facts of her life.

"I understand that you were born in Prince Rupert and moved to Grand Forks when you were five. Your father seemed awfully devoted to you and your three brothers." I pointed to them and read their names as we viewed each brother's photo, "and your beautiful sisters."

Gradually, Laura was able to focus and recall details adding to my commentary. Together, we laughed and shared. Where she had gaps or unclear memories, I filled in the blanks from my memory of clearer conversations with her in the past. The notes and details documented in her life book also served as a guide for those who might be less familiar with her life. By the end of her life book Laura was her charming, good-humored self again.

I suggested we get her into something more comfortable than her torn dress. Together we picked out another lovely outfit. I helped her change, and together we went back downstairs for a manicure—leaving the wheelchair behind and walking this time.

∞   ∞   ∞   ∞   ∞

I suggest that without siding with Laura, returning to the peace and quiet of her apartment, and reviewing her well-planned life book, Laura would have probably taken a serious fall, she may even have hurt the hairdresser or others present. Incidentally, this intervention only took 20 to 30 minutes—time well-spent. The alternative may have been to use medication, to spend the rest of the day reacting to unsettled responses, such as anger or aggression, other situations, or worse—a harmful fall.

Some may question this intervention and identify that such an approach does not always work. This may very well be true, but it cannot be a limiting belief. The effort must always be made to try different approaches and to collect and use the tools available. We must be prepared to challenge our perceptions and beliefs in the interest of quality care. We must establish personal quality assurance measures and apply them accordingly.

Mitchell reminds us that

> diagnosing people based on observed behavior denies the fact
> that every human being constructs personal meaning and makes
> choices based on personal options and individual realities.
> (1990, p. 175)

Our perceptions and beliefs affect our interactions directly. It is important for us to recognize the space the individual is in. In a critical situation we must be prepared to join the individual's journey. The bottom line is that the so-called aggressive resident is not being aggressive for the sake of aggression itself. These individuals are simply defending their reality.

Aggressive residents are defensive as a primal instinct, reacting to stimuli. Something is unfamiliar or unclear and they find it frightening or threatening. Within the limitations caused by damage to the brain, individuals are not able to interpret and respond to stimuli as they may have prior to the onset of dementia. Their response is a measure of communication based on remaining skills. As a result basic instincts kick in and take over as a measure of survival. Knowing this, and recalling occasions in which we have experienced an overpowering rush of adrenaline in a dangerous or threatening situation, we should be able to empathize very well with our residents. Imagine a life experience where control and familiarity were taken away from you. Think of how frightening it is to lose your ability to understand and respond comfortably and clearly to cope with the situation. An example of this would be to consider being lost or injured in a foreign country where you have no working knowledge of the language. You may know a few words but couldn't put them together to save yourself. These are the daily, moment-to-moment experiences of the person living with dementia.

The categories of stimuli (see **Table 6**, pp. 70–71) suggest a starting point for assessing where the person may be sensing a threat. They suggest areas for us to maintain specific awareness. We must routinely examine our actions, our words, and the home environment we are trying to create as well as how we utilize them to the benefit of everyone involved.

A well-planned intervention or improvisation goes beyond the moment of stepping into the scene. The use of props or tools such as life books or life kits, familiarization with the individual's life experience, and siding with the individual's perception of the situation goes a very long way in settling a dispute or calming a frightened outburst. Imagination is the key in using these tools. We play an important role in knowing when to intervene and what to use to be situational change agents. As one recreation worker put it

> When a person comes to us we are presented with the border to a puzzle. The border or frame is complete. However, the puzzle is not. We are also given a jumble of pieces to complete the puzzle. It is how and when we use these pieces that makes us effective at putting the puzzle together to create a beautiful image.

The challenge continues as we are repeatedly called to be detectives, actors, directors, and prop managers. Making use of the tools and resources available to us can appear to make us miracle workers.

Funny what we learn, or relate to, from television. Remember the "good cop, bad cop" routine from your favorite police show? (Now don't misunderstand this analogy, I am *not* saying this should be an intentional practice—just adding situational clarity.) One person may appear to be completely ineffective or counterproductive in their interaction with an individual. Yet, another person may step in and appear to be a miracle worker. We can speculate over many reasons why this occurs. Some say the individual may recognize the "good" person as a positive influence from their past. The apparent "bad" person may trigger the memory of someone they feared or disliked. On the other hand, sometimes the initial approach frightened or disoriented the individual (bad cop). A fresh face (good cop) may be the calming or cueing influence. Sometimes a person seems to need time to consider a request or perhaps needs to be given control of the situation. Yes, timing is everything.

Oh, how we can speculate! Speculation broadens our thinking and lends insight to our approaches and our responses to the individual's own response to stimuli. Keep thinking, be mindful, and get ready to step in and help, or for that matter, back off and defer to another. Success is up to us.

Our willingness to see past our pride and witness the needs of a given moment puts us on this very path. Yes, our self-conscious human nature can interfere with care. We must learn to see beyond ourselves and into the reality of the person whose needs we endeavor to meet. We must be mindful and willing to step out of our task focus to achieve success and ensure comfort, respect, and dignity of the individuals for whom we provide care.

TABLE 6
Categories of Stimuli

Gestures/Approaches

Fine or Gross Movements
Busy, large, or fast movements are confusing and disorienting. To avoid overstimulation or frightening a person, use paced, moderate movement that the individual can follow.

Speed/Pace
Follow the pace of the individual.

Direction of Approach
Never approach from the side or behind. This will startle the person. Walk a wide circle around to get in front of the person. The best approach is from the front while making eye contact.

Number of People Helping
Always defer to one leader or speaker when approaching the individual or asking the resident to complete a task. Too many "helpers" is both intimidating and overstimulating. Be aware of who is helping and step out of the picture unless you are the leader. "Tag-team care" works here if all are aware: step in and out as the facilitator based on your success with the individual.

Environment

Lighting
Make sure the room is bright enough that someone with a visual impairment can manage. Ensure the person is not being blinded by direct or reflected light.

Temperature
If the room is comfortable for caregivers it is likely too cold for care receivers. If caregivers are uncomfortable, residents will most likely be comfortable. Watch for signs of discomfort.

Just the Facts

Understanding how individuals make choices based on personal values and perspectives has clarified the uniqueness of each person's situation.

—Gail J. Mitchell

There is no question that confidentiality is crucial as a matter of respect and preservation of dignity. But how do we offer our volunteers, extended family members, and friends all the "right stuff" to ensure quality interactions with residents, satisfaction for visitors, and the maintenance of confidentiality?

TABLE 6 (continued)
Categories of Stimuli

Crowds
Too many people can generate an overstimulating scenario that is uninterpretable and therefore unmanageable

Noise/Confusion
Speaking loudly in a dining room, shouting down a hall, and talking over someone while providing care and support cause overstimulation and are examples of poor care practice or nonresident-focused care.

Language

Complexity of Request
The words we choose can complicate or simplify a task. Use brief statements with familiar words.

Facial Expression
Nonverbal body language communicates very loudly. Soft, friendly facial expressions; nodding in understanding to show empathy; and eye contact promote success and understanding.

Number of People Speaking
Always ensure only one person speaks to the resident at a time. There is no flexibility in this. Too many voices or instructions is too confusing. Use simple language for clear communication. Defer to a leader, or alternate by speaking one at a time.

Voice Quality
Volume, tone (soft or harsh), pitch (high or low) and rate (fast or slow) of speech all generate response. A gentle, clear, and unrushed voice reassures and builds trust.

Recognizing that volunteers, for example, are unable to review the legal chart document, which is full of social history and facts, we devised a purposeful summary: the personal fact sheet (PFS; see **Figure 3**, pp. 73–74).

For each resident, we compiled data drawn from the chart and/or acquired through conversation with family or the residents themselves. To further personalize the content, the PFS is written in the first person. Each PFS was then given an attractive cover to encourage use of the information. Both volunteers and staff found the PFS useful as quick reference for one-on-one interactions. The format used for a PFS is what I like to call proconversational. By this I mean the facts are basic, yet informative enough that conversation may flow from the content. Although some residents have lost the ability to express themselves, the information contained in the PFS is simple and straightforward enough that they may follow and agree with or add to the data presented in their own way. It is also presented simply so the person initiating the interaction may personalize it with ease to share like interests or experiences.

In the case where presentation of such a useful tool is a challenge, flex thinkers find the solutions. Take the case of the Orr family, where their mother's life kit and PFS would find their way into the back of her closet. The simple solution found by persistent family members was to post her PFS on the bulletin board in her room. The family soon noticed changes. The biggest of these was the continued presence of her kit by her bedside as they preferred. The pleasure for the family increased when staff actively sought them out to share discoveries of things in common with their mother.

Personal fact sheets, as any other tool, are as effective and supportive of our care goals as we make them. Although the example in Figure 3 demonstrates suitable content for the form, there are no limitations to the creativity of the content. Finally, to further offer support to the tools of discovery and life kits, the PFS suggests (among other preferences) which kits are most beneficial for and therefore most appreciated by the individual resident.

Take a minute to get to know me! Much like you, my life has been filled with challenges, joys, sorrows, laughter, and all sorts of adventures. Although I have difficulty expressing my memories of past years, I would love to share them with you. Here are some facts about my life that will help us to visit and to enjoy our time together.
    Thank you for bringing my world back to me.

Name:

Please call me:

Place of birth (village, city, country):

Other places I called home (time frames):

My parents were:

Their careers/endeavors included:

Brothers and sisters (older/younger):

Favorite pets (childhood/adulthood):

Favorite pastimes (books, authors, music, instruments, song, sports teams, special skills or hobbies):

Today I enjoy talking about (news, career, family):

FIGURE 3
Personal Fact Sheet

I married (who, when, where; state year of passing if applicable):

In our life we enjoyed the following together:

Our family included (names and birthdays of children or significant persons):

If we can sit together and read, I prefer (poetry, newspaper, humorous shorts, specific personal items):

I would enjoy a snack or beverage while we visit (state preferences):

Dietary precautions:

I enjoy using (state physical activity or prop that achieves positive response):

My life kit is located in:

The discovery kit I most enjoy is:

Other points to ponder while preparing to visit with me include:

Note: Be sure to list family losses or cautionary areas to be sensitive to the individual's needs.

Rosemary Dunne, Revised 1997

FIGURE 3 (continued)
Personal Fact Sheet

The Bonus Round

The individual is given the opportunity to celebrate himself or herself.

We are always seeking benefits of the tools we use. It is imperative that we justify our tools, our time, and our methods of intervention. Thankfully, it can be clearly stated that there are many benefits to the development and use of the discovery kit. I consider the clear benefits a real bonus to the simple joys of the interactive process. Discovery kits offer four basic benefits or goals.

Preserve Individual Identity and Self-Esteem

Kits specific to a person's career or interests and history acknowledge the uniqueness of the individual. They offer the person the opportunity to revisit their experiences through reminiscence and self-expression. Props contained in kits cue memories and offer the individual a chance to be the "expert" by demonstrating use of or familiarity with specific items. The individual is given the opportunity to celebrate himself or herself.

Develop and Maintain Relationships

In small group or one-on-one interactions the individual is offered the opportunity to discuss and explore common experiences. The individual is provided a setting in which to demonstrate support, to socialize, and to learn from peers. The experience is in the moment and it may or may not continue beyond the group setting. The opportunity to become familiar with others and to develop trust and rapport exists just the same.

Reduce Potential for Isolation

Through proper development of a variety of kits based on the resident population, we address mixed needs. In doing so, we increase the potential to involve more residents. By rotating the contents or adjusting kits based on population changes, we continue the practice of involvement.

Evoke Memories Through Reminiscence and Sensory Stimulation

A creatively assembled kit will touch on all or most senses depending on your specific goals or the theme of the kit. It will offer through varied props the means to cue and to stimulate reminiscence on various levels. The more familiar and varied the props, the greater the success of the kit. Authenticity is crucial—the more original the prop the more likely it will be to cue the desired outcome.

I am reminded of an intergenerational group I once led. We asked the children to bring cherished items (props) which they owned. We supplied items relevant to the resident's cherished pasts if they were lacking props from their day. The plan was that the children would try and guess the senior's prop. In turn, the senior would try and guess what the prop the children brought was used for. I passed around an old crank style meat grinder and asked the children to tell their senior tablemates what they thought it was. The children amazed one and all with their suggestions: a telephone, a periscope, a hammer. When we explained it was similar to the modern Cuisinart food grinder, they looked at us perplexed.

Age is irrelevant when it comes to the effectiveness of familiar props. Keep the concept of overstimulation in mind when developing a kit. Too much can lead to little as residents become unable to focus on an item or theme. Ultimately one of the best aspects or benefits of the discovery kit, from an employer or family perspective, is the opportunity for staff to become more familiar with the resident as a person of experience and adventure, much like ourselves. To find commonality between staff and residents is a valued step toward the highest quality of care. When we can closely relate to those with whom we work and for whom we care, we reduce barriers and enhance the quality of our interactions.

Great Discovery Challenge: Creating Kits

Your creativity could never be challenged more than it is now!

The great discovery challenge is all about the fun and adventure possible in the pursuit of functional discovery kits. Kits are developed based on specific needs, such as

- general demographics
- individual histories
- cultural or social aspects of a community

- gender specific
- seasonal considerations

Imagination is the first step towards success in creating discovery kits. Once you know what you want to make, establish a period—1920s, 1930s, 1940s, and so on. Having established this, your challenge has just been enhanced. Authenticity is a top priority in pursuing a successful kit. In some cases this may be extremely impractical due to cost. Your creativity could never be challenged more than now. I have been asked many times: Can we just buy a kit? I always say, "No." Collect a kit and you will have far more success—leave the niceties of newness behind and the ease of convenience at home. Just as Rome, kits are not built in a day. The easiest approach to creating effective discovery kits is to challenge others to do it for you. Do you have an expert in an area or theme you would like to pursue?

I was grateful to receive the support of a volunteer who is a hunter and a fisherman. He donated an old, worn tackle box, some flies, bobs, weights, and shiners. We added some wooden fish, a plastic frog, and pictures of various fishing experiences. Before we open the challenge up to others for support and input (in the form of a promotion or contest) let's explore the four Rs of discovery kits: recycle, requests, resources, and rummaging.

Recycle

Explore your attic, storage locker, kitchen, and garage. Don't limit yourself to your own home. Seek out your friends, family, and neighbors. There is plenty of "stuff" we never use but keep for decades "just in case." Explore your work site, as "just in case" applies there too.

Requests

Advertise your needs—advertise, advertise, advertise (see **Figure 4**, pp. 78–79). Don't hesitate to make wish lists of the items you would like to see on the unit as part of a kit. Post your advertisements around the facility. Advertise in staff and resident newsletters or even the local church bulletin. Stretch your imagination. As you receive advertised items, be sure to post your gratitude as well.

Resources

As I have said before and will say again, my father always told me it never hurts to ask. We all know someone who can help—our family, volunteers, professional affiliations, and even businesses we frequent. Each of these is a resource, which when used appropriately may provide a fruitful outcome.

Rummaging

A little repetition here perhaps, but the attic, dollar stores, liquidators, auction-eers, flea markets, and garage sales are not only fun to rummage through but also may provide extremely unusual and hard to find items at fair prices. A little tip: It often helps to explain where you are from and why you are in pursuit of the items you are after.

The Challenge

Once you have done your detective work and exhausted your initial resources it is time to get others working for you on a fun and creative level. This brings us to the great discovery challenge.

The great discovery challenge was proposed. Two weeks passed, and out of seven departments we received a total of six kits, not to mention two more at the idea stage—an "E" for effort for everyone. Today all of these kits are in use by the staff on the unit. The promotion was simple:

- Banners advertised the challenge
- Sample kits were placed on display in the staff room
- Posters and signs explained why we offered the challenge

For every problem or question asked, we incorporated it into our adver-tising to simplify the challenge for all. At the end of the two weeks we cel-ebrated our success by offering thanks in poster form listing the kits and the department responsible. We supplied donuts and coffee on the last day and arranged a pleasing display of the kits that had been submitted through the

---

CLIMB ABOARD FOR ADVENTURE

We are going on a journey, a safari, an adventure of sorts.
Beginning today, each department will choose
a theme and together create a Discovery Kit.
The possibilities for kits are endless and
limited only by the imagination.
If you need ideas for Kits, the Activity Department has suggestions.
In two weeks we will gather to celebrate each other's
DISCOVERIES.
Climb aboard and join us for some great fun!

Let the adventures begin...

FIGURE 4
Discovery Kit Advertising Ideas

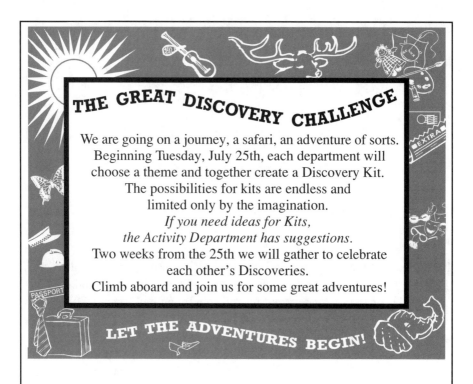

FIGURE 4 (continued)
Discovery Kit Advertising Ideas

challenge. A little coaching, a lot of promotion, support mixed with enthusiasm, and belief in the project resulted in a tantalizing array of options in discovery.

Possibility Thinking: Educating for Action

Purposeful and beneficial use of leisure time builds the self.

If you thought the challenge ends with a drive for kits you are mistaken. There is adventure in this for everyone, including yourself, as you now endeavor to promote the understanding and subsequently the successful use of discovery kits, life kits, and personal fact sheets.

We developed an in-service that focused on understanding the kit, its purpose, and its benefits. We focused on the importance of purposeful and beneficial use of leisure time. This was emphasized through an intriguing breakdown of the 24-hour clock and how our residents spend their time (see **Figure 5**). Through this process, we gained a greater understanding of resident needs as compared to our own. We demonstrated how we could enhance time through discovery and life reviews. We demonstrated the value of enhancing our residents' quality of life through purposeful leisure opportunities and clarified our responsibility to do just that.

Take a typical 24-hour day and consider all occupied time:

How many hours are spent sleeping? _____

How many hours are spent eating? _____

How many total ADL hours? _____

Total the above numbers and subtract from 24 for remaining hours.

Total hours remaining: _____

FIGURE 5
24-Hour Reverse Clock

We taught staff that these interventions were useful not only during periods of potential inactivity and boredom (a source of frustration and frequent reason for wandering and other less appealing behaviors) but also during personal care time. Imagine how the care relationship may be enhanced when esteem-enhancing information is discussed during a bath time or while dressing for the day, thus valuing the person and distracting from what might otherwise be a frightening or humiliating task.

We walked staff through the process of evaluating the value and role of leisure in our own lives and then applied the new thinking to our residents. It was an eye-opening experience. Staff now recognized that residents have a history of and a right to the same leisure opportunities and comforts we hold dear for ourselves and our families.

Begin the thinking process. Ask yourself or your staff the following questions as you lead into the evaluation of a 24-hour period:

1. What do you do when you are not working?

2. What would you like to be doing?

3. Would you rather work or play?

If leisure is a time when we are free to do that which we choose, then:

4. How do we enjoy our leisure when we are no longer able to initiate and make choices?

5. How do we enjoy our leisure when we can no longer remember our favorite pastimes without cueing?

When we take time to explore and answer these questions we can further appreciate the reality of the person with special care needs as well as their 24-hour cycle compared to that of our own. It is imperative to understand that regardless of whom or how old we are or what ability or disability we may have—we have equal rights to a quality of life that includes a quality leisure lifestyle. The awakening comes as we realize the residents are relying on us, as their care team, to help them to live quality, meaningful, purposeful, expressive, healthy, and normal leisure lifestyles. With this knowledge, a new dimension is added to our responsibility.

The reverse clock approach was extremely valuable as the staff became aware of the exact amount of unoccupied or discretionary time the residents had. Staff now understood the impact a lack of direction or opportunity based on the functional, self-directive skill losses residents had experienced.

When taken through the exercise the staff consistently determined that sleep totaled six hours (actual nighttime normal periods of sleep, not "boredom" sleep). Hours spent eating were estimated at three, and ADL hours (activities of daily living), including postmeal toileting totaled three hours.

(Personally I prefer to refer to this time as "freshening-up"—it seems to add a significant amount of dignity in ways "toileting" simply never could.) This brings the total of occupied hours, as determined by the staff providing the guidance and assistance, to twelve. The remaining hours in the day matched at twelve hours.

Imagine that—twelve hours to do what? Suddenly, a whole new dimension is added to the responsibility of the care team. When applied to their own lives the staff found their own remaining time after ADLs, sleep, eating, and work was far less. What do they do during this time? They enjoy a quality, self-directed leisure lifestyle. They enjoy quiet time, social time, or specific recreation. Upon examining the polarized difference between their time and lifestyles and that of the residents they began to realize and value their role and responsibility. They now saw the value of empowering the residents through the provision of purposeful leisure and recreation activities in those many remaining hours. Yes, the responsibility is great, and yes, the tools can be even greater. Appropriate success-oriented recreation and purposeful activity programs, props, and interventions (e.g., discovery kits) mark the way to a satisfied, healthy, and content individual. Providing a meaningful, normal leisure lifestyle in addition to quality care—this is what the special care resident relies on the care team to fulfill as their responsibility.

Leisure In Our Lives

Leisure is a time when we are free to do what we choose to do, or a state of being when we experience personal satisfaction, the joy of re-creation, and an enriched sense of self-worth and inner calm.

Recreation is engaging in activity during leisure time, which may or may not be freely choosen.

If we promote this expectation (there's that wretched word again) with the staff, then we as practitioners must fulfill our responsibility. We must provide a workable framework that will guide, with great flexibility, the activity pursuits of and proactive leadership by the team.

Leisure is something you have—*recreation* is something you do. The pursuit of a satisfying and healthful leisure lifestyle is an ongoing, challenging, and ever-changing process throughout one's life.

—source unknown

PART 3

PROMOTING SUCCESS THROUGH PROGRAM FRAMEWORK

Breaking the Pattern

The escalating behavior pattern must be broken before it is beyond the resident's control.

Quilting requires great patience. It requires us to know the pattern, the direction, the stitches required, and other relevant nuances. This analogy can be applied to awareness levels and our familiarity with our resident's patterns of behavior.

Maintaining awareness of the needs of residents is yet another responsibility of caregivers. We are in control of the quality of the outcome. If we do not actively seek to be aware of resident needs, the outcomes will be negative. Caregiver awareness and subsequent conscious action results in favorable outcomes. It is a simple concept—if the environment is too stimulating, it nags at the resident (unbeknown to the staff). Then the individual becomes restless as new demands (with little communication or empathy) are made of the resident: get up, go to the toilet, change clothes, sit down, eat, do this, do that. Soon the resident becomes frustrated, then agitated, angry, and last but never least—the resident resorts to a final catastrophic measure of frustration to say "stop" by responding with aggression. To prevent this from happening, the role of the caregiver is to be aware, to anticipate, and to break the pattern.

This is not meant to be done in the midst of an upset. By then it is already too late. The behavior pattern must be broken before it is beyond the resident's control. This again becomes an issue of protecting dignity. Think of the times a person is arguing a point, and they realize in some small way they may be wrong. Not everyone is disciplined enough to acquiesce. It can be embarrassing and therefore difficult to retract and "save face."

The concept of *neurolinguistic programming* (NLP), developed by behaviorists and taught extensively by motivational speaker Anthony Robbins (1987), suggests that interrupting a behavior consistently can effect a change in the behavior. Before behavior reaches a critical point, interrupt the resident's movement toward distress by calming, distracting, or appealing to his or her ego through compliments. A compliment goes a long way toward boosting and sustaining a person's self-esteem. It may also serve as an adequate form of distraction from the potential problem. The issue of how the person feels about himself or herself at a given moment influences his or her coping ability and reactions to stimulus or activity regardless of dementia.

By breaking the pattern before it escalates to the least desirable outcome (usually aggression) we protect the dignity of the resident and for that matter the safety of caregivers. Picture the following flowchart (see **Figure 6**) as you observe or recall resident behavior patterns. As you examine the patterns, you will note the escalation as well as opportunities to intervene and prevent aggression by breaking the pattern. What indicators can be observed in an individual which are your cue to break the pattern? Some examples would include a person who refuses eye contact; becomes quiet; begins wandering, banging, rocking, fussing, or vocalizing; or refuses a greeting, a direction, or assistance. These and others are suitable cues often inherent to an individual. The same indicators may be used in care planning as this type of behavior is mostly consistent.

Breaking the pattern does not mean "shocking" the person—absolutely not. It means we must drop whatever it is we want the resident to do and hear them. We must be present to *their* needs. This refers to applying the concepts of improvisation through Needs Response. The simplicity is in appealing to the moment the person is in. By doing so, we appeal to the ego by giving time and showing respect. Certainly it appears as if no work may get done, but by taking the time to break the pattern we not only save the time it takes to intervene and bring back an agitated individual to a state of peace, but also reduce the level of stress of both resident and staff. Does this not seem a far more beneficial priority?

What a lovely quilt of peace, comfort, and happiness can be designed and sewn together when we take the time to examine the pieces and carefully attend to its pattern.

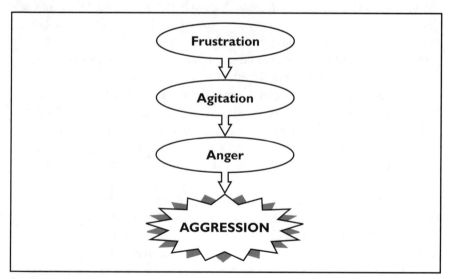

FIGURE 6
Breaking the Pattern

Trouble in Paradise

*Comforts and celebrations cannot be taken from all
for the sake of one or two.*

Awareness is far reaching when we address and respond to the needs of those
with dementia. Throughout the year we discuss, decorate, and celebrate a
range of events and circumstances, such as

- New Year's Day
- Robert Burns Day
- Chinese New Year
- Valentine's Day
- St. Patrick's Day
- Easter
- Canada Day

- Fourth of July
- Thanksgiving
- Memorial Day
- Halloween
- Hanukkah
- Christmas
- Ramadan

Of course, the lengthiest and most drawn out of celebrations is the joyful
season of Christmas. The question is: Joyful for whom? Well, if handled
appropriately, joyful for everyone involved, including the resident.

Prior to the formal opening of our special care unit, the decision had
been made that no Christmas decorations would be on display. This was
believed to prevent sadness, disorientation, and potential agitation or aggression. According to some members of the care team, this seemed a very kind
gesture and was certainly intended to be in someone's best interest. But one
must ask: Is this a normalized approach? If the goal of special care is to create
a normal, homelike, family-oriented, comforting, and supportive environment,
does it also mean that it must be seasonless?

Christmas, Hanukkah, and other celebrations are a part of everyone's
lives. These celebrations are a part of our identities, our histories, our legends.
Certainly there is an element of sadness present for everyone as childhood
memories gain strength and may overwhelm the average person's ability to
enjoy the season. This is particularly true if parts of our happy memories are
no longer present to access. As family members move away, loved ones die,
and society changes, some of those joys may become tarnished. It is important to find the joy again. It is imperative to maintain the celebrations of the
self. Challenges are ever present in special care. Coping with seasonal influences is yet another challenge.

A "seasonless" environment cannot fit the mandate of a special care unit. When the task is appropriately handled the responsibilities of staff look like this:

- Ensure that decorations are not displayed for more than two weeks (a week before and only briefly after works best).

- Make or purchase safe ornaments/decorations (i.e., non-breakable, nontoxic).

- Involve the residents in the creative process (e.g., making ornaments, decorating, counting down the days to Christmas).

- Address resident anxiety with a mixed approach of reminiscing and reality orientation.

> *One day a resident asked, "How was your Christmas, dear?" Her question was genuine, socially appropriate, and season- ally correct...but it was only the 12th of December.*

What was wrong with this scenario? Well, nothing. Bear in mind that this resident was not oriented to time. However, the discussion throughout the building and all indicators point to the season about which she was com- menting. What would be an appropriate response to this?

First, in one's mind one must acknowledge not an error on this woman's part, but accuracy within her own means. She was early in the suitability of her query, but accurate in the choice of discussion. To find the answer, look back to earlier discussions. Refer back to the concept of "displaced questions" and the need to respond in a supporting, validating fashion. At the same time try to orient the individual in a gentle, nonthreatening way to time.

> **Q:**   *"How was your Christmas, dear?"*
> **A:**   *"I am really looking forward to Christmas this year. Thank you for asking. Imagine, it is only 13 days away. What is your favorite memory (or tradition, or gift) from a past Christmas?"*

Taking this approach acknowledges the appropriateness of the resident's question. (Remember that all around the building the residents cannot help but hear staff and visitors discussing the holiday and extending best wishes for the season.) Gently, and without embarrassing the resident, indicate the time frame. Do not dwell on the person's inaccuracy but focus on their ac- curacy by moving into a moment of validating reminiscence. This is an easy formula for resolving these straightforward situations. It is common sense— no one sets out to embarrass themselves. People set out to communicate which is a strong social need and must be supported with care and attention.

But what of those individuals who pack their bags to go on holidays, as was their life habit during the season? One cannot simply stop the person—this would only lead to agitation and potentially worse scenarios. Again, use a gentle approach. Respect where the person is, acknowledge their needs and attempt to validate their desire to travel. Keep in mind that this is a seasonal influence and be prepared to let it go. Attempt to redirect the resident by using past or present clues and the puzzle pieces they provide to you that are relevant to their current reality experience. Improvise and use your creative powers. We cannot control, nor should we seek to control, resident behavior. We should seek to accommodate and redirect the resident based on the moment in which he or she is living—Join their journey.

Depriving resident populations due to the fear of potential negative or difficult responses is a cop-out. The bottom line is that the staff must be prepared to provide a supportive environment for whom they provide care regardless of the season. Anyone can be at least somewhat volatile during times filled with memories and experiences. It is the responsibility of the staff to be prepared to respond in an appropriately stimulating sensory environment. Withdrawing the opportunity to experience the season, festival, or celebration from the entire population for the sake of one or two residents indicates a lack of understanding of dementia more so than a means of protecting the residents. These individuals maintain the absolute right to experience, relive, reminisce, and be treated with the necessary care and attention required to enjoy their lifelong celebrated festivals and seasons. Ask yourself: If it were decided that Christmas will be canceled because it is too upsetting, how would you react? In our practice the question we should be addressing is: How can we make Christmas comfortable and happy for everyone involved?

So the folks are restless during seasonal celebrations. Is there trouble in paradise? What happens when we hear residents are restless generally? How do we explore and cope with their behavior and needs at these times? Do we, in a task-focused mind set, react to the needs expressed or do we respond to the resident's needs? *Needs* is the operative word in this instance, but isn't it always in dementia care? One can easily refer back to the most basic approach of gentle Needs Response. Unfortunately, it can be very intimidating to some caregivers.

One of the best examples of a restless resident was a woman who busied, fretted, and expressed her worry to anyone and everyone she came across. On speculation, the increase in this behavior was blamed on Christmas season decorations. Further exploration discovered something interesting: Earlier that day she had left the building with her son for a medical appointment. Upon return from the outing he rushed her back to the unit, dropped her off, and left. For the remainder of the day she was distressed.

There is a settling period after every intervention that must be respected. Failing to do so leaves the person "hanging"—looking for something or someone. (This is a great example of a trigger for wandering behavior.) When a person is withdrawn from their comfort zone, they need support to reacclimate to their safe environment. Support comes in the form of appropriate Needs Response interventions to reorient the individual to their familiar environment. It is imperative to remember that although the individual has settled into the unit as "home," he or she still needs to reorient after each time away. To resume the same level of independence and coping, they must receive support to refamiliarize themselves. The Connection Continuum (p. 98) outlines means to achieving successful and supportive interventions and important transitions in more detail.

As much as we may endeavor to create a paradise-like living and working environment, this may not always be the case. We must ensure that action as opposed to reaction is our mandate. If the residents are restless, don't look to blame. Take action—look for the trigger, and make use of the information for future reference. Anticipation and planning are the keys to prevention. Communicating outings and appointments is the first step to peace. Accept and be prepared for trouble in paradise, and you may find more paradise than you find trouble. In anticipation of recurrence, the next time this woman goes for an appointment, her son may be asked to plan time to sit and visit or walk about the unit with the resident upon their return. If not feasible, plans may be made to have someone meet her and help to reorient her to the unit.

A gentle hand to guide, calm, redirect, and wind down (relax) following any interaction or event is a necessity on any special care unit. The right approach or program plan can be most successful at achieving a peaceful outcome. The programming approach used is similar to an exercise program: warm up, program, and cool down.

Warm up: Bring the residents together and gently introduce the activity.

Program: Variety of interactive programs led by staff or volunteer.

Cool down: Conclude every program with a period of quiet activity, ranging from a gentle ball toss to reminiscence and discovery kits.

This gentle, caring, attentive approach prevents restless wandering and related behaviors of a cohesive group of residents. Those who do not fit this category may best be served through one-on-one, individualized Needs Response.

∞   ∞   ∞   ∞   ∞

A resident, Betty, returning from a community outing where she had a lovely time was completely disoriented upon her return, this was not home and she had been dropped off here.

"How am I to get home?" she asked the recreation worker.

The recreation worker, who was about to start her premeal wind-down, dropped everything and initiated Needs Response, which successfully helped the resident find her way home:

"Betty, come with me, and I'll show you home," the recreation worker responded. Together they strolled to the door of Betty's room.

Betty hesitated, still unsure of where she was. "Will you come in, dear, and show me?"

"Sure, Betty, here are your lovely paintings." The recreation worker glanced around the room, "Oh look," she said. "I have always admired your beautiful tea service. Now may I help you with your coat?"

"Thank you, dear," Betty said as she accepted the help.

"Let's hang it here in your closet. Are you comfortable now?"

Betty hesitated which prompted the recreation worker to suggest: "Betty, I was just about to start a bean bag toss and I must get back to it now. You are very welcome to join us if you would like."

Betty smiled, reached out her hand and together they left for the lounge and an enjoyable game of bean bag toss. Once again, success through gentle, attentive, caring Needs Response.

∞   ∞   ∞   ∞   ∞

We must attend to the needs on the unit that we are present to meet: those of our residents. When determined appropriately, a well-trained and problem-solving–oriented staff member can resolve virtually any situation. Disorientation, overstimulation, and related behaviors can be successfully addressed with caring and intuition as well as application of these approaches.

Coming Together:
A Framework for Success

Every day is a different reason.
　　　　　　　　　　　　　—*Barbara Moffatt*

When one recreation worker comes to work she is prepared for anything. Her belief is simple: Every day is different for different reasons. This approach reduces the potential for stress and dead-end interventions. What she does, she says, is not teachable. She could not be more correct. Her success comes from an intuition—an openness and acceptance of the *individual* who lives on the unit, not the collective *residents with dementia*. She describes "a connection with the residents" whereby she "reads" the people and the situation and determines her interventions. To sort out instinct and feelings, we must take into consideration the

- person
- staffing variations
- environment
- other unforeseen elements

Each element is a card in a constantly shuffled deck. One affects the other from one moment to the next or not at all. Consider the people, their abilities, and your resources—these then come together to make the program or intervention happen. *Never expect your session plan to have the same outcome.*

For that matter, have several potential outcomes in mind as you plan your sessions. A wise mentor once taught me: forewarned is forearmed. In other words, be prepared. Your preparations may fall short as you learn that predicting behavior is an art, virtually beyond your control. But this is what makes commitment to special care an exciting journey. It is important to remember the differences between special care and general programming. With special care we can set open, flexible goals and objectives, acknowledging the likelihood of change and the unpredictability of the population. The foundation to build your goals on is one of no expectations.

Eliminating the word "expectations" from one's vocabulary is an enormous step toward program success. Essentially, we eliminate the risk of failure for residents by withdrawing expectations for skills possibly lost in the onset and process of the dementia. Once we have successfully achieved this (and this is not easy for everyone) we can begin to plan a loose framework around which to build a program routine. By virtue of the extreme flexibility required for a "routine," this framework is not a structure.

Changing Our Language Means Successful Opportunities and Outcomes

Change from: Structure + Expectation = Failure
                 (for both staff and residents)

Change to: Framework + Routine = Interactions + Outcomes
                 (successful results for residents and staff)

Structure alludes to rigidity and lack of flexibility. Structure exists in ample quantity as we offer consistent meal times and staffing changes. Even their own circadian rhythms, as off kilter as they may be at times, create a structure for the resident. *Routine* suggests a consistency—a flexible, malleable consistency. We plan a framework promoting a routine the residents can rely on. The routine supports residents at various levels of functioning. For those who maintain an awareness of a routine of specific events, tasks, or interactions during a given day or time frame, routine consistency supports their need to know their next direction. For the resident who lacks this awareness, the flexibility provided can address needs as they arise yet maintain consistency within the framework. Each job assignment for a unit must ensure there is sufficient emphasis away from task orientation. Too many folks follow the literal word. A listing of tasks that are the individual's responsibility is appropriate since we must know what is expected of staff. However, a general listing of ways to provide Needs Response, everyone's responsibility on the team, is also essential. To suggest "It's not my job" is to deny the team and the overall goal of the special care environment. Individual members of the team are responsible to contribute to everyone's (including the residents') achievement of the goals of the unit. A summary statement of this might be to provide a safe, secure, homelike environment where individuals are supported and encouraged to maintain their optimal functioning and best possible quality of life. This is achieved through choice, respect, humor, a peaceful atmosphere, opportunities for self-expression and socialization, and preservation of dignity within a framework of care. The specific routine followed by a member of the team may change or stay the same depending on the staffing and programming set out for the period. The exceptions or changes may also occur with seasonal influences. In the case of the recreation worker, programs other than recreation (e.g., music therapy, pastoral care services) are times the recreation worker may build in nonresident responsibilities (e.g., documentation, breaks).

Time and again we see and hear examples of the recreation worker as she stops her program preparation, delaying her start time to provide specific resident Needs Response. Although it may seem disjointed, each time this is done, it is effective and efficient for all involved. The resident is put at ease, and others at risk of being a "victim" of a resident's agitated or aggressive behavior are protected. As a result, staff are relieved of the potentially added stress of an *angry, agitated*, or *aggressive* individual. We could simply call this *diffusing triple-A behavior*. A responsibility of every member of the care team, regardless of role specific responsibilities, these take the back seat to Needs Response.

In the midst of building an arsenal of tools and approaches (e.g., Needs Response) caregivers must attend to one of the most important points of all: Repetition within a flexible framework.

Repetition Is the Path to Achievement and Success

As a practitioner, I am a learner in the caregiver exchange. I am a more patient, kinder person because of my interaction with people with dementia. They taught me that feelings are not a brain function—they are of a different order and I can have my heart opened by them.
—Carol Hansen, Educator

On the verge of the sundowning period, a recreation worker searched the lounge for the beach ball. It was time for a session of ball toss with the residents to bring them purposefully through the transitional period from the afternoon program into the evening meal. As the recreation worker searched, she commented to staff, asking "Have you seen the beach ball?" While she looked, the residents waited patiently, watching and listening to her every word.

Suddenly, without speaking, one gentlemen rose from his seat, strolled over to the storage cupboard, picked up a foam ball and returned to his seat. The group began to toss the ball from one to another around the circle. In awe, the recreation worker stood back and watched her friends enjoying their game on their own, without her leadership or encouragement.

∞   ∞   ∞   ∞   ∞

> **Sundowning**
>
> Characterized by the onset or exacerbation of agitation, restlessness, panic, intensified disorientation, or verbal/physical outbursts in the afternoon or evening.

What could have brought these folks together to manage this difficult period of their day with a purposeful, socially interactive experience without the leadership of the recreation worker? What caused the gentleman to interpret the familiar group setting as needy, to get up, and to implement the program himself? It could be argued on a very complex level with all sorts of insightful hypotheses but, frankly, there is a very simple explanation.

The role of the recreation worker is multifaceted. One of the primary responsibilities is to promote the highest level of independent skill (or functioning) possible for the resident while at the same time promoting the person. This is achieved through a flexible, adaptable approach that ensures continuity in the living environment. It is an environment of interventions that promotes repetition, which is not as boring as it may sound. Through repetition, we create the elements of security, familiarity, continuity, and (most important) relationship building among peers. The valuable practice of using repetition is emphasized by understanding that our relationship is an exchange of feelings and constant learning. Caregiver success comes from the application and interpretation of approaches that promote patience in action. Through attentive, patient exchange we learn how to better interact and support residents as they cope from day to day. One model of approach used by recreation therapists is a helpful measure to guide caregiver methods and interventions.

The Therapeutic Recreation Service Model (or Leisure Ability Model) developed by Peterson and Gunn (1984) represents the three areas of therapeutic recreation: treatment/therapy, leisure education, and recreation participation (see **Figure 7**, p. 96). It is easy for professional caregivers to associate only one phase of the model with residents who have special care needs. However, we are wrong to limit the residents through quick application of this model. Upon examination of the group's functional levels (they are always changing), each area of the model can easily be adapted to the specific needs of this population. With awareness, we take a positive step toward fulfilling needs and celebrating the resident community.

Understanding and interpreting areas of the Leisure Ability Model, such as the treatment phase, generates success when we open our thinking and allow ourselves to be taught by resident responses in the relationship-building phase. With this in mind, and a desire to promote the celebration of the self, we have before us yet another tool for promoting the person with dementia.

Recreation Participation

Developed over the long term once a group has formed; environment has settled; and cohesion, routine, and familiarity have been established

Leisure Education

Promoting the highest skill level possible; continuity, flexibility, and repetition

Treatment/Therapy

Calming, supporting, relationship building

FIGURE 7
Adaption based on the Leisure Ability Model (Peterson and Gunn, 1984) as applied to dementia care programming interventions

Treatment/Therapy

The treatment or therapy phase of the Leisure Ability Model promotes a supportive approach. It encourages the maintenance or enhancement of the functional abilities of the individual. For example, for all three levels of physical, cognitive, and social functioning the recreation worker determines specific needs and addresses them through verbal cueing and environmental adaptations. In special care it is a modality of understanding, patience, calm, support, encouragement, familiarity, and relationship building. In the care of people with Alzheimer disease, we must create an esteem-enhancing environment. This environment must be conducive to the growth and development of a cohesive community. It promotes independence, maintenance of skills, and the pursuit of opportunities that celebrate the individual. Further investigation of the Leisure Ability Model explains how the remaining two components—leisure education and recreation participation—apply to the special care population.

Leisure Education

Leisure education promotes the understanding and development of leisure-related knowledge and skills. In the case of special care, practitioners guide residents through consistent repetition of programs and tasks reinforcing participation with positive support. It is an ongoing process that adapts to changing needs. Through this process the group's familiarity increases, thus contributing to the formation of a cohesive community.

Certainly days come and go where little or no cohesion exists, but the environment can be created. Intuitive staff will be mindful and able to intercept behaviors or risk factors that may disrupt the success of the experience. In the end it is the consistency and quality of the repetition and reinforcement that influences familiarity, awareness, and success.

Recreation Participation

Recreation participation is achieved only after a lengthy period of bouncing back and forth between the first two phases: treatment (support and relationship building) and leisure education (training through repetition and positive reinforcement). Throughout this process, residents experience stages of group development, thus influencing the functional abilities of the community group.

Understanding and awareness of the *group formation process* of

- storming
- norming
- forming
- performing

is valuable to determine at which phase of the Leisure Ability Model residents may be functioning.

Storming occurs before norming, as residents must first find security in their environment. The *storming* phase is experienced as residents settle and become familiar with peers and routines of the environment. Once security is established, they are able to develop a peer network. *Norming* follows as individuals begin to feel safer in their environment. Thus residents seek each other out for comfort, assistance, and social interaction. *Forming* follows suit as they become able to see to each other's needs and to work toward *performing*—together or apart in comfort—either by rote or understanding on a level beyond our rational capacity to understand.

With consistent program and task repetition, the individual or the peer group is finally able to perform. Factors such as illness, environmental variables, pain, disruption in routine, change of medication, and family/friend visits, which may not be concluded in a supportive manner (by either the visitor or through lack of support by staff) can affect the quality of life and success residents experience in their environment. However, mindfulness and consistent support continues to promote recreation participation and community development.

Recreation participation occurs just as it did when the gentleman rose from his chair during the ball toss, with an awareness of the need to participate in the environmentally and socially cued activity. His recognition through repetition, support, encouragement, and peer familiarity created the need, desire, and ability for this man to initiate the process. Whether he truly understood why, what, or how he was performing the task is not the issue. The issue is that through the use of a supportive approach and repetition, he was able to recognize and initiate a successful outcome, not only for himself, but also for his peers.

The Connection Continuum

The process of caring is true, sincere, accurate, and egalitarian, and the communication is congruent. The whole relationship might be described as one of empathic identification.
                                    —*Kitwood (1997, p. 130)*

Programming for those with dementia calls on us to attend closely to group needs and responses. It requires us to be able to turn on a dime and redirect our program focus. We must be flexible and able to sense and observe individual's needs as he or she communicates them to us. Our responsibility is clear: to provide appropriate, supportive, enjoyable interventions. What follows is an outline of the Connection Continuum. This model proposes a flexible approach to life when caring for those with dementia. It encourages us not to see failure or problems when our goals seem to falter, but to see new opportunities.

Program Duration

Much has been discussed of how long a program should be run. In fact, those we serve should guide duration. This requires much energy and attentiveness to the moods, tolerance, and needs of each individual. Limitations can create more problems than they help for those for whom we provide care and service. Suggesting a program or intervention should last only 15 or 20 minutes can create an environment of stress for both caregiver and receiver. Therefore, it is essential that there are stages in our interventions. Applied appropriately, each stage alone may take 5 to 15 minutes or longer. The following stages of the Connection Continuum (see **Figure 8**) are extremely effective and easy to learn with a little repetition and practice. The Connection Continuum is a simple five-stage model by which everyone may guide care. The five stages include initiation, introduction, peak response, closure, and redirection.

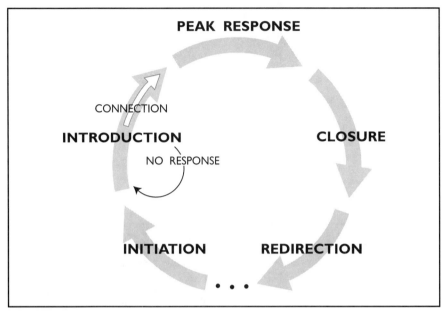

FIGURE 8
The Connection Continuum: A Cyclical Model of Approach

Initiation

The process of initiation for dementia care programs is threefold:

1. Program setup (This may or may not involve residents.)

2. Invitation (A wise approach is to start with those who would not be inclined to wander away and then invite the wanderers. Don't panic if they leave, the odds are they will wander back.)

3. Welcome (Ensure comfort in the environment, adapt seating and environment as required.)

One recreation programmer was able to initiate her programs simply by starting once her community was established. Residents would then join her for a wonderful period of quality interaction.

Introduction

This stage is probably the most complex and demanding part of the model. Observation and attention to the responses of residents are required at this time. Here we look for one of two things: (a) no response or (b) a connection. If there is a poor response or no response to the activity in progress we must reevaluate the choice of the program. Reasons for no response are as varied as the participants for this outcome. Ask yourself the following questions:

- Is the timing off?
- Are the residents too tired?
- Could the person be in pain?
- Is the level of stimulation suitable for this occasion?
- Was my approach clear?
- Did I use an approach representative of best practice? (see *Approaches for Success*)

Approaches for Success

These tactics are an asset to general success when using interventions with people with Alzheimer's disease and related disorders.

1. Always use slow, quiet movements (not threatening or startling)
2. Using a low-pitched voice, communicate at a face-to-face level.
3. In making eye contact, position yourself at or just below the individual's line of sight.
4. Position yourself directly in front, do not approach speaking from the side.
5. Agree with the individual's statement of reality in a given situation. Then take the time to make a suggestion that they may in turn agree to. Involve the individual in the problem-solving process.
6. "May I make a suggestion?" (Try it, it works!)
7. Obtain the individual's permission (ask them and wait for the response) before intervening or directing.
8. Compromise ("Perhaps we could try...")
9. Ask them to "Show you how to..."
10. Speak softly and with care.
11. Be authentic, tell the person how you are feeling if things aren't going well. You will be surprised how the individual's nurturing and caring instinct will kick in.
12. Treat those with dementia as they are: adults with experience in life just like yourself.
13. Treat others as you would wish to be treated.
14. Celebrate this individual just as you would wish to be celebrated.

These are just some examples of the many questions we must constantly ask ourselves as we evaluate the direction our interventions take. We may also ask ourselves if this is the wrong intervention for this time. Although it may have been effective before, this may not be the right time now. Don't give up too quickly, however. Try again. Try two or three approaches and then go to your backup program. By the way, always have a backup plan. We may cycle through many plans before a connection is made. This reality is what ranks flexibility and patience at the top of the skills list for folks working with those living with dementia. Finally, don't give up too quickly. Perhaps the resident simply needs more time to process what we are asking of him or her and settle into the activity. Sometimes a period of observation makes the difference in both comfort and comprehension. A connection will soon follow.

A connection is magical. This is the moment everyone hopes for where both programmer and participant recognize and celebrate through their enjoyment. Little is required to describe the connection. Simply put, the intended goals and objectives are in the process of being achieved. Another way of saying this is that the program seems effortless and worthy of endless enjoyment. That is definitely something worth waiting for.

Peak Response

This is the true joy of a program or intervention. It is the moment everyone hopes for: flow. The program is underway and the caregiver steps back. We may turn over leadership to the residents or individual. (Yes, this is possible.) We have a tendency to "do for" more often than is necessary. When we "do for" (and perceive this as a helping behavior to rationalize our actions), we steal the remaining skills from the individual for whom we provide care. Our role is to enable. Our responsibility is to promote the maintenance of surviving skills for as long as possible.

We must focus our behavior on supporting rather than overtaking for the sake of efficiency. When we seek to experience a peak response, we seek to turn control over to our residents. Participants can subsequently guide the program's duration and mood. At this stage, the caregiver becomes a supporter and encourager. Peak response may have only taken a matter of minutes to achieve and it may last for a brief moment or a lengthy period.

The key to success and determining duration is to monitor:

- satisfaction
- level of participation
- quality of interaction

- fatigue
- interest

Closure

Based on our assessment of individual needs, we endeavor to celebrate participant success and enjoyment. We may quietly remove program props at this point while suggesting a change of plans. Throughout this process we involved the individual in the discussion—this is essential. Often such a conversation is internal as we plan and look ahead to our next action. I challenge you to welcome others and include them in your thoughts. This achieves two things: We share what is happening, and at the same time build trust through communication. These are powerful tools to develop.

> Caregiver: Gee, it is getting close to dinner. Perhaps we should put the ball away now.
> Resident: Oh, yes. I'm hungry.
> Caregiver: Will you help me put the ball in the cupboard? Let's take a walk to the dining room together.

It bears mentioning that even conflicts and challenges during the program are discussed with participants. This enhances understanding of what is taking place, thus empowering these worthy individuals. Not only will participants support the caregiver with their empathy, but also they will participate in problem solving if given the opportunity—a whole other program within a program. Active participation or active observation in this process determines our success at the next stage.

Redirection

At the point of redirection, our goal is to offer an activity of choice, enjoyment, or preference for the residents. This is a *transitional phase*, as they may wait now for the next part of the daily routine to be initiated, thus repeating the ongoing cycle of the Connection Continuum. An example of this would be a meal. Having settled the individuals into their preferred activity or tasks, we can then withdraw from the scene to attend to our next responsibility.

Connection Continuum

This is the Connection Continuum, a cycle of stages that recur over a day. We seek to provide purposeful, age-appropriate, independence-oriented and esteem-enhancing activity. Whether it is a bath, a meal, self-care, or a recreation/social program, our reasons for programming are life enhancing. We program for individuals when they are no longer able to do so on their own. This means we create a process of grounding for residents. We assist them through capturing interest and making a connection on many levels of need, including social, emotional, cognitive, physical, and spiritual.

But who says it all has to be serious? Humor and lightheartedness are essential elements in this recipe for grounding. A fun process is created, which decreases feelings of displacement and restlessness or simply feeling at loose ends. These are intense feelings rarely explored with the individual living with dementia. These folks are usually blamed for other negative behaviors. However, these lost feelings surface in careful and thoughtful, attentive conversations and interaction with folks. These messages do get relayed one way or another. Boredom turns to frustration, which leads to agitation, which can inevitably lead to aggression—a path no one, resident or caregiver, wishes to travel.

We seek to meet many needs in providing support and care, including

- to maintain ADL skills and independence for as long as possible

- to maintain adequate nourishment and hydration to avoid secondary illnesses

- to promote socialization, self-expression, and self-esteem

- to promote dignity and identity recognition

Each of these is of great importance and no one is greater than another. One could argue that one cannot exist without the other...but why? The point of care is that everyone relies on the other for reaching the true goals. We only meet these goals when each area of service supports the others.

Care is just that—no more no less. It is from the heart and to the heart. Caring is sincere, patient, and respectful. It's action and reaction is according to an individual's needs. It is proactive—knowledgeable of the client population and intuitive of the individual. Caring is genuine in every way. The Connection Continuum translates to any daily activity or task to fulfill goals of care. If we choose to adopt this approach on a consistent and comprehensive team basis, our lives as caregivers will change. So too will the lives of the residents change. The final key remembrances for success include

- always have a backup plan or alternate activity

- know that we won't always connect and that is okay

- we are in control of the quality of the outcome

Controlling the quality of the outcome is a simple concept and a good rule of thumb to follow. Whether we achieve what we set out to achieve or not (e.g., bath, meal, program, social visit, dressing, changing, freshening up) the mood or state of mind we leave the resident in following our attempt or intervention is up to us. The resident may reject all our efforts. This is not the end of the world. It is the fact that we are still in control of the quality of the outcome that matters. It mentioned earlier, we offer supportive (controlled) choices to the resident. In accomplishing certain tasks or outcomes our goal remains: leaving residents in the same or better state of mind than before we arrived. Regardless of response, we still control how we respond to the individual's reaction to us, and therefore the state of being in which the individual is left.

∞   ∞   ∞   ∞   ∞

Two staff members approached a "difficult" man (as he was labeled)—each grabbed an arm and pulled him up telling him he was going for lunch. He swore bitterly at them, tugged, kicked, and hollered. They pulled and pulled. *He must get his nourishment.*

Another staff member happened along and stopped the proceedings with a quick wave and the two backed off. This member approached the man with a quiet voice saying, "Gee, Albert, I'm sorry you are upset. The young women were just trying to help. You see, it's lunchtime." She pointed at her watch and motioned to the dining room across the hall. "They didn't want you to miss out."

Albert replied with a courteous nod, "Oh, I'm sorry. Pardon me." He smiled, got up, and went for lunch.

∞   ∞   ∞   ∞   ∞

We are in control of the quality of the outcome. Communication (establishing a common understanding), a gentle touch, and a patient approach will succeed virtually every time.

With these essentials in mind we are on our way, secure in the knowledge that all will be well. Many other opportunities arise each day to connect with care. Don't allow yourself to get stuck. Be prepared to make a detour on this path of dementia caregiving. We never know how truly beautiful the detour may be…if only we allow it to happen.

Making Friends Out of FOAs

A lifetime of experience and skill is a foundation of one's self-esteem. This must be preserved and encouraged when so much else is lost.

We all take pride in something. Our identities are formed from our experience and abilities—take these away and we are lost. The reality is if we stop in at any unemployment line, we see that any lengthy period of not being able to take pride in one's work has an impact on one's self-esteem. Take this thought on to the special care unit and you will find the same impact on self-esteem. The disease process slowly robs people of their skills and abilities, from the complex to the most simple.

Throughout the better part of our lives we discover purposeful activities that contribute to the formation of our identities. We spend most of our lives working not only to survive economically, but also to feel good about ourselves. We wrap our whole identity into our occupational pursuits. Generationally speaking, those who reside in our residential facilities today come from an era focused on work—not leisure. Much more of their identity truly comes from those roles than today. We, the caregivers, are a generation of leisure pursuers. We measure our identity with the degree of risk and social interaction associated with our leisure and recreational pursuits.

Perhaps we have yet to truly grasp the type of programming we ought to offer our residents. Leisure activities can be enjoyed by all, but are a far more important part of our generation than previous ones. Due to the difference in leisure interpretation and practices between the generations, it is again important for us to educate ourselves to clearly understand these differences. Through this understanding we can then work toward striking a balance in the lives of residents. We seek to support a restful, restorative, satisfying, and purposeful leisure lifestyle. This balance becomes increasingly challenging when it comes to our residents with dementia. The most familiar activities may tend to be career focused or task focused. These may be the most restorative and satisfying for one reason: They lend purpose to their existence. A *purpose* creates a healthy self-esteem and self-confidence.

Now, imagine after a lifetime of working and pursuing satisfying, purposeful activities we begin to lose skills. Abilities that shape our identity and contribute to how we function day-to-day begin fading away. This is a terrifying thought. It is difficult to comprehend this without facing some significant, life-altering loss to promote an appreciation of this concept. Yet, it remains only part of what happens to those living with dementia.

Current trends in dementia care encourage us to provide the environment most suitably familiar to our residents. We often refer to the long-term care environment as home, but find it difficult to actually simulate. It is imperative for our residents with dementia to have a genuine home environment, not one that has been simulated. We seek to create less-crowded living quarters (i.e., fewer residents), with meals prepared and laundry cleaned in this environment by staff and residents working side by side. As a team they work together, seeking to maintain remaining skills and strengths while building trust, rapport, and promoting purposeful activity. This is the wave of the future and it is underway. This is *dementia wellness*. Until this is the norm, let us seek to create this pseudo-home environment by making such tasks available as worker roles.

To support our residents we seek to provide purposeful, esteem-enhancing, and satisfying activities for these folks who now rely on us for direction. This is what familiar occupational activities (FOAs) or worker roles are all about. FOAs are purposeful activities familiar to the residents. We know that lifelong learning experiences tend to stay with us by rote in the very least form—a career postal worker will still be inclined to deliver mail, the housewife will clean, the electrician or carpenter will seek out opportunities to fiddle with or fix things. FOAs are the activities or tasks we can direct residents toward to fill their need to be busy, helpful, productive contributors—a need we all share.

The development of the FOA program was a way of formalizing a purposeful, self-gratifying, self-esteem building approach to involving the residents in daily living activities. These tasks and activities could be done alone or as a small group, formally or informally. Creativity is essential for developing a FOA program, along with the understanding that the task must

---

Familiar Occupational Activities (FOAs)

Domestic	Career Related
dish washing	filing
dusting	writing
picking up	stuffing
folding laundry	sorting
sweeping	opening
washing windows	delivering
making beds	adding
watering plants	
weeding	
setting tables	
tidying	

have meaning to the person performing it. It must be purposeful and have an outcome (e.g., folded laundry, a clean floor). It must also lend to the development or maintenance of self-esteem. These are empowering tasks that in the end will awe the nonbeliever on a special care unit.

Our FOA program linked closely to the care plan. Having completed a formal assessment with the input of the resident (when able) and the family, a profile of strengths, interests, and preferred tasks or familiar occupational activities is developed. After trying them with the resident, three of the most successful (you may struggle at first to come up with three) are ranked by preference. Preference may be defined as enjoyment, success, willingness, and a measurable tolerance for the task/activity. This list is subsequently documented in the care plan.

We set up the resident with the task. They may perform the task for five minutes or 55. Task endurance depends on the day, the hour, the mood, the quality of the environment, the pattern of behavior the person is in (e.g., frustrated, anxious, agitated), and what approach is used to set the person to task. Once the enjoyment or the task itself runs out, we move on to preference "B" and implement the same plan. Once this time passes we move into preference "C." What happens next? Back to "A" or "B" or perhaps it is time for a whole new intervention. Essentially what has happened is the FOA care planning approach gives us the means to offer satisfaction and purpose to our residents. It is something normal; a part of everyday life. It is not another program, but a chance to be an expert at something we have practiced all our lives. How do we feel when we are "the expert?" How would our residents feel? Knowing what value there is in these feelings and strengths, one cannot help but seek to implement such a program.

Remember, however, if we get someone started they may not be able to stop. It may appear that they are enjoying the task so much they don't want to stop. Depending on the area of the brain that has been damaged by the dementia, they may not have the ability to stop—just as they lacked the ability to initiate. Monitor residents and use periods of rest after 20 to 30 minutes before changing or restarting the familiar activity. (Rest periods may be as simple as having a glass of juice and a biscuit while sitting down.) If they cannot thank you verbally for this assistance, in the words of Dr. John Tooth, "They are thanking you on the inside."

A basic concept of valuing and supporting individuals based on their identity and skill levels, this is an essential program for any dementia care unit (or nondementia care unit for that matter). Everyone has value and the right to purposeful activity, regardless of ability or age. Until we can provide the environment that promotes living, then providing the activity is our obligation as caregivers.

∞   ∞   ∞   ∞   ∞

The team who took responsibility for the FOAs on our special care unit took great pride in their successes, just as the residents did. Each day after the program, the housekeeper assigned to the unit glowed with pride. She took time daily to invite a group of ladies together to fold the plastic bags that she would later place in the bottoms of trash cans throughout the building as she emptied them. The ladies were such masters at the task that the housekeeper found herself called back frequently to tear more bags off the roll for them to continue their very important job.

As time went by, she got the hang of implementing FOAs and became an even greater asset to the unit as she involved residents in sweeping, dusting, and other related duties. Orders for brooms and dusters came in and the unit sparkled with pride. Today, her housekeeping cart goes everywhere with a personalized duster made for one resident who works by her side quite regularly in a beautiful example of FOAs, not to mention the celebration of herself.

Social Meals Programs and Dining Solutions

Food for thought...

Most of us hold wonderful memories of the family dining table and those delicious home-cooked meals. Restaurant fare, in the company of friends and loved ones, can warm one's heart just as well. What makes these environments so special? There are many theories to be explored. Simply put by one individual who reflects on such positive life experiences

> Every night we gathered at the table to listen and share our
> days with one another. Mother spent hours preparing her table
> and we spent equal time enjoying the food.

Social activity in association with meals is a lifelong learning experience of positive reinforcement. Theories abound about nourishment and what is described as the sensation of warmth in the belly. Combined as a memory, we experience overwhelming comfort and security.

The same is true for those living with dementia. When we combine a supportive social environment with a familiar meal setting, we see the expression of lifelong, not to mention normal, behaviors. Frequently in dementia care we refer to the quality of the environment. It must be safe, calm, quiet, familiar and normal. Much of our dining room practices are far from normal. Consider the following:

> *A group of caregivers move about the dining room quickly inserting and removing dishes full or empty. Little social interaction takes place. Well, that is except the frequent buzz as caregivers share plans for the weekend or the latest gossip. Caregivers stand, talking to one another, feeding individual residents from the side or behind. Or worse yet—feeding tables—great exercises in efficiency, but really, how inhumane and impersonal. One, two, three, one, two, three...the only benefit of which can be seated caregivers "feeding" individuals at eye level.*

Situations such as these are what generated the evolution of social meal programs.

First, we must tackle language. How would you like to be called a "feeder" or seated at the "feeding table" with the "tube feed?" "She's a feeder." "He's a tube feed." Ask yourself, "Is this the language I would use with children, parents, or friends at a favorite restaurant?" Challenge yourself and others to pay close attention to the words chosen when referring to a person for whom we are providing care. If we suggest adopting "She needs assistance" instead of "she's a feeder" just think of what an impact—subtle though it may be—we will have on self-esteem of both care providers and caregivers. We are in this role to provide mealtime assistance and support. Think of what a difference this will make to the overall environment. Think of how visitors perceive the enhanced degree of care as we pay close attention to the dignity of our residents.

By choosing words such as "she requires meal assistance" we do acknowledge a limitation, problem, or need exists. The difference is it is done with dignity and recognition of the person. We do not "deal with" residents—we support them. We do not demean the individual for having a deficit out of his or her control. A skilled caregiver recognizes a need exists and puts her skills to work supporting the individual at his or her level of need in the most dignity enhancing way possible. The key in this approach is in knowing our residents. Again we promote the recognition of the uniqueness of the individual. Because we make an ongoing effort to stay familiar with our resident needs, plus their history and identity, we know what degree of meal assistance is required. A skilled and cohesive team may determine a series of meal assistance levels summarized as MA-1, MA-2, or MA-3. But, if we then make references such as "she's an MA-1," what will we have gained? Slang and demeaning phrases will soon fade away and the person, not the dementia, prevails becoming the focus of our caring energies. Now that is a goal to easily set our sights on.

Our behavior has as much impact on the ability to self-nourish as dementia itself. This is a frank and direct statement meant solely to challenge both attitude and approach. If we view and treat the individual as incapable then so it shall be. In fact, it does *not* need to be so. With this in mind, we seek to create the optimal environment that encourages self-nourishment. The following information, therefore, is based on four premises that a true care environment seeks:

- to *identify strengths* so as to maintain skills for as long as possible
- to create a *normal dining experience* which is supportive reflecting familiar past practices
- to provide nourishment in such a way that *recognizes limitations* as a result of the areas or functions of the brain damaged by the dementing process.
- to *observe and respond* to the individual's response and rates of self-nourishment demonstrated

Identifying Strengths

Identifying strengths incorporates the fundamental process of observation. We must observe and ask related questions to the dining experience:

1. Is the individual able to recognize and manage cutlery?
   If recognition is limited (e.g., uses a knife as a spoon), look for the strength (e.g., able to use a spoon or fork) and make use of it. Therefore, the individual can self-nourish.

2. Does the individual eat slowly?
   If given enough time, without caregiver-imposed pressure, will the individual finish the meal? If yes, what's our hurry? For example, caregiver-imposed pressure creates stress in the environment. It is common and most are unaware that they do it. It is a tough habit to break, as one must first be aware of how one imposes the pressure, but it is a breakable habit. Nourishment—adequate nourishment—is much more important than getting the dining area cleaned up or returning dishes to the kitchen. If need be, buy an extra set of dishes and rotate them (i.e., rotate the cleaning of the dishes into the next shift).

3. Does the individual have difficulty with certain foods or beverages and not with others?
   Establish preferences and ensure that we consistently provide foods of preference or foods that promote independence (e.g., thickened beverages to enable residents to drink adequate amounts of fluid safely and independently.)

4. Is the individual distracted by the noise or too many people?
   Can we set up a separate dining area to promote the social meal environment sans distractions? Are we as meal providers able to reduce stimuli to enhance the existing environment?

Our goal through this process of evaluation and solution seeking is empowerment of our residents. Does this seem so strange when the individual has lost so many skills we would link with independence? Well, perhaps, but there are so many skills and behaviors we take for granted. Among the obvious are more subtle strengths that we may bring forth if the opportunity is presented. We do not expect the person to relearn or recover. Realistically speaking, we expect the caregiver to provide the most supportive environment that allows skills to be nurtured and expressed. Yes, this is quite repetitive—another important behavior. Repetition displays familiar actions and behaviors helping to cue remaining strengths. It also reinforces our own caring behavior. We must reinforce our good habits in support of others.

Normal Dining Experience

What is a "normal" dining experience, anyway? Probably anything outside a healthcare facility. Normal is an environment and meal situation in which anyone would enjoy participating. The challenge of creating a normal dining experience in a care home is to meet specific nutritional needs and to utilize adaptive equipment as necessary while at the same time making one feel safe and at home. If we are not relaxed in someone's home as we sit as a guest at his or her table, what happens? We decline extra servings, we demonstrate certain social graces to emulate our civility, we may starve ourselves to be polite and not to appear rude or a glutton. We may end up with indigestion. Surely, we are not the only ones with this experience.

Imagine not having recent memory to recognize this daily meal environment. In our lack of recognition, we feel we must be polite, hoping for a cue. Imagine, if you will, that you are shy and uncomfortable at another's table. You likely will go away hungry. Imagine if your culture did not eat in this fashion. Rather, everyone waited until the food was served then sat on the floor and ate with their fingers instead of forks or chopsticks. Was your resident the ideal hostess? Always carved the roast or served? Could you create a situation where one person serves another? Can we reduce the stimulation to create a more soothing, relaxing, normalized homelike environment?

Normal meal experience is that which is most familiar to us. It is very simple to re-create in the care environment, thus enhancing nourishment—or better still, self-nourishment. You will be quite surprised by some of your residents upon starting this program. Through the environment and task focus we create in our standard dining programs, we frequently overlook definite strengths maintained by residents. It is the environmental overstimulation that has the greatest impact on use of remaining skills. Again, providing a normalized experience is like providing water and sunshine to a wilting plant.

Normalization, by Wolfensberger's (1973) definition, suggests that the situation is not special to any one need but familiar to all. It suggests that if anyone were to be placed in this environment they can cope and know what to do. This is what we would call an ideal environment for someone with dementia. Cueing the person to respond with appropriate social etiquette is the first step on the path to optimal nourishment.

Role of the Facilitator

The facilitator makes or breaks the program. The facilitator is the one who makes the difference between residents' self-nourishment or self-conscious hunger. Several points have been made so far about successful social meals implementation. None of these will be achieved without a capable facilitator managing the progress of the meal for each participant. Some of the responsibilities of the facilitator include but are not limited to

- creating a comfortable space where interaction and socialization may take place regardless of cognitive abilities
- coaching and cueing participants to the process of the meal (e.g., describing the menu, offering beverages and condiments, other necessities to enjoy the meal)
- demonstrating (modeling) self-nourishment by eating his or her meal *at the pace of the slowest person eating* to ensure they know it is okay to continue eating when the others have finished
- proposing toasts, complimenting the quality of the food, and inquiring of other's enjoyment of their meal to draw the attention of drifting residents back to the purpose of the gathering
- promoting discussion or recognition among participants to promote the social context of the experience

The facilitator is the central point that guides participants to success. In two years of data collection and observation around social meals, we have seen that the facilitative process and environmental adaptations have led to enhanced nourishment and functioning for individuals who do not eat meals at any other time of the day. This is very significant to the health of many, not just the chosen few participants. The role of the facilitator is integral to individual success. This role includes monitoring changes, strengths, and limitations and applying interventions to support the success of the participants.

Recognize Limitations and Work with Strengths

If we can establish what works and what does not work we can further promote nourishment. You might say, after the discussion on normalization, that this is straying from the path. But, if we are achieving the nourishment goal with adaptive practices then we are creating an illusion of normalization in the care environment—a necessity for success. For example, Doris is unable to recognize her cake in the dessert dish. Exchanging the white ceramic dish with 45 degree sides for a clear glass, rounded, and shatterproof dish makes a difference. She can see the cake and grasp the dish to pick it up herself and eat it. She achieves a perfectly normal action occurring through the benefit of a normal yet adaptive device.

Another essential factor in this exercise is creating contrast. While cleaning up after a party in the general resident environment, it was observed that there was very little cake waste this day. After some thought staff realized a difference. Today's cake was chocolate, on white plates, on red tableclothes. What was different? A typical party used white cake, on white plates, on white tableclothes. There was distinct contrast on this day, thus enabling residents to enjoy their desserts with much greater success. Needless to say, the standard party plan now includes careful contrasting of plates, cakes, and table coverings. Imagine how similar scenarios can impact resident nourishment. Try a minicontrast audit and see if you can spot any areas for adaptation. Remember, solid colors are more successful than patterns or floral as it reduces the confusion and overstimulation created by a pattern.

Another example of working with strengths—or creating strengths—is the story of the dry potatoes. Edith had little trouble recognizing and trying to eat her potatoes. However, with decreased salivation she, like others, experienced some difficulty. To solve the concern and further encourage nourishment, staff opted to treat soups like gravy. Served as such, residents responded extremely well and even opted for second helpings.

Observe and Respond

When we observe that someone is a slow eater or has some other identified need, active and creative problem solving can enable both resident and staff. If we know that someone requires more time, try starting early and carry his or her mealtime on beyond the rest. This creates a balance. We give the individual the opportunity to get a successful start at self-nourishment without the added stimuli of a busy environment. Staff reduces any pressure they feel on their role of service by inviting the individual to start early. Finally, the meal does not extend so far beyond the end of a designated mealtime that no one feels pressure on his or her routines. How much of this approach is resident focused versus meeting staff needs? Well, it leans both ways. This is how we strike a balance and successfully care for the caregiver *and* receiver—as is our goal.

Bistro Programs

Programs such as designated "social meals programs" or "bistro programs" encourage us to think and act in familiar ways. We bring about a sense of familiarity and ease for participants. There are those who in spite of our efforts still struggle in the dining room environment. It is a given in dementia care that all interventions do not work for all individuals. As a result we must again adapt our approach. The wonder of adaptation is seen in a resident whose overall health and well-being is enhanced. The result for caregivers (we always hope for a benefit for ourselves, too) is that the individual retains/regains strengths that enable them to maintain self-care longer. Our support to sustain these strengths means decreased demands, reduced frustrations, and more moments of celebration as we support residents to achieve their needs.

One such supportive program is known as "Marguerite's Bistro." This program targets one or two residents whose nourishment intake is at risk. Marguerite's Bistro is a special setting to encourage a safe social meal environment with no interruptions or distractions. In a private setting away from the dining room, the staff member sits with her own plate of food to enjoy the meal with her companions.

Eating with the patrons of the bistro is imperative. Their lifelong learning has taught them to share and not to eat in front of others who are not eating. Central dishes are placed on the side or middle of the table to serve the meal as one would do at home. It is amazing how folks will take repeated smaller servings and in the end consume two or three times the amount normally eaten in the dining room. There is no stated duration to this program. It certainly calls for a time commitment. However, when we weigh the time spent against the health dollars, stress, and life-threatening illnesses associated with dehydration and malnutrition—time is of little concern.

∞   ∞   ∞   ∞   ∞

Three women sit at the dining table far from the din of the large cafeteria-like dining room down the hall. Their hostess is a lovely young woman who seems to know them well. The women recognize her face but can connect no name, only trust—they know they are safe.

The hostess smiles as she brings the cart closer. She seats herself, lifts a dish from the cart, and begins serving. As each dish is served, the ladies exchange verbal and nonverbal pleasantries. The language is somewhat beyond interpretation, but the intent is there. When offered second and third helpings, the ladies accept, and their hostess eats with them. She sits as the hostess and as a guest. The ladies periodically observe that she lacks food. Polite offerings of different dishes are made, and gratitude are expressed. Each takes care of the other.

This group shares a mutual purpose clear from the outset. Once satiated, they all sit back for tea and coffee, conversing as comfortably as they are able. When all is said and done, those who are able do their best to help clear dishes. Those who cannot wipe the table, support the others with polite observations. Another satisfying meal for this little social meal club.

∞   ∞   ∞   ∞   ∞

Bistro programs are not only nourishing but also lots of fun and a marvelous way to get to know and build trust with your residents. One way to help members of the team build trust and rapport is to rotate bistro hosts/hostesses to facilitate the trusting relationships. It is worthwhile to mention again here that trust in the caregiver relationship is essential to achieve successful outcomes.

With the success of social meals programs well-established in our research, we now promote the entire environmental social meals dining experience. This suggests that the need to remove residents to a private space would not be necessary if we could facilitate the process generally. This would require the implementation and/or rotation of service staff and facilitators. For example, if the staff were to be divided down the middle as Group A and Group B at the beginning of a shift, Group A would serve today and Group B would facilitate. They may rotate roles the following week. Spacing the rotation out is important to facilitate the development of trust between caregivers and receivers.

While one may consider the facilitator role the easier of the two because the facilitator is sitting down to eat a meal with the residents, I assure you the opposite is true. If the facilitator is hosting the meal correctly, he or she should be quite exhausted after. The facilitator must eat at the slowest resident's pace—not an easy task in spite of how it sounds. This concentration—accompanied by making sure everyone has what they need, remains focused, and receives cueing or assistance as need arises—is exhausting. It takes time and practice to know individual needs and to meet these needs without succumbing to the temptation of taking over or doing for the person. This is no walk in the park. However, the benefits of increased self-nourishment, increased self-confidence, and enhanced rapport with residents in and among themselves is more than worth it. Stress goes down and caregiver–receiver interaction is greatly improved.

There is much to be said about the social meals program. To summarize it would be to say that the benefits far outweigh perceived costs. Staff meals are inconsequential to the cost of rehydrating someone in hospital or treating someone who is suffering malnourishment, delirium, or injury, as is perceived extra time to facilitate the program. The average time spent in a dining room meal is 20 minutes when served by staff. The average time in a social meals program is 40–45 minutes. The significant difference is that in the longer mealtime, the residents consume their entire meal. (It takes time to reach this point when beginning a social meals program.) The practice of ensuring adequate nourishment in dementia care is essential when considering later-stage metabolic changes. A 10 to 15 pound buffer of weight is essential to maintain a person through late-stage increased metabolism, which causes the body to burn away much needed calories to sustain life.

The social meals program is a proactive means of meeting needs while addressing the challenge of providing quality care. There are many challenges and problems we see in the provision of a healthy and supportive care environment, as we have seen evaluating the meal experience. There are, however, useful tools that can help teams facilitate challenges of care through creative problem solving.

Creative Problem Solving

Over the years I have observed a strong tendency of dementia care units to be *reactive* instead of *proactive*. Although we are unable to predict an individual's course or the pattern that the dementia will take, we do know what potential behaviors or losses to expect. Appropriate assessment, such as the use of the Global Deterioration Scale (Reisberg et al., 1982), and reassessment over time does show at what levels residents are functioning and what is expected at each stage.

Behaviors observed over the years have resulted in many common and uncommon solutions. Creativity, flexibility, and spontaneity are integral factors for successful interventions by caregivers. We know what may potentially take place; therefore, we have a responsibility to prepare for it.

Proactive behavior on our part demands that we observe and act. We don't look for quick and easy solutions to help *us,* but for solutions that benefit *everyone involved.* Creative problem solving, as you will see in the following flow chart (**Figure 9**, p. 118), can be much fun. It promotes brainstorming and flex thinking (Dunne, 1997) as participants consider the options.

Flex thinking demands that caregivers apply three behaviors as they review a problem or as we interact with peers:

- First, we *are mindful of the language we use.* We seek to use appropriate, professional, and positive language to represent our residents and our team.

- Second, we *look for the benefits of a scenario.* In every situation, there exists the good and the bad. We must simply look for them.

- Third, we *talk and listen positively.*

Listening positively encourages us to be open to what is being said. We try our best not to have negative internal dialogue, which shuts out others' ideas. Each of these behaviors has an impact on the quality of the outcome. We may have to relinquish some of what we believe is best to accomplish our mutual goal. Letting go usually puts us much further ahead as we seek to solve a problem together. Flex thinking is similar to brain storming in that it welcomes all possible creative solutions to challenging situations.

The *Creative Problem Solving Model* considers the residents, staff, others involved, and environmental concerns. The premise behind this model is this question: What is the consequence if I/we don't do something? In other words, if I/we don't act on the problem what will/will not happen? This is also known as the "pain or pleasure outcome measure" (Robbins, 1987). Robbins suggests that we evaluate situations, problems, or things that we procrastinate over by determining whether there is more pain or pleasure involved in action or inaction. Proactive behavior has greater potential to alleviate stress than procrastination or conflict resolution at the time of occurrence.

When transferring this perspective to caregiving we must consider the needs of all involved, evaluate safety factors, and review our care goals. What is the consequence if we don't take action to protect both resident and staff as we pursue our care goals? A big question, but one which we must constantly integrate into our daily routine of care. Following is an example of evaluating the desire to act in the best interest of both residents and caregivers.

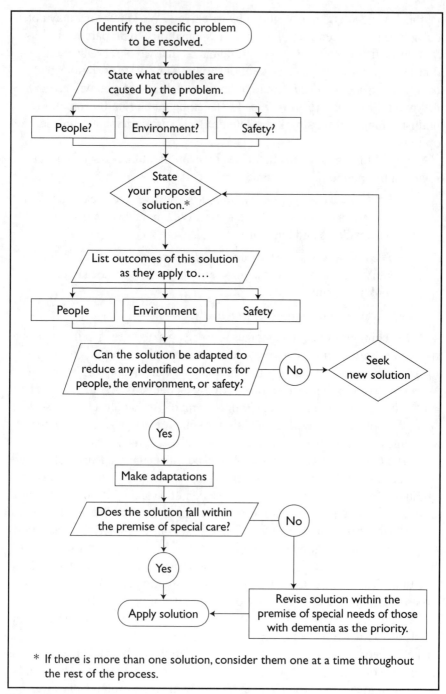

FIGURE 9
Creative Problem Solving in the Dementia Care Environment

Repeated problems with a woman who used a wheelchair challenged the team to find a solution. The problem was that she would pull herself along and up a slight ramp in the dining area toward a balcony garden door. Going up wasn't the problem. It was coming down. The *specific problem* (concern) was that she would roll backwards uncontrolled down the ramp, which on one side was a blind corner, and crash—injure herself, other residents, or staff. Due to the physical layout, individuals with wheelchairs or walkers required assistance to safely ascend the ramp to get outside. Once this was recognized, the group began searching for a solution.

A session of creative problem solving proposed a *quick solution:* place a rope across the balcony access that can be unhitched if staff needed to access the balcony. Great idea, but what about safety concerns? Could residents climb over? What if someone pulled on or fell against the rope? Anchored to drywall, the odds were that the drywall plug would be forced out of the wall causing a fall. So, back to the drawing board. A *new solution* was proposed: a gate—a secure and safe idea. Again, someone could try to climb over. At the same time, this as the other idea restricts access to the secured balcony garden and walking path. This defeated the purpose of the special care environment. The team proposed a *final solution*. A removable, partial gate was installed. This gate allowed ambulatory residents the freedom to pass through to the balcony while it protected one and all from free-flying wheelchairs, yet allowed assisted access. This is just one way in which we can create a positive working and living environment for caregivers and care receivers.

The keys to successful creative problem solving are

- Be concise and clear in establishing the exact problem to be solved.

- Be open to all suggestions or solutions.

- Take each solution through the process with careful consideration to all factors (residents, staff, environment).

- Do not skip any steps—do a complete evaluation/assessment to ensure the solution is viable.

- Ensure it meets the parameters of the "special care environment" as your team has defined it.

- Follow through to ensure all members of the team are aware of the process and the outcomes.

- Make sure everyone participates in applying the solution.

- Evaluate the solution after a predetermined period (30–90 days) and make appropriate adjustments as need be, or celebrate your success as a team.

At the End of the Day

Isolation brings sadness and steals the magic within—
the celebration of the self should be public.

As we seek to meet needs and resolve problems, at the end of the day each of us hopes to have made a difference. In special care the difference we hope to have made is in the quality of our residents' life experience that very day. The game plan changes daily with our residents based on their individual needs and experiences. Should this limit or expand their opportunities for social interaction and expression? The answer to this question—like so many others—is no.

As we built our collection of approaches and interventions, we realized the breadth of our responsibility. We pursued our mission of a warm, comfortable, and safe environment vigorously. We promoted the special, secure, and protective new care unit within the whole care facility to inform and bring everyone along on our exciting journey. Suddenly a new reality began to creep out, as we learned that residents who did not require "special care" interventions were misinterpreting the concept of a "secure" environment. Their misguided perception was that once one moved onto the SCU one would never be seen again. It took some convincing to reassure these good folks that our intentions were to provide a genuinely safe living environment for those at risk. Their "never to be seen again" belief was false.

The world of special care does not intend to replicate incarceration—it intends to represent safe, secure, and supportive nurturing care. It intends to promote identity and self-esteem within the capabilities of the resident. It does not intend to withdraw them from the community in which they have lived the greater part of their lives. It is absolutely without question the provision of a normalized lifestyle that celebrates their identity through socialization and integration. If we withdraw the individual from the community, we run the risk of imprisoning them in a world of limiting beliefs. What we create, as a result, is someone who is or becomes increasingly dependent on us as caregivers. This leads to behaviors of learned helplessness.

Learned helplessness is the inability of the individual to believe that he or she can control events and behaviors (Howe-Murphy & Charbonneau, 1987, p. 46). In the case of the individual with dementia, the belief is less theirs and more that of the caregiver. This seemingly benevolent caregiver practice results with the caregiver gradually taking over tasks for the individual. Doing this while the individual still maintains the skills, though they may be slow and require cueing, steals the skills prematurely. To stay as independent as possible the skills must be encouraged, not discouraged. Creating helplessness ultimately creates more work for ourselves. We must encourage and support our residents, allowing them the right to experience the dignities of risk. The right to succeed, and not succeed, must be afforded in spite of the dementia. Who are we to decide that an individual cannot continue to experience the ups and downs of life simply because a process called dementia has complicated their existence—or perhaps further challenged our own existence? We must be mindful and willing to implement and support programs that fulfill the goal of a normalized lifestyle that celebrates identity through socialization and integration.

To be mindful is to be aware of our own and other people's behavior in a situation—it is to pay attention to communications taking place. Mindfulness suggests three characteristics. First, it involves creating new categories to eliminate broad generalizations and labels and to remain open to individualized interpretation. Second, we must be prepared to receive new information about the individual or situation. Finally, we must be open to and aware of more than one perspective. We must "consciously seek cues to guide our behavior" (Gudykunst, Ting-Toomey, Sudweeks & Stewart, 1995, p. 27) and our decisions.

In the case of special care, to be mindful of our residents is to be aware of their level of ability from day to day, moment to moment. It is also to make decisions and implement interventions not based on the diagnosis or the secure nature of the unit alone. The message here is simple: We not only provide a secure, safe living environment, but also ensure our residents maintain the highest level of independent physical, emotional, and social functioning possible as they continue to live their lives. These people are alive.

How can we continue an integrated approach to socialization within the facility? Four guidelines suggest a safe, individualized, and supportive process of determining social goal planning. The following guideline questions help us to determine a resident's ability to cope and safely participate in what we termed "off-unit program participation." The resident must meet all of the criteria or a specified variation to participate in off-unit programs.

Off-Unit Question Guidelines/Criteria
Is the resident at risk when off unit?

Is the resident a persistent wanderer, unable to sit through a given program? Is he or she occupying the supervising staff person's time, thus placing the safe supervision of a program in jeopardy? Without adequate one-on-one support, this individual is not appropriate. Support offers the person the opportunity to get up and wander through program areas or the building for that matter. They may return to the program and settle, they may not. It is the "may not" which creates the risk. It is the support we provide which reduces or eliminates it.

Is the resident disruptive to the success of the program for the other residents?

When a program clearly no longer has meaning or value to the individual and his or her behavior is measurably disruptive, it is time to reevaluate. It is for these residents that the programs of the Special Care Unit itself were ultimately created. A memorable example of this type of situation is that of a talented woman whose life had been filled with music—her identity was music. As dementia invaded her world she hummed and hummed and hummed and hummed. Armchair travel videos, enjoyed by others, were no longer in touch with her reality as she sat looking straight ahead, rocking and humming. While she appeared to do no harm and was certainly at no risk to wander away, everyone around her became increasingly annoyed with her nonstop humming (of which she really had no awareness). She was discharged from the program. Her needs were met more appropriately on the unit through music therapy and other related interventions where this behavior would not seem out of the norm.

Is the resident's personal safety in jeopardy?

This really is common sense and requires no explanation. Could the individual potentially harm himself or herself someone else? Be mindful.

Is there no measurable benefit to the resident?

The intent of a supportive unit is just that—to support and encourage success within the resident's means. Why bring someone to an environment where clearly they will not benefit from the interaction or activity? It is at this point that we must recognize the strengths of the individual and make the utmost of them to allow the individual to maintain their strengths, skills, and personal dignity.

Mechanism of Support

There will always be those, just as we discussed earlier, who will say, "She can't leave the unit because when she comes back she is disoriented and upset." What should be at issue is not forced segregation but an investigation into our mechanism of support. We must allow the individual every opportunity to live in the moment. Therefore, if the individual is successful in the off-unit programs, we must endeavor to support their participation. Not only is this value-enhancing for the individual, but also we support the maintenance and expression of skills for a greater length of time. This may not otherwise occur if we do not encourage the use of social and other functional skills in the general facility living environment. If there is a problem upon return, we must look at our interventions and approaches. It should be expected that disorientation may occur upon return. (I'd rather expect a problem and feel disappointed at not experiencing it than to be naive and not anticipate disruption at some point.) These people may be struggling with the most basic skills. By developing our mindfulness, using the creative problem-solving model, and applying Needs Response, we prepare ourselves with the tools necessary to address the resident's needs or disorientation upon return.

One approach we have used with success is to stagger our programs so the residents who are able to attend programs off-unit return to find a low key program such as a discovery kit exploration, ball toss, or one-on-one interventions with the recreation worker in place. A bonus to this staggered framework approach is that it affords her the luxury of working with residents unable to go off unit in a quieter and uninterrupted setting. We have created a win–win situation for everyone involved.

When family or volunteers take residents off-unit, as in the example with Betty and her son, they must build time into their visit planning to remain with their loved one for up to 20 (or more) minutes on the unit after they return. During this time frame they may wander the unit with the resident, help them to hang up their coat and settle in their room or freshen up after an outing. It takes time to reorient oneself to the change of environment. We must be mindful and willing to support the resident through this important transition. This mindful approach leads only to further success and comfort at the end of the day.

A final reflection on creating a mechanism of support: The more our special care residents interacted with our general resident population—under the support and guidance of the recreation worker—the more they themselves have developed support skills. It is amazing how quickly they have come to empathize, support, and protect the interests and welfare of their less fortunate peers. We can be truly proud of this mechanism of support at the end of the day.

Silence Is Golden

If music be the food of life, play on.
—William Shakespeare

The use of auditory stimulation, such as radio or television, provides the same opportunity for problematic situations and responses as any overstimulating activity or approach. Television may have less negative response than radio because the individual *may* be able to focus and determine the source of the "noise" or "disturbance" through the visual element. However, this is not to say that television is the lesser of two evils. Due to the complexity of the auditory sense, a high level of interpretive ability is required to interpret and understand the stimulus of either TV or radio. A hearing impairment, and the addition of a visual impairment in many cases, further complicates the cognitively impaired individual's ability to interpret unfamiliar stimulus.

Bowlby supports the issues relating to auditory stimulus and interpretive ability and stated

> Audiotapes of discussion or contemporary comedy would probably be lost on individuals with moderate and advanced ADRD [Alzheimer's Disease and Related Disorders]. There are simply not enough cues to make it meaningful. (1991, p. 167)

She suggests that the use of old-time comedy/drama audiotapes (pre-TV) in the correct and familiar context offers suitable cues to be an appropriate intervention. Imagine how effective a group session (or a one-on-one session) would be if we create a setting which takes the memory back to the days of the family enjoying the evening as they sit around the Philco freestanding radio. If an authentic radio is not available to your unit, reproductions are on the market that further facilitate the process. These reproductions look like the old radios but have cassette players built in. There are numerous places a resourceful recreation therapist or care team member can locate taped copies of original radio music, drama, and variety shows. If you do have an authentic radio—set up the environment in such a way as to mirror the comfortable and relaxing family room or living room just as the residents would have known it. Using a tape recorder in a strategic position near the radio, and with a suitable population, a wonderful program is in store for all involved.

There are those who suggest that playing the radio or television would be great to occupy, distract, or divert the residents so that staff may be freed to attend to meetings or other duties. This is a dangerous belief. Watching or listening to the television or radio are passive activities. For the person with dementia, the lack of ability to interpret stimuli from either TV or radio can generate a frightened or overwhelmed response. Because of the unpredictable behavior associated with persons with dementia, more harm can be done if residents are left to their own limited interpretive skills without someone to interpret the situation. Facilitated use of such equipment is the only dignified means of using these technologies with our special care residents. A facilitator may cue, guide, support, calm, or redirect an individual who is or is not being stimulated by the sensations and messages communicated through the equipment. Bowlby emphasizes the importance of a facilitated process:

> Be sure to provide ample reality reassurance information before, during and after—so that the setting does not result in further disorientation. (1991, p. 167)

Likewise, a program of music is provided for the benefit of the residents. Therefore, when considering music selections, first consider the resident's ability to interpret music as familiar or unfamiliar, disturbing or pleasurable, and thought provoking.

Music therapist Lois McCloskey of Seattle reminds us that music need not be ever present in the environment. She poses the question: "Do we have music on for ourselves at all times of the day? Quiet, silence is okay." We all need a break, whether cognitively impaired or otherwise.

Audiotapes of music should be selected based on their texture, tone, and ability to create pleasure or a desired mood. Texture involves the voice and sound quality. Tone and other qualities such as rate and pitch affect our listening endurance and mood—it may be soothing, stimulating, or agitating. The ability of music to create pleasure is certainly individualized. However, in special care we cannot assume that our residents or clients like or prefer something without a solid basis to build on. This may seem like a rigid approach to planning for special care, however, in the case where an individual is relying on others to protect interests and well-being, a degree of rigidity must be viewed as protective. Err on the side of caution when considering music for residents. The underlying belief is that if the resident is not familiar with the type of music, then most likely it is not suitable as a selection. Music types are generationally associated (one can assume familiarity based on demographics).

Unfamiliar music can cause disorientation and agitation, as indicated by Bowlby. Residents cognitively impaired at a mild to moderate level are not able to process information presented randomly without supportive guidance as provided by a facilitator. Therefore, random presentation of radio news broadcasts further provide opportunity for increased disorientation. Based on this information the use of a radio as an open and unstructured program or diversional medium is not considered appropriate. In an ongoing effort of any special care unit the radio, and likewise the television, is not considered to be a purposeful or acceptable tool.

If you are looking for a solution or a preventive measure that will be effective, align your unit with a local music therapist. These wonderful professionals are the absolute authority on appropriate selections of music, including type, time of day, or activity through which to play or not to play music. Music generally recommended includes light classics, familiar period music (e.g., the War Years), or even the occasional nature recording. The general perspective held by music therapists is that resident response is greatest when familiar, repeated songs and phrases are used. Frequently, successful interventions make use of music from the formative years of a person's life. As one professional puts it, "do the math." In some cases, music of the parent's formative years is the influential music in the lives of their children. These were the songs sung by mother to child during an influential (early childhood developmental) period in this person's life. (I love songs from 1950s musicals, big band music and Harry Belafonte thanks to my mother's tastes.) The song A Bicycle Built for Two (Daisy, Daisy) was a hit around WWI. This song could have been sung to a child born in 1942 as a favorite of his or her parents. This same song may have meaning for someone born around 1900. A song can transcend generations yet we cannot assume so. A person age 75 in 2002 was 15 in 1942. The radio played forties dance music, and that person went to dances where music performed by big bands and dances like the Jitterbug were prominent. Be aware of what is relevant to a person's life and why. This thoughtful approach to music presentation results in responses ranging from emotional, cognitive or even expressive musical responses. Unfamiliar music often results, as stated before, in agitation or withdrawal. Do your music math.

Before concluding this segment, a word to the wise: Noise in the environment is not limited to music, television, and radio. The sound environment includes the contributions made by staff and visitors as well. For this very reason our facility restricts nonessential tours and visits by outsiders on the unit. In some dining rooms, clearing the dishes and cutlery may be extremely disturbing. Try using a cloth in the bottom of dish or cutlery bins to lessen the noise. While such practical or external noises may be easy to control, it is difficult for some to resist bellowing down the hall "I'm going for lunch now." These not so subtle orations are extremely abrasive in such a sensitive environment. Each and every one of us must be mindful of our contribution to the quality of the sound environment, be it verbal or in the use of equipment and other potential noisemakers. One Vancouver care facility wisely posts a clear message to raise consciousness of all those who enter their special care unit. At every place of entry a sign, is posted which notifies staff and guests that they are entering a "Sound Sensitive Environment" their cooperation is sought in maintaining a calm and supportive atmosphere. Approaches such as this are both creative and proactive. Proactivity in special care is much easier than reactivity. As with the toys discussed previously, if audio and visual entertainment have been a regular part of the individual's leisure time it is certainly appropriate that they continue this practice for their pleasure and enjoyment in the privacy of their own "suite." Simply consider the functional skills of the individual in this effort in order to determine the type of support the person may need to successfully and pleasurably enjoy these pursuits.

ATTENTION!

You are now entering a

Sound Sensitive Environment

Loud sounds, loud voices, and abrupt movements may trigger agitation and discomfort for residents.

Your sensitivity is appreciated.

Sound Sensitive Environment proactive poster notice created by Sally Howard, Music Therapist. Reprinted with permission from The Yaletown House Society.

A final note on noise in the special care environment comes from Dr. W. M. Clemmer, author of *Victims of Dementia: Services, Support and Care* who reminds us that

> A nursing home is not a hospital. The pleasant sounds of people living and doing should not be eliminated. But you do need to reduce noise—the distracting, annoying noises of machinery (e.g., ice machines, air conditioners, cleaning equipment, carts), paging systems, continuous piped-in music, TVs, traffic, shift change activities, dish washing and dining room clatter, and so forth. Noise can prevent the hearing-impaired from participating in every day activities and interaction. Furthermore, it has been found that increased background noise may elicit wandering, calling out, and other "aberrant" behavior. (1993)

Try designating one or two staff at different times of the day to sit out of the way and write down the sounds they hear. Better still, have them wear a blindfold for part of the exercise to heighten their auditory sensory awareness. When they report back with the results, be open and creative in your approach to improving your sound environment. Be flexible in your approach and commit to regular noise audits. You may just experience a whole new special care environment.

Finally, keep in mind that when using music selections that exceptions to the rule always exists. Let us not forget the enjoyment provided by specific "themed" programs where, out of context, the music would be determined as inappropriate. Christmas tunes and Mexican, Portuguese, or Polka types of music can be extremely effective and enjoyable for all—when used in an appropriate and directive context.

A Little Soft Shoe Goes a Long Way

Who's on first?
Exactly.

—*Bud Abbott and Lou Costello*

I would be terribly remiss if I did not include one of the most valuable tools available to each and every one of us—resident, family, professional caregiver alike: the enduring and contagious qualities of humor.

Perhaps only two words are necessary to convey the message of this little chapter: Norman Cousins. No one before or since his marvelous book *Anatomy of an Illness* (1981) has captured the enormous importance, value, and physical and psychological benefits of humor. Rich, deep laughter cures the deepest blues and relieves the most tense of moments. We know that with the person with Alzheimer's and related dementias the link to polite, supportive behavior sustains itself into the disease process. Experience has demonstrated that when we ask permission and seek input and involvement from those for whom we provide care we are greeted with polite response. It is also true that the ability to laugh may be sustained through encouragement, support, and gentle use of humor.

Not only is humor important to the resident, but also to the caregiver. Are we taking ourselves too seriously? If we are unable to step back and find the humor in the little things and even some of the bigger things each day, we are headed for a sorry state. It is in our best interests not only to be able to laugh at ourselves, but also to be able to bring out the natural sense of humor present in those for whom we provide care. This is not to promote ridicule or teasing on a destructive level. This is to say that one quality that always remains is humor. For each of us the gift of humor comes from a greater power or spirit within us.

Admitting our mistakes, checking in with the person whose needs we are addressing, and duplicating a small *faux pas* (i.e., mirroring a mistake made by another, thus showing that anyone could make the error) shows our own human frailty. In our interactions, each is a supportive element when used with love and good humor. It is now common knowledge that chemical reactions in our physiology (the release of endorphins) have proven benefits on physical and emotional levels. What better way to have a positive impact on another's well being, not to mention our own.

Whether it is a little soft shoe in the corridor (no excuses, I can't dance worth a lick but I always get at least a smile), a pun, or a funny face (well-timed, of course) amazing things can be accomplished with a little comedy. Laughter truly is the best medicine.

∞   ∞   ∞   ∞   ∞

Once I took a rather crowded elevator ride. One of the gentlemen standing quite close to me (who happened to reside on our special care unit) reached forward and tapped out my name on my nametag.

"Rosemary Dunne," he said in his beautiful Irish brogue.

"Yes, sir," I replied with a friendly smile.

"Well now, that's not a name for you," he chuckled.

"It isn't?" I responded both curious and surprised.

"No, it's not." he replied with a laugh and a nudge.

"What makes you say that?" I queried.

"Because that's not a name for a guy," he answered smartly as I stood before him wearing my dress pants and short summer hair cut. He reached up and punched me on the shoulder in a friendly sort of way, quite assured of his belief.

I was surely defeated by his confident smile. I bowed graciously as the elevator came to a halt, backed out and replied, with a wink to one and all, "Just call me Mike."

∞   ∞   ∞   ∞   ∞

Too often the temptation to correct or change behavior or situation is so great we lose track of the lighter side of life. Being able to laugh at ourselves and the situations presented us is essential to maintaining a balance in special care. No one values humor more, from my experience, than those with special care needs.

Wrap Your Mind Around It

Think big!

In *Attitude of Discovery* (p. 35) we discussed the importance of a positive attitude. Here we explore the complementary traits of flexibility and openness. These traits are essential to the success of any caregiver.

Singer Rita Coolidge is quoted as having said, "Too often the opportunity knocks, but by the time you push back the chain, push back the bolt, unhook the locks and shut off the burglar alarm, it's too late." Here Coolidge recognizes that inflexible attitudes can result in a missed opportunity. Her recognition underlies the goal of the flex thinker: eyes and ears sharp, ready to bend at a moment's notice—opportunity cannot be missed. Our willingness to be flexible enhances our ability to be creative and open. It would then make sense then that "if we give up some of what we believe to be true or think is best we end up much further ahead in the long run" (Willis Zoglio, 1997, p. 93). We must be mindful and willing. This is a flex thinker.

Flex thinkers are open thinkers—flexible and open to any change or disruption in routine. One astute nurse who regularly works the night shift is known to say, "Any time is tea time on our unit whether it is two in the morning or two in the afternoon."

Here is a caregiver who does not miss the opportunity. She examines the situation and responds to the need of the resident. Not only is she a flex thinker who is listening and observing to meet the needs of her resident population, but also she is an abstract thinker. The task-oriented linear thinker may be drawn at 2:00 a.m. to view a wanderer simply as someone out of bed. True, but the flex thinker asks the questions:

- Why are they wandering?
- What do they need?
- What can I do to meet that need?

Returning or redirecting the individual back to bed may not resolve the situation, and it may in fact agitate it. We must open our eyes and ears as flex thinkers. What is their real or actual need? Did they in fact get out of bed to use the toilet and get lost going back to bed? Or are they actually trying to go home? Is loneliness a factor? Are they cold? Did something frighten them? Do they simply need a glass of water? What could the need be?

Through care, attention to detail, and stepping out of our task orientation we move beyond the glossy portrayal of a "special" care unit. We move past the slogans (which in their own right, as a shared belief by a given team, have value) to action. The flex thinker is ready to change point of view—to see a whole new picture. In using this approach, change becomes less threatening. A successful flex thinker is secure in himself or herself and able to abandon traditional thinking. Try it next time you have a problem or challenging situation. Skip the obvious solution and consider the ridiculous; this may very well trigger an answer to the problem. Although not related to health care, this example of flex thinking has always impressed me.

Years ago, British Columbia Transit was faced with the enormous expense of replacing worn out trolley buses whose electrical systems were shot. One engineer, it is said, proposed the solution to the problem. The bus chassis' were in fine repair they simply needed new power sources. The engineer proposed to remove the electric drives and replace them with diesel-powered engines. This abandonment of traditional thinking is described by some as stepping out of the box. This quick thinking fellow saved the transit company hundreds of thousands of dollars.

Flex thinkers are action people who believe they can make a difference and demonstrate this belief in their daily practice. And that is just what it is— practice. For the most dedicated of flex thinkers, practice makes perfect. It also makes for a grand adventure. This model is a step toward examining our whole set of priorities and may well end in a complete paradigm shift. Flex thinking could be the best thing to happen to your world. Think big and wrap your mind around it.

PART 4

SHARING THE PROGRAM MAGIC

Care versus Control

Ask yourself: How would I feel if all the facts of this incident were played out by the media?

People choose their career paths carefully. Mine chose me, at least that is my explanation. My grandmothers and their personal needs in long-term care set my heart afire, and I sought my career knowing what I wanted to do but not knowing what it was called. I found the field of therapeutic recreation. As a recreation therapist, I have been able to promote life, dignity, identity, happiness, and general well-being through the promotion of—among other things—recreation and leisure. This path brought me to the discovery kits, FOAs, and suitable frameworks for providing programs and care on special care units. My greatest desire is to maintain in each resident the person they have been most happy with and proud of through the course of their lives. I believe that I am called to care, and since I know my own experience best, this is why I relate it to you. Your choice and the choice of others to provide care in the arena of geriatrics, specifically in dementia care may, of course, be similar to mine or unique to your own experiences. The bottom line is that if you have read this far, in your heart of hearts, you care. You care deeply for those to whom you provide assistance with making each day a joy filled journey and a happy reality, wherever it may be. This is the elemental difference between caring for and controlling the needs of an individual.

When a distressing situation presents itself to staff, what takes priority: caring or controlling? Do we immediately kick in our care-focused mode, or are we inclined to try to maintain control of the individual to achieve our own desired outcome? If we maintain control, are we fulfilling our mission as caregivers in long-term care? Control is an element to be used carefully and with greatest caution. When control over a person is used to maintain power and to dominate the vulnerable individual, it becomes a form of abuse. Abuse perhaps of the worst kind, as this population is unable to defend itself or cry for help. This is a heavy topic and one to which an entire book may be devoted; certainly the subject of elder abuse is well-explored. However, the area of special care requires distinct attention. If presented with a situation where care versus control becomes an issue, how can we sufficiently advocate on the resident's behalf?

For example, a resident desires a bath which staff consider to be too hot. The staff decide that a regular temperature is sufficient. However, when requesting a hot bath the resident perceives she is receiving a cold one as it is not the temperature to which she is accustomed. She refuses her bath boister-ously, each time frightening the staff. Their desire to maintain control has created a dilemma.

We are presented with an ethical dilemma as we investigate the mandate for care and the type of care that is being provided. An effective method of evaluation and problem solving is one that could be termed "ethical brain-storming." The questions we must ask are as follows:

1. Who are the primary stakeholders?
   • residents
   • family
   • staff
   • facility

2. What are the ethical issues relating to:
   • quality care?
   • aggressive behavior?
   • resistive behavior?
   • communication problems?

3. What are the relevant facts? (May or may not relate to 1–2)

4. What are the practical constraints surrounding 1–3?

5. What does each stakeholder have the right to expect?

6. What are the possible solutions?

7. What possible constraints to solutions may exist?

8. What are the ethics to the alternatives?

9. What are the implications of long-term and short-term solutions?

Using these questions in a frank discussion that considers, without bias, the needs of all involved, a solution or series of solutions may be proposed. (Maddux & Maddux, 1989, pp. 51–53.) When all is said and done, the follow-ing three questions should be used to test the waters of the decision-making process:

1. If all the facts of this situation/discussion were made available to and published by the media, how would you feel?

2. How do you feel in your "gut" about this decision?

3. How will your self-esteem be affected by this decision?

In the end, this woman received her hot bath. How did they determine the temperature and address her care needs? A pool thermometer (much more familiar than the digital gauge on the tub) was purchased from a supply house at a minimal cost. The resident and her daughter ran a hot bath to her liking and together they took the temperature. The nurse documented the temperature in the resident's care plan. The thermometer was designated as part of her care when running a bath. The tub was subsequently run at her preferred "hot" comfort zone and everyone was content. She had her hot bath, the staff felt safe, and her care plan was followed without question. A dilemma resolved through discussion and problem solving by a team of caregivers.

The threats to ethical behavior (caring vs. controlling) include an unwillingness to take a stand when cost is involved, always looking for simple solutions and being satisfied with quick fixes, or ignoring or violating our own individual ethics and values. These threats are not to be taken lightly. A responsible professional is willing and determined to see such issues through to the best of her ability.

Be mindful of the choices you make in providing care. One of the simplest rules to follow is the golden rule: Do unto others as you would have done to you. This is part of caring, exploring, and understanding ethical approaches and decision making. These are wise goals for those who seek to ensure that the journey special care residents are making is a safe and joyful one.

Seasonal Scheduling

I was "baby-sitting" and not giving them credit for what they can do! They want to help and the more they do the happier they are!

—Barbara Moffatt

We must ask permission—gather their favor and proceed with care and respect.

Many people have hours they prefer to work. It is very handy to be able to set one's schedule to one's own preferences. However, the reality for most recreation therapists and recreation workers is that to provide a normalized routine of programming the schedule varies to accommodate program needs. The 8:00 a.m. to 4:00 p.m. recreation department does a lot for the staff, but what of the residents?

A recreation department may generally offer a 8:00 a.m. to 4:00 p.m. schedule which allows staff to offer up to three programs, perhaps more, during the course of a day. Each special care unit is unique and must apply programming appropriately. In special care, program scheduling has even more applications as residents' natural clocks fluctuate with the season and their needs with the time of day. A dual season schedule, with flexibility for special events, has proven extremely effective. Keeping in mind that staffing is funded per resident need, so should hours be set. This is an exercise in flex thinking.

A "summer/winter" routine accommodates the light changes brought on by daylight savings time. In summer, with the long daylight hours, we found the residents up and about much longer. Thus residents required later program interventions to address their needs for purposeful interactions. We ran the schedule successfully from early afternoon to between 8:00 and 8:30 in the evening. Although at one point we considered running even later, we realized that not all solutions could come from the recreation staff. The remaining members of the care team were introduced to programming possibilities, including the use of discovery kits, which could be utilized late into the evening to accommodate resident need. Regardless of the success of this schedule, the day shift complained somewhat, saying how busy they were and how much they needed assistance. Their time would come.

As the summer rolled by the days grew shorter. At the switch back from daylight savings time the recreation worker's shift switched with it. The shift started late morning, to accommodate the care team's desire to help the residents to rise slowly without rushing and agitating them in the process. The recreation worker would begin her day with an easygoing program, which warmed up participating residents for the day. This would be followed by an easy cool down that prepared them for the transition into the noon mealtime period. The winter shift ran into the late afternoon so the recreation worker would be able to accommodate two specific criteria: a second mealtime transition (to supper) and the elements of the sundowning period.

Sundowning takes place approximately between 3:00 and 6:00 in the afternoon (mid to late afternoon). It is a period of restlessness and wandering which can lead to severe agitation and upset generally on the unit. It may occur with one or—heaven forbid—all of the special care resident population. It is a strong need or desire to get home, to return somewhere to care for someone, for example. It may be a desperate need or an easily pacified one, it is unknown and unpredictable in its measure. However, many who experience a period of sundowning do so consistently, or do so by way of the same triggers. While it may not be entirely preventable, we can ease the presence or potential for sundowning by

- eliminating or reducing the triggers
- providing purposeful tasks or programs over the transitional time frame

Or, failing these, we have one remaining solution:

- intervening with appropriate Needs Response directed to the specific individual

Having switched to a day schedule, we continued to address needs of the midday, meal times, sundowning, and disruption often caused by shift changes of the care team. Not to mention the fact that we also appealed to the cry of the day shift who wanted so badly to have the recreation worker addressing needs during their time on board. You can imagine who would have been less happy with the change: the evening shift.

Although the resident's tendency is to head for bed shortly after nightfall, the evening staff still found some difficulty coping without the assistance or presence of the recreation worker. All is fair as they say—a valuable resource must be shared. There is a strong benefit to the operation of the recreation department by using this approach. As a result of the haves and have nots of a summer/winter shift, both day and evening shifts hold the role of and the valuable assistance provided by the recreation worker quite highly. This is some of the best free PR a department could ask for. If we had it our way— regrettably budgets rarely allow—we would certainly staff days, evenings, and weekends. However, in the reality of economics, we must work within budgets and accommodate where needs may be greatest. If this approach means a summer/winter shift is the most effective way to benefit our resident needs, if this approach helps the residents to function optimally within their remaining abilities, then let seasonal scheduling be the norm for therapeutic recreation programming and services on a special care unit.

Programming Guide

The tables presented in this chapter represent the challenge of identifying and analyzing a set group of programs. The programs do not replace staff inter-action or minimize the undeniable importance of purposeful roles and activi-ties. These intend to augment a well-rounded care environment. We consider the entire team's role in maintaining a quality living environment (i.e., home-like environment) without placing pressure or responsibility on recreation or activity staff to entertain, play with, or distract our most worthy residents. These are programs meant to fulfill the leisure lifestyle component of our resi-dents based on their abilities and strengths. This is just one part of the whole.

Table 7 (p. 140) is a surprising collection of potential programs and ac-tivities. In fact, all are not even listed! Those listed were evaluated based on

- when they were most beneficial (*time of day*)
- if they were *calming* or *stimulating*

- whether or not they served to *burn energy*, thus promoting fatigue and sleep (This was considered apart from stimulation, as activity versus sedentary existence is preferred for overall wellness regardless of dementia.)

Based on the programmer's approach and environmental conditions the results achieved may vary. Consideration was given to which domains were targeted and the time of year programs were implemented (e.g., Are they seasonal or anytime programs?). This analysis provides greater insight into program appropriateness and participant suitability.

TABLE 7
Potential Programs and Activities

Activity	Time of Day	Calming	Energy
Armchair Travel	A	Y	L
Arts and Crafts	P	Y/N	L
Baking	P/S	Y/N	H/L
Ball Toss	A	Y/N	H
Bean Bag Toss	M	N	H
Bowling	M/P	N	H
Bus Outings	P	N	H/L
Dancing	A	N	H
Discovery Kits	A	Y	L
Entertainment	P/E	Y/N	H/L
Exercise	M	N	H
Five-Card Bingo	P	N	L
Gardening	P/S	Y	H
Group Talks	A	Y	L
Happy Hour	P	Y	L
Ice Cream Making	P/E/S	Y	H/L
Intergenerational	P	N	H/L
Manicures	A	Y	L
Pet Visitations	A	Y	L
Putting	P/S	Y/N	H
Puzzles	P/E	Y	L
Reminiscing	A	Y	L
Social Tea	P	Y/N	L
Stamp Pad Club	N	N	H/L
Theme Parties	P/E	N	H/L
Walking	A	Y	H
Word Games	P	N	L

KEY

A = anytime; M = morning; P = afternoon; E = evening; S = seasonal; Y = yes; N = no; H = high; L = low; Y/N and H/L= depends on an individual's functional abilities and level of participation in the activity

The domains considered in **Table 8** include physical, social, emotional, and cognitive. Spirituality is addressed from a parallel perspective through stories and insight. Humor, I believe, has the potential to be set aside as a unique domain with great necessity to be nurtured. Dr. John Tooth summarizes the value of humor and laughter in his wonderful words: "Where you have laughter, you haven't got fear anymore" (personal communication). Until we wisely add a classification on humor for emphasis, the domains are explored using the following considerations or criteria.

TABLE 8
Potential Programs and Activities—Domain Involvement

Activity	Domain Involvement/Stimulation			
	Physical	Social	Emotional	Cognitive
Armchair Travel	L	H	H	H
Arts and Crafts	L	H	L	H
Baking	H/L	H	H	H
Ball Toss	H	H	H	H
Bean Bag Toss	H	H	H	H
Bowling	H	H	L	H
Bus Outings	H/L	L	H/L	L
Dancing	H	H	H	L
Discovery Kits	L	H	H	H
Entertainment	H/L	L	H	H
Exercise	H	L	L	H
Five-Card Bingo	L	L	L	H
Gardening	H	L	H	H
Group Talks	L	H	H	H
Happy Hour	L	H	L	H
Ice Cream Making	H/L	H	H	H
Intergenerational	L	H	H	H
Manicures	L	H	H	H
Pet Visitations	L	H	H	L
Putting	H	H	H	H
Puzzles	L	L	L	H
Reminiscing	L	H	H	H
Social Tea	L	H/L	H	H
Stamp Pad Club	H/L	H	L	H
Theme Parties	H/L	H	H	L
Walking	H	H	H	L
Word Games	L	H	H/L	H

KEY
H = high; L = low; H/L = depends on an individual's functional abilities and level of participation in the activity

Physical

Involving gross motor movement, the physical domain focuses on activities or tasks of a physical nature. Some fine motor involvement is present in most tasks and may be a primary focus for certain activity. Physical activities promote restoration, maintenance, and/or increase of overall physical strength and endurance.

Social

Social interaction involves both verbal and nonverbal communication within a group. Quality and types of interactions vary depending on group size, environmental elements, and program goals. Social interaction promotes self-expression, self-esteem, and self-confidence. It offers an opportunity to build community and general familiarity.

Emotional

As emotions range so do opportunities to evoke or to stimulate them. Expression of emotion is a valuable means of addressing needs, pain, and individuality. Facilitating appropriate expression of emotion is a challenge in special care due to the nature of the disease process; however, we can adapt the situation to meet the emotional needs of the individual through Needs Response.

Cognitive

The individual's level of cognition affects all of the previous domains. The following cognitive elements influence complex skills and behavior: attention, concentration, orientation, recent and remote memory capacity, praxis (movement), language (expressive and receptive communication), and visual/spatial skills. We often refer to this domain as intellectual. For the purposes of the programs outlined and the complexity of the disease process, cognition was chosen to increase skill emphasis instead of knowledge.

Spirituality

Spirituality is an essential part of human identity. You will immediately observe that the spiritual domain has been omitted from the programming lists. Often overlooked as an integral part of the makeup of individuals living with dementia, describing spirituality is essential to ensure a basic understanding.

The human spirit is not a domain easily measured, or for that matter, agreed on. Within the world of dementia care, spirituality becomes all the more essential to identify. The human spirit evolves throughout our lives. It is all that makes us loving and brings us to love. This is the one part of our humanness that cannot be touched or stolen by the disease of dementia. There is no lobe in the brain identified as the spiritual lobe or source of spirituality or humanness. We see the truth in this statement through the expression of humor and empathy by our residents at different stages of the disease, often when we least expect it.

The only limitations of the spirit are those imposed by observers or caregivers. See not the disease but the spirit of the individual and you will know the identity trapped therein. This further validates the magic of dementia care. So often we are blessed with surprises—a thought, a word, a look, a smile, or a gentle touch coming from one thought to be incapable. Nothing can erase the spirit of a person—only those who choose to disregard the humanness and spiritual context of a person experience that erasure by their own doing.

A spiritual component encompasses all caring relationships. Therefore, spirituality is identified in each program through the stories and experiences of residents and caregivers. The spiritual domain is the magical self that generates and sustains the life force in each of us.

Off-Unit Program Criteria and General Programming Guidelines

Candid Resident Words
I'm not sure, but, I think the reason I'm here is because I don't think!?

Program success is based in our ability to ensure several things:

- preservation of dignity
- orientation to successful outcomes
- presence of choice
- dignity of risk (respecting ability)
- appropriateness of program or intervention

Through careful thought, knowledge of participants, and anticipation of potential outcomes we mindfully present residents with the most suitable environment to meet their needs. In this process of integration, the more special care residents interact with general resident population—under the support and guidance of the recreation worker—the more they have developed support skills. It is amazing how quickly they come to empathize, support, and protect the interests and welfare of their less fortunate peers. We can truly be proud of this mechanism of support (Dunne, 1999, pp. 187–192).

- Bonnie spends her days on the unit because that is where she chooses to be. Staff respect her choice not to leave her comfort zone.

- Sam prefers to be alone. When most residents are off unit enjoying a general program Sam walks the halls enjoying the peace and quiet.

- Nan also prefers to be alone. She enjoys playing her own version of solitaire privately in her room.

These are a few examples of the individual need, in spite of dementia, for quiet and privacy. One need not always be busy keeping up with the Joneses. Every program is not for everyone. This is the value and rationale of appropriate assessment. We must seek to know our clients and their needs. We strive to provide opportunities for success, interaction, self-expression, and satisfaction. Sometimes a program just doesn't cut it. Sometimes we serve our clients better by respecting his or her decision not to participate and ensuring he or she is not presented with a situation outside the realm of comfort, need, or ability to succeed.

Meeting Needs Prior to Programming

Betty worries about her unpaid bills, Conrad wants to return to Ireland, and Alice doesn't want to leave her room. Once we determine the context of the worry (the first time is always the longest time spent deciphering), the next step is a breeze. After determining the source of worry, we can anticipate the need and our ability to respond promptly to decrease anxiety. Over time the period spent addressing needs and concerns diminishes and the opportunity to initiate the program is increased. Of course, it is also important to recognize that we cannot meet all needs all the time. Sometimes we must let them go: "I wish I could help, but I just don't know what to do for you."

Frequently the result of such empathy and gentle attention is unexpected success through distraction. Alternatively, the fact that we are puzzled and troubled at the other's worry can frequently net genuine empathy in return and change the focus. One student's goal was "to answer the resident's questions." Time quickly adapted this magnanimous goal to her revised purpose: to empathize and validate residents as they expressed their worries and needs. This goal is much better—less stress, greater success.

In the Part 6 (p. 161) you will find program content lists with the letters GP after the program title. This will refer to programs held off the special care (dementia) unit. These are programs offered for residents neither residing in nor requiring special care support. Therefore, the criterion are a valuable resource to help programmers determine the appropriateness of individual participation in these programs. Where possible, individuals should not be cut off from others. Carefully facilitated integration can help to support and individual's maintenance of social and other skills. The goal is to ensure we can provide a supportive environment by which individuals can maintain their identity, self-esteem, and life skills for as long into the disease process as possible.

Use the criteria previously described to determine and support participation for residents in programs appropriate to their individual needs. Adapt according to your own needs and add quick thoughts or statements made by residents (recognizing confidentiality, of course). These statements, as you will read in examples throughout the book, are precious eye-opening words that really tell us how we are doing as caregivers…don't let them slip away. Jot them down as a reminder of whom we serve, and how they witness the experience.

PART 5

MEETING THE CHALLENGE

Real, Honest, and True

Studies in Care

In her inspirational and thought-provoking classic story *The Velveteen Rabbit*, Margery Williams offers children and adults a vision into the truest spirit of humanity. Between the wise Skin Horse and the worse-for-wear Velveteen Rabbit an inspirational discussion ensues prompting one to challenge one's whole value system. The conversation inspires us to view the torn ears, splitting seams, bald patches and unappealing stains as elements of experience and wisdom. The scenario presents itself much like those folks who have, for better or for worse, survived the ravages of time. We see and honor the elements of experience and wisdom in the scars and trials of their unique lives as we endeavor to support their daily efforts just to go on.

> "What is Real?" asked the Rabbit one day, when they were lying side by side near the nursery fender, before Nana came to tidy the room. "Does it mean having things that buzz inside you and a stick-out handle?"
>
> "Real isn't how you are made," said the Skin Horse. "It's a thing that happens to you. When a child loves you for a long, long time, not just to play with, but really loves you, then you become Real."
>
> "Does it hurt?" asked the Rabbit.
>
> "Sometimes," said the Skin Horse, for he was always truthful. "When you are Real you don't mind being hurt."
>
> "Does it happen all at once, like being wound up," he asked, "or bit by bit?"
>
> "It doesn't happen all at once," said the Skin Horse. "You become. It takes a long time. That's why it doesn't often happen to people who break easily, or have sharp edges, or who have to be carefully kept. Generally, by the time you are Real, most of your hair has been loved off, and your eyes drop out and you get loose in the joints and very shabby. But these things don't matter at all, because once you are Real you can't be ugly, except to people who don't understand."
> (Williams, 1983, pp. 3–5)

The key point in this expression of love and insight is the honesty and truth surrounding the last line "…once you are Real you can't be ugly, except to people who don't understand." This is the calling we accept: to see beyond the disease, to see the Real person within, to acknowledge the struggle, and to move forward with love. This is all that is real, honest, and true for the professional caregiver, family, friend, and each individual with special care needs. As you read the following two sections, you will see and feel the understanding in the journal of a loved one. Here is the story of Daniel, one individual made Real.

Daniel's Journey

Journal Entries of a Loved One

> *"I hate the word 'funeral,'" he said.*
> *"What do you prefer?" I asked curious.*
> *There was a pause and he said, "Nothing."*
> *"How about 'peaceful good-bye'?" I posed to him.*
> *He responded, "Yes, that's perfect, peaceful good-bye.*
> *She would like that."*

Journal Entry: Winter 1996
"What the hell are you doing?" Daniel raised his voice as the church fell silent. Embarrassed, I thought: good question! After all, everyone in the church had just stood up to participate in the next phase of the liturgy. Why would I be stopping Daniel from standing…only to protect him from tumbling forward over the foot plates of his wheelchair? Yes, it was important to stand now. However, he had forgotten he was now sitting in a wheelchair. His frustration out, he promptly returned his attention to the priest offering the Mass of Christian Burial …it was his sister's funeral.

∞   ∞   ∞   ∞   ∞

I was on the telephone, very tense, the shock of her death —so sudden and unexpected— had us all reeling, still. "That is fine, you break the news to Daniel. Ok. Now, I certainly hope you plan to offer him the choice to attend her funeral?" This was met with great hesitation. I could see the person at the other end of the phone. Certainly he sat shaking his head. Determined, I carried on. "He is clearly capable of making this choice. Daniel knows what he wants to do and what he needs. He simply needs to be given the opportunity to make the decision."

∞   ∞   ∞   ∞   ∞

Quietly they gathered, three of them as brothers."Danny we have sad news for you," said one. "Our sister, Frances, has died suddenly." Silence befell the trio of men. They waited for a response. Did he hear them? Did he understand the news? Did he care what was going on or even know who they were?

Yes. As any would respond he felt the grief and shock silently hearing it over and over again in his head. Said the other, "Do you want to go to her funeral, Daniel?"

Their hearts skipped a beat, startled by the strength and determination in his voice as he responded abruptly, "Of course I am going to the funeral," as if to say: Don't be stupid; she was my baby sister!

∞   ∞   ∞   ∞   ∞

Daniel stood in the corner of the elevator as we rode down to the car. Now that we were in privacy and away from the noise of the 40-plus bed special care unit, I offered my condolences: "I am so sorry about Frances, Daniel."

He looked at me and said, "It was a stunner. A real stunner."

The conversations in the car as we drove to the church were humorous, reflective, honest, and eye opening. Daniel quoted himself as a boy, as was handwritten in a leather bound dictionary he had made in school, "Too clever a man for ordinary people to understand." He laughed out loud, proud of his ability to fool folks…something he had done so well over the years. He spoke of how close he and Frances had been. Sure, we all knew how these two unmarried siblings, living in close proximity of Vancouver's West End for over twenty years, had fought, teased and joked with each other over the phone and in person every day all this time. Did we know how close they really were? No. His sadness today told the story in volumes however. An expression of emotion, even in his few words, subsequent head shaking and quiet reflection, so overpowering was this it is difficult to capture on paper. This man, this forgetful, "aggressive," confused man knew exactly what he was experiencing. He knew his loss and reflected deeply on their life together — now over. He was neither forgetful nor aggressive. Confused? Perhaps only in the furiously human inclination of grief as we question God's hand in such a theft. His sister was gone. Any confusion would be normal. However, none was apparent. He sat quietly as the long drive rolled by. He asked questions: Who will be there? What parish is it? How are various family members? Every question accurate and clear. He grieved his losses, not only his sister but also his capacity to verbalize and communicate clearly. "I can't find some words," he said with resignation mixed with anger, even struggling to get this message out. I helped and he thanked me. It seemed that he was grateful someone had the time to understand.

I counted. Including the brief church episode, only three times over the four hours I was with him that day—only three times—he lost his focus.

"What are they doing over there?" he asked, laughing at the strange group of people standing quietly around the casket as final prayers were offered at the cemetery. Every moment was clear. Each loss of focus could be explained: out of auditory range, facing perpendicular to the group (out to the grounds of the cemetery instead of toward the service, due to seating), he could neither hear nor see what was going on at the moment. He had made the choice to attend the burial. He knew as we followed immediately behind the black hearse where we were going. He asked questions to clarify.

Daniel lost focus again as he observed the beautiful greenery around him. "Do you take care of the grounds here or do you have someone come in and do it?" Perhaps he hadn't lost focus! Perhaps he was simply addressing the wrong person! He was content to continue his observations and needed no response. I continued with the prayers. He was content to look around. Afterwards, he expressed his pleasure in having attended the interment at the cemetery. He joked about his nephews—too many to know who was who. He looked at the picture of his sister in the memorial card. "She always had a giggle on her face. This is her. That smile is her," he said staring intently inspecting the picture just as I had done the evening before. I knew and felt, I believed, exactly as he did at this moment.

Daniel had experienced a great loss. This was truly evident in his reflections as we drove from care home to church to cemetery to reception. It was a long and exhausting day, but it was necessary. Daniel needed the closure. Daniel was grateful for the closure. Daniel said good-bye to his sister—with the love of a devoted big brother.

The Visit

A Quiet, Rich Exchange between Loving Family

The phone rang and Jackie said "Sheila, the baby, and I are going to visit Daniel. We are coming after lunch. Is that okay? I know it may not be the best time of day but that's the only time we can make it." She continued on by asking some very important questions. Questions which would not only affect Daniel during and after their visit, but also her own and Sheila's comfort and enjoyment while visiting with their uncle.

"Where should we visit? What do we say? What do we do?" she asked patiently. The answers were easy, the challenge was hers.

"Turn the visit over to Daniel," I suggested. "He may wish to visit in a large common area. Try walking with him to a quiet area where there is less environmental stimulation. Perhaps take him to his room to visit quietly.

"Before determining where to visit, you might want to avoid the infamous 'quiz.' We never want to present a situation where he is bombarded with questions, or thinks he's being tested. He would enjoy being put on the spot and drilled just as much as you would, kid," I told her with a hint of sarcasm.

"Introduce yourself completely. Never assume Daniel will remember your name or identity. He *may* very well remember, but why risk putting him in the potentially embarrassing position of asking," I continued. "Further, it may also be confusing to him to attempt to identify his 'mystery guests'—and that's not fair. Try a complete introduction like: 'Hello Daniel, I'm your niece, Jackie, your brother Patrick's daughter.' In doing this you have created two links to his long-term memory. You may need to mention your identity several times over the course of the visit, but really, that is *not* a problem.

"Generally, the problem is *our own discomfort* with repetition or lack of recognition. These are unfortunate realities but the key word is *reality*. In the course of the visit remind yourselves why you are there. Is it for your own benefit or for the benefit of Daniel? Assuming that the intention is to benefit Daniel, your whole focus will shift.

"Trust yourself, Jackie—you will be fine," I assured her, "And so will Daniel."

∞   ∞   ∞   ∞   ∞

Jackie, Sheila, and baby Grace arrive to visit Daniel. Daniel has decided he's had enough of the noise and "those people." The four of them walk back to his room. All the way along Jackie and Sheila listen patiently to his stories of what is going on in "this place" where he lives. It makes little sense to them. Out of respect, they listen. Periodically they agree with him, clarify, paraphrase.

Daniel hears Jackie incorrectly, and the story takes another turn. She tries to clarify by repeating what she said again. It doesn't work. Once everyone is in his room, he shows them around and offers them a gift. It is a library book belonging to the care home. They accept it graciously. Rather than trying to correct him, they plan to drop it off at the nursing station on their way out. They succeed in preserving his dignity.

Daniel asks about the baby. He knows how old she is and that she is Jackie's child. He can't recall the relationship exactly, but he is recalling accurate details of having met the baby at his sister's birthday party a year ago. His mixed memory is confusing them. He asks who this other person is.

"This is Patrick's daughter, Sheila," Jackie replies. He thinks of his sister Sheila, but corrects himself after a moment of thought. He compliments

Sheila on how well she looks and then begins to crack a couple of jokes about their family. His humor shines through the tarnish of all his losses.

Jackie isn't sure what to do next. She looks around the room, and spots his life book. Aha! It is a beautiful compilation of pictures (originals and copies, including enlargements for ease of visibility) created with love by his sister-in-law. Jackie and Sheila sit down beside him while Grace explores his room. They ask if he would like to look at it with them. Daniel, being polite and equally eager to have something to do with his guests, agrees.

Page by page they reminisce together. Grace joins them and helps turn pages. One at a time they take turns pointing to a picture and describing who is in it. Daniel nods, acknowledging the scene. Sometimes he recalls a detail they know or don't know. Other times he just nods. Once in awhile they find he isn't connecting with what is going on around him.

"Are you tired Daniel?" Jackie asks. Daniel shakes his head no. The visit continues for 20 or 30 minutes, maybe less. Jackie and Sheila begin to realize how exhausting it is to try to support and guide him through a visit. Thank goodness for the young grandniece who breaks the moments with her curiosity and vitality.

After Shelia cues some stories that she knows he enjoys telling and tells well, Jackie suggests that everyone is tired.

Perhaps it is time to say good-bye, she thinks. Now what? A touch of panic and guilt sets in. When we leave, what will he do? Jackie recalls the phone conversation:

"Don't you worry about leaving. The truth is that Daniel spends the better part of each day with few family around him. This is not to say he is neglected. He is in the competent care of those with whom the family has placed their trust. The key to your departure is to avoid creating a sense of abandonment. It is overwhelmingly disorientating and frustrating. Finding something interesting and enjoyable for Daniel to do as you say your farewells is the most effective means to a temporary end. Even though it may seem deceptive, *not* saying good-bye is gentler. 'I'll be back' may communicate the same idea without communicating the finality of a 'good-bye.'

"By doing this, you accomplish three valuable things. First, you provide Daniel with something purposeful and meaningful to do for the time being. Second, you provide yourself with a comfortable, quiet, guilt-free and stress-free departure. Third, by making this effort you create an environment that is less volatile for the staff. Often when families come and go, it is literally a coming and going. Good-bye is so final and disturbing that it triggers a range of emotions and situations with which the staff and residents must attempt to cope.

"Build a farewell into the visit. For example, if twenty minutes is a pleasurable experience for everyone visiting, then divide that time to allow for a successful closure. It's to everyone's advantage. A ten to fifteen minute visit benefits from a five to ten minute 'settling up.' This is the time to get comfortable with the departure. It's time to say 'I'll be back' instead of 'good-bye.' As a result it avoids creating a sense of abandonment."

Jackie, Sheila, and Grace walk Daniel back to the lounge. A picture book of Royals sits on a side table. Together they make themselves comfortable and begin to look through the book. Daniel enjoys reflecting on the history of the Monarchy and his interest and expression become more focused. Grace begins to fidget with her own need to explore. Sheila gets up while saying that she and the baby will be back shortly. Once they have left, Jackie mentions what a lovely visit she's had with him. He agrees, "We should go out to lunch together sometime."

Jackie nods in agreement, "It might be a good idea to wait until the weather improves though." Daniel agrees.

After a few more minutes pass Jackie excuses herself. Daniel acknowledges her polite request, and returns his focus to the book.

∞   ∞   ∞   ∞   ∞

It is a funny thing rarely communicated to families. When one crosses the threshold and takes in that lungful of fresh air, it is hard to reflect back on the unit and what may be taking place. To be a fly on the wall, as it were, creates a whole new understanding. This not always being possible, let us then take the approach of a gentle, settled and quiet departure.

The polite nature of an individual may outshine us all. Daniel, Sheila, Jackie, and the baby had a lovely visit—a quiet, humor-filled, rich exchange between loving family members. Those nieces never had it so good! Forget all the losses he has experienced, the point is—Daniel is some guy.

Rules of the Game

Rules were made to be broken... that is part of their fun! However, the most essential rule is this: Do unto others as you would have done unto yourself.

The First Rule

There are no rules. Actually, for anyone seeking some summary solutions without delving through the entire text: This is your chapter! Read on and find the right information to share with concerned and active family members. These pointers may go a long way in reducing distress and enhancing celebrations.

The Magic Answer

We are always searching for the magic answer, the rulebook, the best way to avoid conflict and to be healthy or happy. We look for the fastest and shortest line at the grocery store or the fastest route to the nearest drive-thru. The truth is never what we *want* to hear. The truth is that there is no magic answer.

So now that we have got that out of the way the pressure is off and you can kick back and take it easy! What's that you say? You still don't know what to do when interacting or visiting with someone experiencing the losses of dementia? You feel uncomfortable and guilty? Aha! Isn't it true that when we think we are doing something for someone else it often has a hidden agenda: A little feel good action or attending to a sense of obligation or guilt exists for ourselves. Well, the fact that you are reading this book or even this chapter suggests this is not your agenda. You want to do the best you can for someone who has done and would continue to do the same for you except for a nasty turn of events.

Much like in "The Visit" the quality of the journey you embark on with each visit is up to you. Rather than a set of rules (Why attach more guilt to an already weighty situation?) I offer you a set of guidelines to which you may refer. This book has been full of suggestions, but here are some more specific summary suggestions to assist the process for you:

- Be sure to incorporate greeting and good-bye ("I'll be back") time into your visit by breaking it down: *n* amount of time to reacquaint and settle, *n* amount of time to visit and *n* amount of time to settle the person into another task before you make your quiet exit. (Don't make a scene about saying good-bye.)

- Make use of tools/props available, such as discovery or life kits.

- Create a personalized kit for the visit. Remember the benefit gained is not only intended for the individual who is being visited but also for the visitor. After all, the quality of the visit impacts both in very different ways.

- Find out what time of day is best or worst for you to visit or spend time with the person. For example, right after lunch people tend to be more exhausted from the degree of concentration required to eat in such a stimulating environment; this may not be a time to ask for someone's attention and expect recognition or success.

- Time your visits with the programs a facility offers. (Check with the recreation worker as to which programs are suitable and success-oriented for the person before diving in.) If the individual enjoys and succeeds in the social and recreational programs offered, it may be beneficial to visit and interact during program times.

- It is wise to communicate with the program leader to understand the goals of the program, skills of the person with whom you are visiting, and how you can be of help. In taking this proactive role you are helping not only the individual you are visiting, but also yourself, the program leader, and the other participants. There are many benefits to this approach, including enhanced quality of visits, insight into the interests and abilities of the individual, and reduced guilt or discomfort when visiting. Although it may take a couple of tries for you to gain personal comfort and security in the program situation, you may be greatly surprised and pleased with the outcome.

Remember the value, role, and importance of *choice* and *decision making* for the individual. It is true that cognitive skills in this area are lost over time. However, we can present situations and decisions in such a way that the person is treated with respect and valued through the presentation of options. This relates directly to seeking permission from the individual rather than bulldozing ahead and telling the person what is going on without involving him or her in the process. Remember and use the steps of the Connection Continuum (p. 98) to enhance your success. We may already have a pretty good idea of what the outcome is going to be, but there is absolutely no reason (except perhaps safety) that we cannot involve the individual in the process. The bottom line here is to keep in mind the losses mounting for the person we are supporting. By providing outlets for self-expression or decision making, we reduce our contributions to a build-up of stress waiting to blow. In doing so, we create a greater chance for success.

Discovering Humanness

> Two roads diverged in a wood
> And I, I took the one less traveled by
> —*Robert Frost*

Throughout the process of providing care, support, and love to those living with the losses experienced through dementia, there is one factor still to be recognized: remembering the humanness of the person.

The greatest challenge of professional caregiving is preventing oneself from becoming overwhelmed and controlled by a task orientation. When caught up in such a way of thinking we cease to recognize the human element in our provision of care. No meeting, no break, no wall, no floor, and no bed is more important than a moment, however brief, of recognition and acknowledgment. A moment of caring communication—until we can console, answer, or support whatever need is being expressed—can prevent catastrophic outcomes.

Yet to accomplish this we must be willing to be present for and aware of the people to whom we provide care. We and they are one in the same: humans with emotional, social, physical and spiritual needs. We are still one as we consider our differences—nearsightedness, the desire to sit and rest, confusion, anger, fear, hunger, thirst, forgetfulness, frustration. We remain one and the same in that our needs may vary but we still seek to be safe, happy, healthy, loved, and reassured.

Healthcare promotes a natural task orientation. We perpetuate this task orientation by a task-oriented language. Previously we discussed the language of meal support: "feeder" versus "he or she needs assistance." One word suggests action or task while the other *recognizes a human need*: "I'm going to 'do' Mr. Willy" versus "I'll be helping Mr. Willy get ready now." These follow the same distancing and impersonal orientations of *action/task versus supporting a human need*. "John needs to be toileted" versus "Could you help John use the toilet?" or "John needs to freshen up," or whatever suitable wording we choose. Neither is English as a second language an excuse for such poor communication. The effort must be present on the part of the entire team to ensure a common respectful language is in place to protect the dignity of our employers: the residents. This type of language is a pervasive plague promoted throughout healthcare and the educational system. It is one of a medically focused, task-oriented origin that tramples humanness. It is time for this to change.

The difference we seek to promote is one of *changing our language* to be not only age appropriate but also *person* or *human needs oriented* rather than *task oriented,* which has the unpleasant potential to be dehumanizing.

Discovering humanness relies on us to promote the recognition of the person within their surviving capacity. Having got to know the individual through other means of assessment and interactions, we now seek to enable folks by encouraging their self-expression. We remember that these people are doing the best they can with what they have in terms of brain function. When we seek to provide a consistent, loving, and supportive environment, it seems that this is what we experience in return. This is a reflection of Secret #4: We receive what we give. The following story is a wonderful example of the benefits of Secret #4.

∞   ∞   ∞   ∞   ∞

Brenda, the recreation worker, arrived for a busy day to find the ladies wandering without purpose. Upon seeing and recognizing this friendly face, the ladies one by one came to greet their familiar friend. Together they walked to the dining room. Brenda sat as the ladies joined her.

She began to tell them of the weather she encountered on her way to work that day. The ladies marveled at her story with supportive words of awe and appreciation. One woman stood rubbing her back, while another stroked her hair as she listened. Still another woman laughed at this delightful story and her tablemate sat listening and watching attentively.

From a distance this happy group seemed like a reunion of girlfriends from days gone by or neighbors gathered to gossip and share while a favorite pie baked in the oven. Upon a closer look and listen, it was a different scene. Brenda told the story of snow in her neighborhood as she marveled at the beautiful sunny day before the group. As the ladies touched and listened to this familiar and soothing voice, no one was rushed and everyone was equal. No one spoke cohesively and coherent thoughts were far from evident.

It was a time of warmth, love, and community. A moment of being one, together, with no consideration for the disease they shared in common. Brenda participated by supporting them and they existed peacefully in the moment. A connection took place. Not only did they share their humanness, but also they contributed joyfully to sharing the magic.

Journey's End

In the end is my beginning.

—Mary, Queen of Scots

I hope you have enjoyed this journey as much as I have taken pleasure in relating it to you. It is my hope that you have experienced both familiarity and kinship as well as a few "aha" moments.

Dementia care truly is an adventure. My fondest hope for you as you embark or continue on your journey in the world of dementia care is that you will find new challenges daily and that each will be filled with discovery.

Intuition may make a difference for some, while others supplement with education. Training serves to further enhance and create understanding of care. With a commitment to ongoing learning, each will make an equally valuable impact on the lives of those living with dementia. It is a commitment of the heart not only to preserve the dignity of the person but also to encourage residents to continue to celebrate themselves (and their identities) long into the onset and thievery of dementia. Dementia care requires an ethical commitment to promote dignity, relationships, and communication. It demands that caregivers listen to feelings, support retained abilities, and encourage independence for as long as possible. In this we succeed at recognizing the person with total respect and dignity. Dr. Tom Kitwood suggested that

> The best dementia care is, paradoxically, a paradigm for human life. The excellent caregiver is, so to speak, a moral artist, and sets an example to all of us as we search for the right and the good. (1998, p. 34)

Seek out every opportunity for celebration. Take the road less traveled, have an adventure, step up to the challenge of genuine care, and have a joyful journey in every reality you explore. Now as your reading comes to an end, your caregiving journey embarks on a new beginning. Bon voyage!

PART 6

A TO Z:
PROGRAMS, STORIES, AND
CONTENT

Read on for a selection of programs, stories, and content that can guide anyone from novice to expert, recreation therapists and other care staff to home care workers through a valuable program or interactive exchange.

Candid Resident Words

When invited to participate, a former teacher stated:
  "No, I don't care for your technique. It's obvious that the children do, that's the main thing."

"You're not supposed to be understandable because you are an old buck.

"You just take everything they shove to you."

"I've decided I'm going to grow old—but I'm not going to grow up!"

Armchair Travel

Imagine starting a new job where the schedule is not entirely clear. Well that is how this armchair travel program came to be. A recreation worker misread the calendar and thought the program was for the special care unit when in fact it was a movie program for the general population. Finding no session plan she urged on her creative self. Gathering a bundle of postcards and magazines, she sat down with a small group of residents, opened her travel agency, and the journeys began. It's just that easy.

∞   ∞   ∞   ∞   ∞

It was a beautiful day to travel as we set upon our journey. Destination: London.

With preparations under way, we set out for jolly old England and talked of our method of travel. Which would be better: a quick flight or a relaxing journey by boat? In the interest of time, we opted to fly. Upon arriving we discussed our tour plans. Where will we go? We scanned the tourist brochures and made a plan for exciting visits to Buckingham Palace, Big Ben, Piccadilly Square (the most popular choice, with by far the most colorful postcards). Though a bit out of our way, we next journeyed to Stonehenge.

It was about this time that Doris' daughter entered the room. She sat quietly enjoying our travel with us. Stories flowed as each participant acknowledged their experiences in one way or another—a nod or a story kept this lively trip moving. Teatime was announced and we came in for a happy landing.

The next day Doris' daughter returned. She had so enjoyed our trip abroad that she returned with the hopes that we would consider a trip around our beautiful province of British Columbia. With lovely picture books in hand she turned them over to us wishing the group a bon voyage…she told us to watch out for stowaways, as her heart was ready to travel, too!

∞   ∞   ∞   ∞   ∞

Great adaptations are always possible. Pictures are marvelous cues. Consider the likes and personal histories of participants. Perhaps the Italian resident would enjoy a postcard of the Leaning Tower of Pisa? That lovely Irish poet is always eager to travel home to the Irish countryside. Max has always enjoyed life on the water, so his eyes always go to the boats first. For those folks who find difficulty following the conversation, picture matching can take them on joyful journeys. Take the pile of postcards from your journey to Holland and encourage them to match the windmill pictures all shapes and sizes. Everyone can be a part of these satisfying journeys.

Life kits and other carefully prepared albums or collections can have a lasting impact. One resident's family remembered their mother's travels to

Arizona. They lovingly created a beautiful album containing the old 15¢ travel books filled with rich color pictures and details of the area.

Although this lovely woman has since died, her memory lives on in this beautiful book enjoyed and shared by others. What a great way to involve everyone...collections of postcards clutter everyone's drawers. A good cleaning goes a long way, not to mention it does a good turn as well. Losing postcards to hoarding residents isn't all that bad when we have a regular source of family, staff, volunteers, and friends who can contribute to a most worthy cause.

Never let yourself be stopped for lack of a concrete plan. This is why we were born with our imaginations and creative selves. Celebrate your creativity at every turn. You may end up hearing this resident's wonderful response: "Hey! I've been there before!"

Program Content for Armchair Travel

Participants
GDS Rating: Levels 3–6

    Target: Verbal, high-functioning individuals able to communicate stories of past travel

    Others: Those who might enjoy listening or viewing sample postcards, brochures, pictures, and souvenirs

Equipment
Postcards, travel brochures, travel documents (e.g., passports), pictures, souvenirs; food or beverages relevant to a destination

Social Domain
Everyone loves to share his or her stories of travel and familiar experiences; can be very exciting

Emotional Domain
Self-expression; sharing; validation by others

Physical Domain
None

Cognitive Domain
Stimulating the memory; cueing stories; focusing; attending; responding

Strengths
Promotes self-esteem; most folks have traveled in their lifetime so this program is far-reaching in the number of participants it can potentially touch

Challenges
Getting participants to return postcards; retrieving items from participants with hoarding behaviors

Adaptations/Special Considerations
Carefully select items to be given to residents who hoard so potential loss is not too great (a good staff stress reducer, too!). Monitor safety concerns with souvenirs—sharp, breakable, or toxic items should be omitted or used with supervision only.

Notes/Ideas:

Arts and Crafts

Candid Resident Words
A resident reflects on the successful completion of a
group craft project:
"See how clever we are... and we were so dumb at first!"

A resident sorts through donated gift cards for a craft
project and comments:
"I like these cards, but they keep on getting my name
wrong."

From the sublime to the ridiculous—this is the range of potential craft projects to consider for dementia care. Safety precautions for scissors and other sharp objects, toxic materials, and potential for ingestion are just some of the things we worry about as we set out to create a craft program.

Most concerns require a common sense approach. When reviewing a list of supplies, ask yourself: What could possibly go wrong with this item? Is there a potential for danger if I am suddenly called out of the room or distracted? How would we plan around essential supplies like scissors? (Keep them with you always and store under lock and key.) Sessions which raise concerns should have adequate volunteer support even if the primary responsibility is monitoring equipment and supplies.

Need a list of quick craft projects? Bingo markers as paint pens to dab color on artwork. Watercolors to paint the monthly calendar (theme colors like green for March) before writing out the activities. Photocopy symmetrical line drawings (e.g., flowers, hearts, butterflies, shamrocks), sponge paint, fold, dry, and cut out shape to adorn bulletin boards. Yes, these activities have been used for children, but the approach used and goals following completion influence whether it is appropriate or not. Each of these listed crafts is manageable for all skill levels if interest prevails. Two dabs or twenty—it doesn't matter if the person is actively participating in the process. Some folks coach, others stabilize work, still others observe and compliment their peers. Cleaners are part of the process and can be one of your biggest assets.

Program Content for Arts and Crafts

Participants
GDS Rating: Levels 3–5
   Target: Craft specific; a core group will often be at hand

Equipment
As required

Social Domain
Supportive, assistive (one holds, the other ties, paints) and interactive

Emotional Domain
Self-expression

Physical Domain
Manual dexterity: Fine motor skills, hand-eye coordination, skills specific to craft

Cognitive Domain
Selection of colors and tasks (choices); following instructions (one, two, or more steps as able)

Strengths
Choose items that may be completed in the designated time frame; truly success oriented

Challenges
Gluing the wrong side of an item…does it matter?

Adaptations/Special Considerations
Flexibility gets us through anything! Glue on the wrong side? Discreetly put the piece to the side and slip in a new one—tact is everything. Bingo markers are a super low budget way to go. There are water soluble, nontoxic "paint pens" on the market as well.

Notes/Ideas:

Baking

Candid Resident Words
A resident comments on an activity, as her turn to play
once again comes up:
"Oh, but I've never done that before!"

If the program plan calls for one person to mix the dry ingredients and one person to mix the liquid ingredients, then so it shall be. However, when the delightful little lady who had reverted to her language of birth no longer understood it was time to stop to avoid overmixing, what did the recreation worker and her industrious volunteers learn to do? Well, Margaret received her own bowl and her love of mixing continued. A bit of this, a bit of that… she mixed and mixed to her heart's content. All the while the rest of the gang produced their favorite: blueberry muffins. At the end of the session, Margaret sat both pleased and proud with the rest of the bakers as they sampled their tasty goods. Must have been in the mixing!

∞   ∞   ∞   ∞   ∞

Consider also the fruit salad. It may be hard for some to believe, but even the men will peel oranges and be part of the act. Those with fine motor skills cut apples, while others pull grapes from their bundles. Of course, quality control includes the tasters! It is particularly amazing that the quality control group, our lovely tasters, are the same folks who refuse to eat at meal times. Needless to say, there are many benefits to a program such as this.

Carrots. Not enough on the menu? Well, so said one resident. If nutrition services isn't readily able to oblige, don't worry. When this finicky eater complained of the lack of her favorite vegetable, a solution was found in a one-on-one cooking session. Together the recreation worker and the resident sat in the kitchen, resident peeling, recreation worker "visiting." This finicky woman got her carrots: she peeled, cleaned, and cooked them to her hearts content. Funny thing was that she had actually stopped eating sometime before. This was her first meal in a long time. This is an excellent example of successful Needs Response.

Let's not forget an apple exercise. Hand each able participant an apple and a paring knife (if safe) and watch what they do. Some take a bite and enjoy that apple—mmmn good! Others see how many different ways there are to peel an apple. What a great discussion comes of this little experiment.

Possibilities are endless as is the potential to link other programs. A healthy herb garden, both safe and edible, draws the gourmet group out for a harvest.

∞   ∞   ∞   ∞   ∞

Our multitalented baking gardeners spent an afternoon out in the sun pulling pieces off their plants. Rosemary, thyme, chives, sage, and oregano contributed to the cause. Inside again, the group prepared for a canning session. Bottles sat in the ready as the participants began to drop in their branches and leaves.

The magic of the moment came when they poured in the vinegar, which released the fragrant oils and memories in concert with them. Everyone came from all around and joined in the process as the canning came to a close. Baking is more than just a recipe book.

Program Content for Baking

Participants
GDS Rating: Levels 3–7
    Target: Anyone…especially those with noses

Equipment
As called for in recipes or spontaneous, creative plan

Social Domain
Sharing baking secrets; supporting and encouraging one another

Emotional Domain
Childhood or life memories cued by smells (olfactory stimulation); confidence enhancing

Physical Domain
Fine motor skills: Chopping, measuring, peeling, pulling, washing, and all the other relevant baking tasks (including licking spoons!)

Cognitive Domain
Sensory stimulation

Strengths
Versatility; seasonal flexibility (baking in winter, fruit or other salads in summer); able to meet individual needs

Challenges
Overmixing…we solved that one!
    Hygiene: Ensure hands are clean (a washing program prebaking); colds and other germs; monitor participant food handling
    Safety: Be mindful of sharp knives and who is using them. Be sure to key-lock or secure the oven; keep eyes on the oven while preheating, too

Adaptations/Special Considerations
Precut items if safety is a dominant issue due to any resident. Look for recipes that do not call for a Mixmaster or have a volunteer or leader do this type of mixing away from the group.

Notes/Ideas:

Ball Toss

"Give the ball to the turn-up man," she said.
"Who is the turn-up man?" Barb asked.
"You know, the one who always turns up!" She
chuckled at the joke she had just made.

Andrew wanders his path around the unit. Each time Andrew passes the lounge where the folks play ball toss he stops for a turn or two. Andrew is the turn-up man and he enjoys the game.

∞   ∞   ∞   ∞   ∞

Imagine a program that meets and challenges everyone's needs on one level or another while at the same time targeting all domains. This describes perhaps the ultimate dementia program experience.

This program offers the greatest opportunity for self-expression, communication, social interaction, supportive behaviors, physical activity, emotional satisfaction, creativity and countless other benefits. Everyone can be involved from active participation to observation and enjoyment.

Here is a quick list of different activities with which residents initiate or respond:

- the former soccer player who uses his head to butt the ball back to the group—delightfully self-expressive
- the woman who catches but cannot throw back
- the woman who holds her own small exercise plan of repetitive bouncing before passing it on to the next person
- the outside observer who watches carefully from beyond the circle and kindly gets up to retrieve the balls gone astray
- those who can't catch or throw, but they can sure kick!
- the woman who can catch the ball, but won't decide to whom she should pass it

∞   ∞   ∞   ∞   ∞

"Whom should I throw it to?" she says over and over, responding to the group leader.

"Throw it to me" the leader says.

"Why do you always get the ball?"

"Well then, throw it to Ellen," says the leader, "She has the blue sweater." Two things happen in this interaction. The holder is cued to throw to another participant, and the receiver is cued that the ball is on its way.

∞   ∞   ∞   ∞   ∞

Take the individual who relates the program to a previous life experience. For example, the woman who told her daughter she was back in school and the ball toss was an exercise program to strengthen her arms and wrists. "Yes, this was true," said the recreation worker to the daughter, "I did tell her how it would help her arms and wrists." She has made some connection to a past life experience and this is how the program remains with her.

Imagine the power of observation and discovery within such a program. Doris' ability to communicate verbally is long gone. However, her nonverbal communication speaks volumes. Each time the ball came to her she turned the ball so its "belly button" was precisely on top and then threw. Another resident shared this behavior. What did these two women have in common? The more easily observable of the two, Ellen, has the regular habit of cleaning the unit. A place for everything and everything in its place. We asked Doris's family if she had been an organized and neat woman throughout her life and received a positive response. We learned the truth through the power of observation.

Volunteers come in every shape and form. Resident volunteers are the crème de la crème. Imagine having an on-call volunteer present for virtually every program or intervention. Take Shirley, whose agility and awareness in spite of her resident status make her dream come true:

> It's ball toss time again and no one is around. Shirley and
> the recreation worker set up the room in ready for the game.
> The recreation worker begins to toss the ball back and forth
> with Shirley. All warmed up, Shirley takes over and passes the
> ball to folks as the recreation worker invites them into their
> seats. The game under way, the recreation worker supervises
> from the side as she cleans shelves and cheers participants
> on offering her guidance and support as necessary.

This program is a fill in. When all else fails, the ball toss can capture energy and bring together a community of folks who otherwise would be lost.

Program Content for Ball Toss

Participants
GDS Rating: Levels 3–6
  Target: All residents can participate if they choose to do so

Equipment
Circle of chairs or like situation; soft ball to be thrown or kicked (e.g., punch ball or sponge ball); extra ball

Social Domain
Give the sponge ball to a participant unable or unwilling to throw the ball once caught, he or she may spend a few minutes examining it and then move on. This allows for the experience of inclusion without extreme disruption.

Emotional Domain
An accidental hit to the face, head, or upper torso can be supported through gentle laughter to lighten the situation. Acknowledge the individual's momentary discomfort or startle with suitable concern. (*Caution:* Be aware of resident mood as this situation may backfire.)

Physical Domain
Individual needs are met through stretching, reaching, kicking, catching, throwing, and passing depending on flexibility, agility, balance, and fine and gross motor skills

Cognitive Domain
Attention; visual spatial skills; concentration

Strengths
An all-inclusive program that can be done anywhere and anytime. High or low energy depending on the facilitator's goals and approach. Brief or lengthy program depending on the intent, and resident mood or focus. Once started, it is a short time before the participants "take over" (peak response) and run the program. In time and with familiarity, little leadership is required to begin the program. A great fill-in program: minimal equipment needs and no prep time. Makes an excellent back up program (see The Connection Continuum, p. 98).

Challenges
Some seating arrangements may not facilitate the program well. Hoarding may be an issue, but hoarding problems (or "I own this ball") may be overcome through use of a backup ball, or by obtaining permission to use the ball from the "owner."

Adaptations/Special Considerations
Soft versus a hard ball; brightly colored for vision; one bounce of the ball allows enough time to cue some individuals to prepare to catch or anticipate the ball.

Notes/Ideas:

Bean Bag Toss

Candid Resident Words
"That's what happens to me sometimes, I just can't get started."

"Good heavens, I'm a winner!"

Of the bean bag toss, Shirley says in jest, "All we are doing is amusing ourselves with a bunch of holes." The group responds to this lighthearted observation with their own smiles and laughter. Style is of Olympic caliber for many in this group, yet remains noncompetitive. For example

- The British athlete whose sporting history allows him to stand way back and use a beautiful underhand to toss the bag straight into each hole.

- A frail woman surprises all with her powerful overhand, which has caused many a bag to be replaced for their ruptured sides.

- The shortest in the bunch slides forward on her chair as they call her up for her turn. She takes her walker and shuffles to four feet from the board. In position, she takes each bag by the very corner, swings it back and forth releasing it to land in the holes every time.

- Ellen has poor depth perception so her goal is not to throw— although she does—her goal is to retrieve. At close proximity she can hit or slide the bean bags into the holes. Whether the bags are on the floor or otherwise she follows directions to slowly retrieve each one. Literal instructions can slow the process, however. Cueing the round red hole with its color description allows Ellen to retrieve her bean bags. If all else fails a couple of taps on the edge of the red circle draws her attention to the location for pick up. A bag that has gone beyond the board (we would describe this as behind) causes her to turn around and look behind her own self for the missing bag. This is resolved by saying, "Turn around again, Ellen. Over here," and a visual cue by the leader guides her to success.

- One of the beauties of special care is the inclusion of anyone and everyone who passes by. Staff, families, and other passersby cannot escape without an invitation to try.

Program Content for Bean Bag Toss

Participants
GDS Rating: Levels 3–6

   Target: Ambulatory or in wheelchairs, limited to those whose comprehension of the task allows them to let go of the bean bag.

Equipment
Basket with 6 bean bags. A frame plywood board painted white, with five holes cut out with red painted circles (2" thickness) around each hole for definition. A portable board makes it easy to bring the board to a person in a wheelchair.

Social Domain
Encourage one another; discuss methods; cue each other

Emotional Domain
Self-expression; self-esteem; peer support; validation

Physical Domain
Balance is encouraged for those who can stand; hand–eye coordination; bending and lifting (retrieving bags). For those normally sedentary participants, simply the act of getting up from a chair is a significant and necessary pursuit.

Cognitive Domain
Concentration; attention; memory; visual spatial

Strengths
Noncompetitive (optional). The lack of a "throw line" allows participants the freedom to determine from where they throw, thus encouraging success.

Challenges
Monitoring individual balance and movement requires constant attention to ensure safety.

Adaptations/Special Considerations
Attach margarine containers to the back of each hole to enable residents to pick up their bean bags following the toss. *To attach containers:* Cut a hole in the lid and glue the rim to the container. The lid lip acts as stabilizer to support container. Affix a container behind each hole in the plywood board.

Notes/Ideas:

Bowling

An adapted program, this definitely requires volunteer support or an agile resident to help. There is much up and down for everyone involved. Assign different roles to different individuals based on skills and limitations (e.g., pin setter, ball catcher, cheerleader).

Program Content for Bowling

Participants

Global determination scale (handwritten)

GDS Rating: Levels 3–5
   Target: Physically agile, mobile individuals. Others as adaptive equipment is available.

Equipment
Bowling pins; carpet to define lanes; a barrier to create a contrasting backdrop to enhance visibility and to catch stray balls; safe balls for handling (sufficient weight to knock over pins)

Social Domain
Supporting and encouraging one another. A noncompetitive focus helps to build community just as in the ball or bean bag toss.

Emotional Domain
Satisfaction from success

Physical Domain
Balance; gross motor skills; assisting with the pin set up (if able); ball chasers; hand–eye coordination

Cognitive Domain
Concentration

Strengths
A win–win situation. Keep trying until success is achieved. There are no restrictions in a supportive environment like this.

Challenges
Safety concerns regarding balance. May require volunteer support to avoid exhausting oneself by chasing pins and balls if residents are unable to help.

Adaptations/Special Considerations
Explaining to some that the "little milk bottles" (wooden bowling pins) are not going to break. Change from a limited number of throws to the number required to be successful with at least one pin (the group will generally understand). If someone knocks out a head pin, a back pin may be brought forward to its place making success easier. Carnival pyramid-style stacking works well as skill levels decrease which allows one pin strike to take out all pins. (Much more exciting but a bit more work!) A ball ramp is an option for those in wheelchairs or those less steady on their feet.

Notes/Ideas:

Bus Outings (GP)

Candid Resident Words
On frequent visits to the toilet, one resident said:
    "Nature was very sloppy in calculating what our
needs would be."

Frankly, I don't recommend bus trips for late stage dementia clients. At least, choose them carefully. I will never forget the long-time argument I carried on with a very fine nurse. I was so stubborn. I look back with some shame today. Thank goodness (if I could attribute a reason for my ignorance) it was before the advent of "special care units."

The issue revolved around taking one woman—whose entire life mission was to get home to the farm—out with us on the bus. The museum and restaurant were pleasurable for her—it was the trip home that started the nightmare. She was so disoriented to time and place that for every intersection we crossed she wanted out at the "next stop." For the most part, I could console her on the ride back. Little did I know or, should I say, would I accept, that I was creating a time bomb. Upon our return and after bidding her good day at her room (which was in a permanent state of packed and ready to leave *now*) the trouble would start. You can use your imagination from there.

Our argument centered on the fact that "in the moment" she had a wonderful time. A former teacher, she would take pleasure in instructing or facilitating our adventures quite appropriately. This seemed a most important practice to promote. A wiser woman now, I realize that I can help her to do the same at home.

Certainly, restaurant outings can be helpful to promote nourishment in a normalized social environment. Overstimulation (not to mention disorientation) is a direct risk, however.

The trip to assess and to implement carefully is "the drive." Most everyone has taken a scenic drive around the city. Already disoriented, just think what sort of agitation and frustration we have the potential to create. A strong caveat is needed here.

Program Content for Bus Outings (GP)

Participants
GDS Rating: Levels 3–5
    Target: Varies depending on orientation

Equipment
Support supplies as required; transfer belts; medications; juices as appropriate to individual needs

Social Domain
Community integration; normalization

Emotional Domain
Can be overstimulating; memory-evoking; disorienting

Physical Domain
Select destinations suitable to the strengths, tolerances, and needs of residents; ambulating on/off buses safely

Cognitive Domain
Processing environmental stimuli

Strengths
Goal-oriented outings (e.g., farm, meal) can benefit participants on many levels. Opportunities for social cueing and normal interactions are presented with adequate support and understanding of individual needs.

Challenges
Overstimulation or disorientation in an environment away from the nurturing safety of home

Adaptations/Special Considerations
Very individual—mindfulness is required

Notes/ Ideas:

Dancing

"I can still dance!"

Such wonderful words to hear from someone whose insight tells her she has limitations in so many other areas! Her true joy shone through in these words.

It is such a pleasure to dance with someone whose children tell us (if that very individual hasn't already) that they met their spouse on the dance floor in New York during the War. A romantic image giving us deeper insight into that individual's life.

Dancing has meant so much to so many over the years. Styles have changed in both the music we dance to and the steps to which we slide, shuffle, and glide. Dancing is a great way to promote familiar physical activity among folks without going to a formal class.

People come alive when dancing. They show us completely different sides of their personality and identity. To enable our residents with dementia through movement and dance is for many a gift of love. For some, the steps may be gone, but the music moves hearts and moods in wonderful ways that even a simple shuffle may constitute a wonderful dance extravaganza.

Program Content for Dancing

Participants
GDS Rating: Levels 4–6
    Target: Anyone

Equipment
Suitable music (may consult a music therapist); CD or cassette player; safe space with places to rest; water or other refreshment for rehydration

Social Domain
Social interaction at its best! Staff with residents, residents with residents, family, volunteers

Emotional Domain
Memory-evoking music; self-expression

Physical Domain
Balance; gross motor movement; range of motion

Cognitive Domain
Concentration; memory (steps); coordination

Strengths
Energy-burning. Everyone can participate at their own level and follow their own rhythm from tapping and clapping to swinging and swaying.

Challenges
Overstimulation at the wrong time of day; overexertion; inappropriate choice of music may be disturbing

Adaptations/Special Considerations
Monitor for safety risks such as balance. Identify individuals becoming too enthusiastic or tired and therefore taking unnecessary risks. Redirect groups with more calming music, which might encourage seated movement to reduce stimulation and prepare to wind down program.

Notes/Ideas:

Discovery Kits

As explored previously in the text, this is a whole new ball of wax, string, tricks or whatever your chosen theme calls for. Reminiscing or discovery boxes have been around for awhile in various forms.

Program Content for Discovery Kits

Participants
GDS Rating: Levels 4–7
> *Target:* Anyone

Equipment
Name that theme and compile a kit. Suitable props combined together create a thought-provoking, multidimensional, interactive kit.

Social Domain
Opportunities for self-expression and demonstration either one-on-one or in small groups; promotes interaction depending on contents of the kit; shared experiences (Oh, the stories you will hear!)

Emotional Domain
Memory-evoking, reminiscing; sharing; supporting; verbal/nonverbal self-expression

Physical Domain
Skill demonstration of props

Cognitive Domain
Concentration; attention

Strengths
Cue and offer opportunities for recollection and demonstration of lifelong learning and skills or interests. No limits to themes or possibilities.

Challenges
Having sufficient kits to target a variety of interests and needs; keeping kits together

Adaptations/Special Considerations
Sturdy containers help to maintain kits (as opposed to cardboard or shoe boxes). Label items to recover from hoarders.

Notes/Ideas:

Entertainment (GP)

Candid Resident Words
"I wish I had some music. But you can't put it in there,"
said one resident, tapping her head, as she reflected
on the talent of an entertainer.
    Another resident observes a gifted piano student
and notes: "She's going to wear herself out!"

Such thoughts and observations are great gifts for us to experience, as residents choose to share their private thoughts and ideas out loud. Such wise observations of talent and effort. Oh, that we should be so innocently candid!

It is something we experience from our earliest years. For our residents it was often the family sharing music. Mother on the piano, brother playing the viola or saxophone, and sisters singing or playing the violin. Before television, times were simpler and talents were cherished and celebrated.

It is of great value to encourage and support the arts within the world of dementia. Not just in the form of music therapy (a program of such immense yet undervalued merit), but performance and expression through a variety of entertainers needs to be promoted. A touch of community brought to the care environment as the world reflects on the lives of our residents and their varied pasts. Tastes may vary and considerations must be given to degrees of ability and tolerance, but everyone enjoys music and other forms of entertainment in one way or another.

Program Content for Entertainment (GP)

Participants
GDS Rating: Levels 4–6
    Target: Residents able to participate off unit

Equipment
As required for the entertainer. Sound systems, however, are not recommended to prevent agitation and overstimulation.

Social Domain
Gathering together enhances sense of community; social interaction with peers

Emotional Domain
Memory-evoking

Physical Domain
Movement to music or participation (e.g., sing-a-longs)

Cognitive Domain
Attention; concentration

Strengths
Normalization: concert-like attendance is familiar and evokes socially appropriate behaviors.

Challenges
Inappropriate behaviors may be stimulated, such as clapping throughout program, or other distracting outbursts.

Adaptations/Special Considerations
Prepare entertainers for possible unsettling behaviors. Remember, join the residents' journey! Monitor stimulation levels and be prepared to taper the program: warm up, program, cool-down, end.

Notes/Ideas:

Exercises

Journal Entry: Spring
I agonized greatly over exercise programs. What was the perfect exercise routine for seniors, in chairs, with dementia, all at different physical and cognitive levels? What was the perfect music? Old, new, upbeat, slow, soft, rousing, or a mixture of these? I tried several routines. Every new student that came in tried their routine. Nothing seemed to translate well and keep the interest of the residents. The residents' physical and cognitive levels are constantly changing. No one routine seemed to work. Yet all the information I had read kept saying "repetition, repetition, repetition..." I wanted a one size fit all routine that I could use forever. I never found it. What was I thinking? After reviewing the programs offered our residents, I realize we do many physical exercises just through daily activities and regular programs.

∞   ∞   ∞   ∞   ∞

Evaluation of physical activities offered on a dementia unit, including programs such as walking, gardening, and ball toss, will give the programmer some direction. Activity analysis guides us through an assessment of domains, degree, and type of physical activity required to perform the task. Through this type of analysis, we can determine areas of need for dementia residents.

Movement and skill maintenance concerns can be addressed through various alternative activities instead of a designated exercise program. However, for some residents whose involvement is sketchy, specialized "movement to music" programs substitute (if by fancy name alone) for more structured exercise.

Program Content for Exercises

Participants
GDS Rating: Levels 4–5
Target: Limited to those who can copy or follow complex movements independently

Equipment
As preferred by facilitator for successful outcome of the program (e.g., music, scarves, chairs, balls, balloons)

Social Domain
Interaction with peers

Emotional Domain
Self-expression

Physical Domain
Balance; coordination; strength; resistance; cardio or simple relaxation

Cognitive Domain
Requires ability to follow cued or observed instruction and demonstration

Strengths
All the traditional benefits of physical activity, as outlined in the four domains above.

Challenges
Frustration by those unable to follow instructions or copy movements

Adaptations/Special Considerations
Needs may be met in the following programs: ball toss, bean bag toss, walking, bowling, shuffleboard bowling, dancing

Notes/Ideas:

Five-Card Bingo (GP)

Candid Resident Words
As a volunteer endeavors to assist a resident in turning
over her playing cards, she is asked:
   "Hey, why do you touch my cards? Don't you have
your own?"

I'll bet this is a game few have heard of and yet it is one of the most popular programs we have added to our vault of resources. A simple game and it's fun for everyone.

Take one oversized deck of cards as your "callers' deck." Mix three or four other decks of cards together. Deal out five cards per player. Players line cards face up in a row. As the caller reveals and calls a card, players turn over their card if it has been called. Through the use of multiple decks for dealing to players, it is possible that a player may have multiples of the card called…turn them all over! This is what makes part of the fun for the game. Yes, it is an honor system. After calling five cards, a player could feasibly call bingo and you would only know they have bingo if you go through the previously called pile of cards to confirm. We don't do that. This is a form of bingo for those who have essentially lost the ability to recognize bingo on a true game card. It is a game for all levels of skill.

Probably one of the nicest things I have observed about this game is that many players often watch over peers' cards and cue them, too—great cooperative play. We charge 25¢ to play for the afternoon and use the money to pick up novelty prizes. Other prizes are also donated to the cause.

We definitely consider this game to be an off-unit program for many; however, let's talk hoarders. Lessons come at the most unpredictable times for caregivers.

Frances is a card hoarder and at meal time, we discovered why.
Pulling cards out of her pocket, she asks, "Is this enough?"
   At first it was thought she was talking about some kind
of card game, then it clicked. Frances has a constant con-
cern about paying for her meals. To Frances, it seemed, the
cards represented money, which she now gladly uses to pay
for her dinner. Two problems solved! She is without further
concern and we play with a full deck.

Program Content for Five-Card Bingo (GP)

Participants
GDS Rating: Levels 4–5
> *Target:* Those who can identify different playing cards
> *Others:* Those who recognize shapes, colors, and numbers and receive volunteer support

Equipment
Multiple decks of playing cards; oversized cards for the caller to display while calling; prizes (optional)

Social Domain
Supporting peers designated as "card turners;" cooperative playing

Emotional Domain
Excitement of winning; self-esteem; self-confidence

Physical Domain
Fine motor control; manual dexterity involved in card lifting and turning

Cognitive Domain
Recognition of symbols; memory; concentration

Strengths
Promotes ability to follow instructions and attention span; simplification/variation of several previously learned games (e.g., bingo, bridge)

Challenges
Clarity of language in instructions (e.g., "turn" may be confused with "rotate"). Recent memory impairment may result in cards previously called and turned over to be turned back or frequently inspected.

Adaptations/Special Considerations
Play only one or two hands for a small group of special care players so they may succeed cooperatively. Turning a card up can be coached back over by saying "It's okay that we have already played that card." (It is their game, so it doesn't matter in the end, does it?) All cards can be replaced (keeping the hoarders happy). This game is an adaptation of bingo and may be further simplified to colors, numbers, or suits. For that matter, five cards left in a player's hand makes an apparently delightful game of their own choosing.

Notes/Ideas:

Gardening

Candid Resident Words
A reflection on happier childhood days:
"This is like an old, fine time."

There are few things as soothing as a messy dig in the garden—grasping and tearing out weeds and watering. The diversity and potential of edible gardening programs is endless. As our goal is to outline the "fit" of programs for dementia care versus writing a gardening book, we offer you the following:

> *Irene is a hoarder when indoors. When outdoors she becomes Weed Woman. Her concentration is unbreakable and her task accomplishment is always successful...sometimes too successful if an eye does not roam with her. A few lovely flowers, roots and all have seen their day thanks to Irene's dedicated efforts.*

I assure you also, that your dietitian will not endorse eating dirt as a mineral supplement. Ah, the challenges. But, what benefits as your nutritionist may agree that sun-infused vitamin D is as beneficial as the task.

Program Content for Gardening

Participants
GDS Rating: Levels 4–6
    Target: Those with related life experience and interests
    Others: Individuals oriented to the outdoors; those who show interest

Equipment
Assorted hand-held garden tools, watering cans, gloves, pails; adapted raised beds/planters; **sun hats and sunblock—monitor sun exposure**. Your local Poison Control Center should have lists of toxic and nontoxic varieties of plants available.

Social Domain
Promotes peer assistance and interaction, as one might hold a plant or implement while the other is encouraged/supported to dig or otherwise.

Emotional Domain
Memory-evoking, story/skill sharing (Recall, "How many ways to peel an apple?")

Physical Domain
Lifting, digging, watering, carrying, bending, balance, walking. Fine motor: weed pulling, seed planting

Cognitive Domain
Gardening techniques may be shared

Strengths
No right or wrong. Individual may pull flowers instead of weeds—no problem, they grow back (monitor carefully!). Familiar activity. Benefits: fresh air, enjoyment of the outdoors (change of environment is always positive).

Challenges
Individuals eat dirt or other items. Coaching and explaining what you are doing and what you are eating can alleviate the problem "This is soil/dirt for gardening, we should wait to eat our snack later." Offer something edible as an alternative since some individuals may lack comprehension to adjust behavior. Some folks may not want to return inside after the program (only a problem if the garden area is not secured). Review suitability for involvement.
    Ensure hoses and other items are tucked away to prevent trips and falls.
Caution: Ensure nontoxic plant varieties. Edible garden concepts are widely available (e.g., herb garden techniques)

Adaptations/Special Considerations
A large bucket of water and several plastic cups may serve as watering implements with supervision, gardening on a smaller scale indoors using pots and trays, half barrels and other like containers give flexibility in setup and further adaptations.

Notes/Ideas:

Group Talks (Spontaneous)

Candid Resident Words
"Isn't it funny, everyone's talking and I don't hear the
words." Says one resident to another whose constant
foreign, conversational chatter is a source of amazement:
"How do you remember all that?"

Group talks differ from reminiscing in that they are conversations in the present. The content of the discussion is about today. This is not a current events or news and views group; it focuses on interests and experiences. Questions are posed to the participants, such as

- What would you do if you won a million dollars?
- What body part would you change?
- What is your favorite meal?
- Would you rather fly a kite or go fishing?
- Where is a place in the world you have never been that you would like to visit?
- Would you like to go up in a hot air balloon?

Each question leads the group on a joyful and unpredictable path of discussion and exploration.

∞   ∞   ∞   ∞   ∞

One day a group sat waiting for lunch when the recreation worker commented on what a beautiful day it was. A perfect day to go to the beach. She asked the group, "If you were at the beach, would you go for a swim in the ocean?"

The subject turned to how they would enter the cold water. She asked them, "Would you go in very slowly to let your body get used to the water? Or would you run and dive in all at once?"

The answers came one by one, some would run and others would tiptoe into the brine. Margaret announced without hesitation that she would run.

"Margaret," said the recreation worker, "You surprise me, I thought you didn't like the water?"

Margaret replied, "Oh, I would run all right—in the other direction!"

Program Content for Group Talks (Spontaneous)

Participants
GDS Rating: Levels 4–6
     Target: Anyone

Equipment
Imagination; a picture or two to help cue

Social Domain
Self-disclosure; affirmation; validation; camaraderie

Emotional Domain
Memory evoking; humor

Physical Domain
None

Cognitive Domain
Memory; concentration

Strengths
Calming; may be used as a transition program while individuals are waiting for meals or other events; passes time and supports residents while being validating at the same time

Challenges
One or two residents may have a tendency to dominate due to skill, strength or personality. Facilitator must maintain control of the group by asking direct questions and using participant names. Responses may vary with verbal ability—closed questions are appropriate, but nonverbal answers are equally powerful and should be interpreted back to the individual for recognition and communication to the group. Nonverbal messages may also serve to guide the discussion further. For example, if someone cringes at a question about Halloween, the discussion may turn to discomfort or fear.

Adaptations/Special Considerations
Choice of tense for questions distinguishes between reminiscing and group talk: "Have you ever climbed a tree?" (past life = reminiscing) versus "Would you like to climb a tree?" (current life = group talk topic).

Notes/Ideas:

Happy Hour (GP)

Candid Resident Words
Of a visitor dressed in a suit: "He is a man about town!"

One day a woman caught the attention of staff with a curious twinkle in her eye. When asked what she was up to she replied sheepishly, "I'm feeling a little tipsy." She had just finished her wine glass filled with ginger ale. Any program is adaptable!

Looking for a topic of discussion and a way to connect folks? Try a discussion on how to give a toast. I like to say cheers when I give a toast—what else could we say? Bottoms up, here's to you, skoal, here's mud in your eye, down the hatch, and a favorite: Here's to us, who was like us, damn few, and they're all dead. Most everyone enjoys the humor and it can be hard to stop as those around begin to share or make up their own.

As a general program this is an enjoyable social opportunity to reintegrate with the rest of the residential population. It also serves as a relevant, age-appropriate, and socially familiar experience.

Program Content for Happy Hour (GP)

Participants
GDS Rating: Levels 4–5
> *Target:* Evreyone. Bear in mind doctors' orders and concerns regarding consumption and tolerance of alcohol

Equipment
As required for beverage service

Social Domain
Socially appropriate behaviors are cued in familiar environment

Emotional Domain
Self-expression; humor

Physical Domain
Manual dexterity; hand–eye control. In the case of hand tremors, try a different style of glass (e.g., beer mug) or other adapted glass.

Cognitive Domain
Memory; familiar activity; lifelong experiences referenced

Strengths
Familiar. Families may easily participate. No skill demands made. Easy to "bluff" social skills to decrease risk of embarrassment.

Challenges
Memory loss sometimes means individuals are unable to recall that they have had their allotted beverages (Many programs have a two-drink limit)

Adaptations/Special Considerations
Ensure alcohol consent is evident within doctors' orders or that recent changes, such as antibiotic treatments, are known prior to serving alcohol. For those whose intake is restricted, ginger ale or 7up are good substitutes in wine/sherry glasses. These can also be used to dilute alcohol. Provide diet beverages for diabetic needs.

Notes/Ideas:

Ice Cream Making

Bowls, cones, and cups of ice cream—it doesn't matter how you serve it, eventually you wear it! Yet despite the occasional mess, almost everyone loves ice cream. Summer garden parties should not be without it. A less than perfect day can greatly benefit from it. That's why ice cream makers have survived the test of time. One item that all dementia care units should have in their inventory is an ice cream maker. Crank-style or electric, they are not inexpensive, but the results can be priceless.

> One hot summer day ice cream was served in the garden. Everyone had either a cone or a cup. The preoccupation was so intense that the silence spoke volumes about the sheer enjoyment everyone shared that day. An added benefit is how it enhances fluid intake—after eating ice cream thirst increases and so does the demand for iced tea, juice, or water.

Program Content for Ice Cream Making

Participants
GDS Rating: Levels 4–7
    Target: Everyone! Thank goodness for opportunities like this program. Both makers and tasters may enjoy the sensory stimulation provided.

Equipment
Ice cream maker; ingredients or ice cream; cones, cups, bowls; spoons; beverages; extra napkins; damp cloths

Social Domain
Potential for great interaction, sharing and fun

Emotional Domain
Fun and memories

Physical Domain
Depends on type of equipment: crank or electric ice cream maker?
Gross motor: Lifting, arm rotation, fluid intake

Cognitive Domain
Sensory stimulation

Strengths
Encourages reminiscing and sharing

Challenges
Monitoring diabetic needs; lactose intolerance

Adaptations/Special Considerations
Some have never eaten from ice cream cones and may have difficulty; others lose the skill. Cups, bowls, and spoons substitute. Sorbets resolve dietary challenges for diabetics and those who are lactose intolerant. Many great recipes using fresh fruit can be found.

Notes/Ideas:

Intergenerational Program (GP)

Andrew circled the room showing everyone *his* valentine! There in the middle of the beautiful red heart was *his* name. Andrew spoke no English, but he recognized his name. Someone had carefully created this precious work of art to recognize and celebrate him on Valentine's Day.

That someone was part of a sixth grade class of students who visited monthly. What a gift! This was a true celebration of identity for this bright and cheerful wanderer. And so he continued to wander the room showing his prized Valentine.

∞   ∞   ∞   ∞   ∞

Children give back youth, connect to memories of loved ones, and have a magical quality that any entertainer or conversation cannot manufacture. Intergenerational programming is a tonic for the aged and a teacher for the young.

Program Content for Intergenerational Program (GP)

Participants
GDS Rating: Levels 4–5
    Target: Students and residents who enjoy one another's company; must be able to tolerate potential "high energy"

Equipment
As designated activity requires

Social Domain
Interaction between generations

Emotional Domain
Memory evoking; comforting; saddening

Physical Domain
Hugs abound—makes for a good stretch

Cognitive Domain
Reminiscent of child-rearing days or childhood. Requires concentration for communication depending on age group and activity

Strengths
Almost everyone benefits from interacting with a different generation

Challenges
Has the potential to be overstimulating

Adaptations/Special Considerations
Rotate children's seats so they may interact with different individuals over time. Some folks are able to communicate better than others; this approach lends balance to the program. Seat children in pairs to help those who are shy.

Notes/Ideas:

Manicures (GP)

Candid Resident Words
Following her manicure, a resident returns from the
program to show off the student's work, saying:
"It's pretty good, I did it myself!"

As she moved her hand, sparkles glistened like diamonds set
in bright red nail polish. This was a most pleasing sight for
one devoted family. They knew immediately that this creative
manicure was made to order for their mother. Her newly
adopted pastime was to sit for hours and carefully inspect
her nails!

Not everyone wants to see Mom in glaring polish. Neither does every woman
wish to wear bright red, or for that matter any nail polish at all. Awareness is
essential if we seek to keep a happy balance. Asking families always pays
off. Inviting the resistant family member(s) to watch their Mom receive her
manicures is a great way to achieve buy-in. One daughter was concerned,
and rightly so, that her Mother's polish would be allowed to wear off and
look shabby. A promise was made to monitor the state of her nails between
manicures. At the same time this daughter was shown where the polish remover was kept. This provided her with a wonderful and literally "hands
on" opportunity to spend purposeful, quality time with Mom.

Program Content for Manicures (GP)

Participants
GDS Rating: Levels 4–7

Target: Everyone who loves to be pampered and can tolerate close contact/ touch. This includes the men whose eye for a beautiful woman is often still intact!

Equipment
Invite a beauty school in and they will bring the tools of the trade. Great way for young students to learn the trade. For staff who may need to remove polish later, there are nonacetone products that are easy to tolerate. Consider "dip sponge" containers, where one inserts a finger into the sponge and it comes out virtually clean. Once dry or full, the sponge can be rinsed out with polish remover from a bottle and refilled.

Social Domain
Great opportunity for one-on-one interactions. Wonderful stories are exchanged and only the manicurist knows for sure what was whispered.

Emotional Domain
Relaxing; enhances self-image

Physical Domain
Touch; massage; reduce stress and soreness

Cognitive Domain
Minimal. Ability to maintain focus and remain seated is helpful. For those who cannot remain focused or seated, a "mini manicure" of soaking, massage, and hand holding may be all they need to feel the pampering of a manicure.

Strengths
Relaxation; enhanced self-image; dignity-enhancing; physical contact is stress reducing

Challenges
May not understand the need to keep hands still when polish is applied or until it is dry. Hoarders may help themselves.

Adaptations/Special Considerations
Nail filing, cuticles, soaks and massage may be suitable as a complete manicure for some. Make spares supplies available for folks to help themselves, thus avoiding the "borrowing" of manicurists' equipment. Set up essentials out of reach/sight.

Notes/Ideas:

Pet Visitations

At 99, with poor hearing and eyesight, Margaret comes to life when the pets arrive for a visit. She chooses not to involve herself in any programs, but this is one thing she doesn't hide from. Usually on the periphery, she's front and center to share her love and affection with those who return the same unconditionally. The energy runs high as residents are heard making wonderful observations—a luxury not always afforded someone with dementia.

As one resident strolls the hall with a visiting dog on a leash she is heard to say, "We are in a hurry to go somewhere!" On they go, together going somewhere undisclosed and equally unimportant as the pair connects in a joyful moment of walking the dog. As the barking draws a small crowd, someone notes, "They are all talking to each other!"

Another asks happily, "How long can I keep him?"

"Oh, how I love dogs!" exclaims one woman of few words.

"These dogs are fine. We love them."

"They bark too much," observes another participant seriously.

Yet another individual notes astutely, "They are always eating."

"Look at that dog," beckons another, "He loves that petting."

Finally, these moments are not for everyone as a woman states "I'm going to be scared." But after a moment's thought she decides, "They chase away the bogeyman!"

∞   ∞   ∞   ∞   ∞

Cuddles, kisses, wagging tails, purring kitties, and soft rabbits. Attention to resident interest and tolerance is paramount. The safety of the animals is of equal importance to the comfort and enjoyment of the residents. There are those who will stay on the edge, as with any program or interaction. There are those who humble us with their love and affection when we least expect or believe it possible. Animals bring out emotions and responses no other intervention can elicit. There is magic under that fur and a few gentle strokes always uncovers something!

Program Content for Pet Visitations

Participants
GDS Rating: Levels 4–7
   Target: Residents who enjoy or are comfortable around animals; those who had to give up their pets prior to admission

Equipment
Pets; snacks; cleaning supplies; equipment to wash resident hands as required for health and safety

Social Domain
Social interaction and stimulation

Emotional Domain
Memory evoking; calming; humorous

Physical Domain
Relaxing; stimulating touch; some gross motor movement in stroking

Cognitive Domain
Opportunity for self-expression

Strengths
Excellent forum for those less verbal to find comfort and familiarity with others who share like interests (often an unspoken interest of great importance to the individual's life).

Challenges
Fears; farm perspective ("We never allowed animals in our house.")

Adaptations/Special Considerations
Ensure those with less comfort or fears are accompanied, or find a safe, private place to be during the visit.

Notes/Ideas:

Putting (GP)

Yes, putting. A wonderful way to normalize an activity especially for our men. Take a look at the garden and consider a three, two, or one-hole putting green. Can't beat getting outdoors and putting on the real stuff. Better still, I can't say I've heard recently of anyone falling on the green and breaking anything.

Putting has a particular bonus that makes it a favorite: It is failure free. There is no set par on the course, and therefore, no limitations on participants. You play as best you can until you are satisfied. This is one program that has given me the greatest sense of satisfaction. Anyone can do it and feel success. Some of the gentlemen who have played have demonstrated great skill and penchant for the sport. The beauty of such an exercise is that a long-learned and well-honed skill may be demonstrated by one who otherwise seems unable to complete any task sought of them.

Program Content for Putting (GP)

Participants
GDS Rating: Levels 4–5
Target: Residents with past experience/interest; those who enjoy the outdoors

Equipment
Hole flag markers; putters; balls; chairs surrounding putting green

Social Domain
Cheering; supporting one another

Emotional Domain
Feelings of accomplishment

Physical Domain
Gross motor skills; balance; hand–eye coordination

Cognitive Domain
Understanding the object of the game; directionality; two-step instructions

Strengths
Physical activity for those less inclined; normalcy from past life experience (particularly for men)

Challenges
Uneven surface on putting greens; climate; relevant balance and mobility concerns

Adaptations/Special Considerations
Shorten distance to holes for those experiencing difficulty. Spontaneously change designated hole when the ball is headed in the wrong direction. Alternate, staff then resident and so on to assist those with difficulty managing to achieve the ball-to-hole task. Different styles of putters are available for those who might have trouble stooping, although lack of familiarity with such putters may add difficulty.

Notes/Ideas:

Puzzles

When Doris arrived on the unit, a table was set up in her room to enable her to continue working on her jigsaws. They were large puzzles with small pieces. Gradually, over time, her skills changed and smaller puzzles with larger pieces were exchanged for the others. Soon she was offered sponge puzzles. In a short while a further adaptation required that only one or two pieces of the puzzle were removed at a time. Doris still enjoyed working on her puzzles even in their most elementary form.

Adaptations such as this continue to move us on the path of empowerment, dignity, and respect of individual needs in spite of the thievery of dementia. Alphabet puzzles can provide alternate sources of enjoyment and self-expression for small groups of residents or individuals.

When attempting to piece together a sponge alphabet one day, a resident began to stand the letters upright prompting another resident to spell her own name. And so the group continued this self-initiated program adaptation.

Program Content for Puzzles

Participants
GDS Rating: Levels 4–5
    Target: Those with interest and/or past experience

Equipment
Variety of wood, cardboard, and sponge puzzles in various sizes; larger puzzles with less complex imagery are most beneficial (individual preference is a consideration)

Social Domain
Group puzzle projects are possible, but experience the same challenges of other programs (e.g., hoarding)

Emotional Domain
Self-satisfaction; confidence

Physical Domain
Fine motor control; hand–eye coordination

Cognitive Domain
Conceptualization; problem solving

Strengths
Ongoing enjoyment of past interest; opportunity for problem-solving exercises

Challenges
Frustration (residents may find even the simplest of puzzles too challenging). Adult-oriented or age-appropriate themes in larger piece sizes may be difficult to find.

Adaptations/Special Considerations
Sponge style of puzzles are beneficial when residents resort to oral fascinations.

Notes/Ideas:

Reminiscing

Candid Resident Words
"Sometimes my memory slips in, sometimes it slips out!"

Reminiscing is one of the most successful interventions of support and care offered to those with dementia. It is success oriented because long-term or remote memory is most easily accessed by residents.

Group talks, although focused in the present, involve a component of reminiscing as they acknowledge life experience and self-expression. The pure form of reminiscing reflects goal-oriented skills, interests, moods, preferences, and personalities from the resident's overall life.

One of the more valuable elements of reminiscing is that it is an activity that anyone can facilitate, at any time, in any location. This is a form of supportive, social interaction that can enable caregivers to accomplish important daily tasks such as dressing, bathing, or eating. The bottom line essential for successful reminiscing with our residents is sincere interest in the discussion and knowledge of the person. These two factors help to determine our success. One is not required to be an outstanding orator to reminisce. Care is what creates the success. Neither do we need to do all the talking. Allowing both silent moments of reflection and pauses after questions or statements gives the resident time to process data and put together a response.

Program Content for Reminiscing

Participants
GDS Rating: Levels 4–7
   Target: Everyone. Even our nonverbal, late-stage residents benefit from reminiscing.

Equipment
Props and pictures relevant to resident life experiences

Social Domain
Self-expression; sharing with peers

Emotional Domain
Reflection of long past memories; validation of personal history, losses, and experiences

Physical Domain
Specific activities chosen may require various fine or gross motor skills

Cognitive Domain
Listening skills; concentration; communication

Strengths
Support and validation of individuals in spite of dementia-related losses. The benefits are recognition, contact, stimulation, love, and respect.

Challenges
Diminished ability to focus. Potential to draw out bad memories and experiences. Takes time and patience. Must allow residents to find the words needed to communicate rather than answer for them, or give up too soon assuming a lack of understanding or interest on their part. At late stage severe dementia, the process is more one-sided, and leaves the responsibility in our hands.

Adaptations/Special Considerations
Support and comfort residents expressing loss or pain. Facilitator may require strong group management skills to allow all participants to successfully express and experience process.

Notes/Ideas:

Social Teas

Candid Resident Words
One woman's words upon seeing the table laid out for
formal tea: "Lovely, it's so lovely."

Well-timed, this program usually follows baking to encourage the social experience surrounding the ritual of afternoon tea. The appeal of this program is multifold. Residents arrive on their own, drawn by the aroma of fresh baked goods. For those residents whose overall nourishment is diminished, this is a wonderful opportunity to offer a familiar social activity while enhancing their intake through the provision of dainty sandwiches. (Finger foods and sandwiches are always on hand in the refrigerator for just such a moment.) The table is set to create the authentic atmosphere of afternoon tea.

∞   ∞   ∞   ∞   ∞

Fancy cups and saucers are placed elegantly on a lace tablecloth. The crystal creamer and sugar bowl sit on a silver tray in the center of the table beside a tray of fresh, delicious goodies. The mood of the room suddenly changes. The ladies sit comfortably around the table. Tea is served and the garnishments are offered.

"Would you care for one lump of sugar or two?"

"Yes, one please" and so the question goes around the table. The last of the ladies is served. Before the words can be uttered, however, a quiet woman, who speaks little English, holds up two fingers. Two sugars, her smile tells us.

Program Content for Social Teas

Participants
GDS Rating: Levels 4–6
Target: Everyone

Equipment
Crystal cream and sugar bowls, china teapot, and other relevant supplies to make the tea as authentic as possible

Social Domain
Like a time warp, it draws out all old learned behaviors and socially appropriate interactions. Great opportnity for insecure family or loved ones to share in social interaction without fear of discomfort or failure.

Emotional Domain
Humor; self-expression; memory evoking

Physical Domain
Fine motor and hand–eye coordination if residents participate in tea service

Cognitive Domain
Communication of preferences and desires

Strengths
Familiar, lifelong experiences which address resident needs to experience inclusion. Success oriented due to generational familiarity.

Challenges
Hot beverage and fragile china—caution is warranted.

Adaptations/Special Considerations
To adapt program for safety concerns would reduce or eliminate authenticity, thus reducing effectiveness. Simply be aware and use caution to ensure program success. A volunteer or family member, seating arrangements, and other similar interventions can help to reduce risks.

Notes/Ideas:

Stamp Pad Club

Candid Resident Words
An expression that when used by staff to a resident is
frowned upon, but when used by a resident to staff is
very endearing: "Can I help you, dear?"

As the resident stepped back from the desk, her smile grew from ear to ear. The unit clerk wasn't quite sure what she was being told but it was clearly a very happy thought being expressed. She smiled back and graciously thanked the woman for her kindness. The group of residents left the clerk's office and continued on their way, making other cheerful notepad deliveries.

∞   ∞   ∞   ∞   ∞

The stamp pad club has its own unique origin but wherever it goes new twists are always added. Like all programs they can only get better with creative fuels burning. A simple concept: Recycle paper when only one side has been used. Have the residents tear the sheets into four pieces. Another resident stamps them "from the desk of," or "to do list," or "thank you!" on the top edge of the paper. Yet another individual, if enough folks have the skills, counts out ten or so sheets to make a notepad (otherwise some folks double up or certain tasks are eliminated). Finally, the most dexterous individual operates the stapler and staples the papers together. A member of the club collects pads and they place them in a fancy basket with a carrying handle.

After a break and some refreshment, the members of the group who are up to the task take a stroll around the building. Together they deliver and share their notepad creations. The adventure is exciting for the creators as well as the recipients of these marvelous gifts.

This is a wonderful way to promote the maintenance of skills and the enhancement of dignity. Purposeful roles such as these, mixed with contact with other members of the care team environment (outside the unit itself), win support and promotes the appreciation of residents.

Everyone enjoys a reward, and the rewards from this program are plentiful—from celebrative refreshment after a good day's work to peer support as they travel the building to share their efforts with others. The group goes from office to office meeting adults, like themselves, who express excited appreciation for having been selected recipients of such a treasured and useful gift!

The implementation of this program fluctuates with the functional abilities of residents. As in any program, one must be very attentive when assigning tasks to participants to ensure success. Remember too, that skills vary from day to day depending on individual mood, fatigue, and previous interactions. Partnerships with other residents can impose challenges as well. (We don't all enjoy everyone's company—that is just a reality.) As some residents live through their dementia experience, they are at times triggered to see others as they are not (e.g., a former neighbor they never trusted, a relative they were not fond of) prompting us to stay attentive and supportive.

Program Content for Stamp Pad Club

Participants
GDS Rating: Levels 4–6
    Target: "Doers" and "watchers." Task breakdown enables more residents to participate

Equipment
Reusable paper; theme rubber stamps; stapler; basket; a ruler to help fold or tear

Social Domain
Encouragement by the "watchers" promotes social visits through delivery of the product after official tasks of the program are complete

Emotional Domain
Satisfaction of task completed; gratitude expressed by staff receiving the product is esteem enhancing

Physical Domain
Fine-motor control and hand–eye coordination; delivery of the product enables residents to gain some exercise while distributing booklets

Cognitive Domain
Following two-step process directions; counting pages (Ten pages is manageable for stapling)

Strengths
Sense of accomplishment as resident creates a usable finished product to be shared with others

Challenges
Ink on fingers, clothes, and table; preventing residents from stamping a page multiple times

Adaptations/Special Considerations
Use plastic tablecloths to protect table. Gloves if preferred by resident (gloves don't work that well). But, the truth is everything is washable! (Washable inks are available at a cost.)

Residents do as much or as little stamping as they wish. Pull out unusable pages later. After all, this is recycled paper—no great loss here.

Notes/Ideas:

Theme Parties

When the music therapist announced she was leaving to get married, ideas began to flow. Soon enough, the theme party was in the works and preparation included a marvelous array of creative ideas. A wedding shower was proposed. The ladies were to wear their finest dresses and straw hats with flowers. A craft project was launched and bridal pictures were cut from magazines and glued on poster board to decorate. The group began reminiscing about their own weddings. A grand wedding skit was organized by the all female staff. A mock wedding was performed with a bride, groom, and minister.

"Do you promise to love and obey and do everything your wife tells you to do?" asked the LPN/mock minister. "Yeah, and put down the toilet seat!" shouted a female resident. Humor prevails!

∞   ∞   ∞   ∞   ∞

Another theme could be pajama parties. This one started out as a reminder to the team that too early to bed more closely resembled a pajama party, not the time many adults would choose on their own to go to bed. With big rollers in their hair, housecoats on, reminiscing, overnight cases, popcorn, dancing, music—everyone participated and had fun.

There are no limits on themes—only imagination. Try a BBQ or May Day races with wheelbarrow races demonstrated by staff, simple relays such as taking turns walking with a cup of water to deposit in a bucket or passing a balloon from person to person, or bean bag or ball toss. Anything is possible, as demonstrated when residents, planned with the guidance of staff, organized a baby shower for an expecting staff member.

In the process of celebrating themed events, conversations abound while everyone enjoys the theme and unique input from residents. For example, at one gathering residents were asked for their memories about Christmas:

- the kids' homemade ornaments from school
- lots of snow on the prairies
- a china doll from Germany
- poinsettias
- putting silver tinsel on trees
- New Year's was the big event
- French Christmas traditions
- Dad dancing around the Christmas tree and telling jokes

Program Content for Theme Parties

Participants
GDS Rating: Levels 4–6
   Target: Everyone who is willing and interested

Equipment
Varies with the theme; suitable props to cue and promote the theme among residents

Social Domain
Great social interactions; reminiscing; thought provoking

Emotional Domain
Memory evoking; self-expression

Physical Domain
As the events within the theme require, such as races for May Day; decorating requires dexterity as we stretch and reach to hang and hold things

Cognitive Domain
Varies with theme: Memory, concentration, language, communication

Strengths
Everyone has a great time

Challenges
Risk of overstimulation depending on activity selection and mood of residents who participate

Adaptations/Special Considerations
Be aware and flexible to adapt accordingly. Age appropriateness and opportunity for self-expression must be promoted.

Notes/Ideas:

Walking

Candid Resident Words
One resident's observation of wanderers:
"Some of them just always go for walks."

Journal Entry
In my naivete, I would escort seven or eight folks out around an unsecured, large garden. After several near incidents the ratio of 2:1 was clearly safer and more appropriate for all concerned. Now was the time to reach out to volunteers for their treasured support.

∞   ∞   ∞   ∞   ∞

Determining the true value of volunteers is easy after a note like this. Family and other staff or student involvement is of tremendous importance. Yes indeed, volunteers are worth their weight in gold. The more assistance that is available, the greater number of needs may potentially be met at once. Volunteers have the ability to take a little more time to listen and be present for residents even while enjoying a peaceful walk together. Again, conversation isn't everything, as being present for someone is as calming as the fresh air and sunshine.

Prearranged visits to the kitchen for "resident cooks," to offices for the career women, or to the laundry for our homemakers makes all the difference in the world. Contact with the familiar enhances the esteem of residents as well as staff who share their working environment. This is a powerful way to promote the joys of dementia care with others, and a great way to get up and move around in the bad weather or during those lengthy Eastern winters.

Daisy would walk slowly, stopping at every distraction: Someone talked, she stopped; a passerby, she stopped; a picture on the wall, she stopped. It was a long, slow process. The trick was to keep her moving and to keep her mind on the task at hand: walking. If we sang her favorite song "Where Have You Been, Billy Boy?" the rhythm gave her a beat to follow. She would concentrate on the words to the song, which kept her mind on one thing. Around the unit we would go in record time!

Program Content for Walking

Participants
GDS Rating: Levels 4–7
   Target: Everyone—fast and slow walkers, wheelchairs, everyone! Fresh air and a change of scenery is beneficial to all regardless of ability.

Equipment
Appropriate footwear and walking clothes suited to the season or weather. Don't forget sunscreen even on a cloudy day.

Social Domain
Sharing in the beauty of the garden; meeting familiar faces in the building if the weather is not in your favor.

Emotional Domain
Exercise helps to burn off excess energy and frustrations

Physical Domain
Flexibility; mobility; balance; strength

Cognitive Domain
Recognition; way finding

Strengths
Fresh air and sunshine; change of scenery; mobility

Challenges
Different needs mean different speeds for individual residents

Adaptations/Special Considerations
Match speeds of walkers together so that one staff or volunteer can accompany a group.

Notes/Ideas:

Word Games

Peter Piper picked a peck of...
Jack and Jill...

Each elicits familiar and quick responses. Remote memory plays a strong role in this successful program. Fill a container full of slips of paper with these sayings and have your participants pick them out. If that is a challenge, you pick them since you will likely read them anyway. The actions of mixing up the papers and picking from the container promote focus on the game, thus helping participants to maintain attention.

Here's how this program got off the ground. In the beginning, pages of sayings were copied and cut into strips: one for each saying. Next they were placed in a clear, plastic jar. One at a time we drew from the jar and read a saying to elicit a response. As you will read, however, much humor and personality prevails in this exercise as individuals provide their responses.

Later, recipe cards in different colors were used. Categories of games were listed on different colors to address different skill or frustration levels. This enhances the success rate of the program and the comfort of the participating residents. This is a great program anyone can do to pass the time day or night. This is also a good table to table activity while waiting for meals. A lounge or other quiet environmental space is beneficial.

Yet another spin on this program uses alphabet letters on bright cardboard. The question: What words do you think of with this letter? One resident would list a word; another would spell the word.

Here are some examples. The anticipated response is in italics. Resident responses follow:

- Don't change horses in *midstream.*
  - ... midnight
  - ... midday

- As blind as a *bat.*
  - ... mouse—you know, three blind mice!
  - ... ghost
  - ... horse, born the baby (eyes shut)
  - ... me! (a visually impaired resident)

- As warm as *toast.*
  - ... oh, yes, tasty warm!
  - ... a kitten
  - ... everybody here

- One rotten apple *spoils the barrel.*
  - ... is no good to anybody
  - ... throw it out quick
  - ... spoils the, um, atmosphere
  - ... spoils people's feet, makes them smelly!

Program Content for Word Games

Participants
GDS Rating: Levels 4–6
   Target: Varies depending on complexity of language pursued

Equipment
Recipe cards with phrases on one side and answers on reverse. Use bold, black print allows residents to read the cards if they wish.

Social Domain
Sharing; interactive; self-expression

Emotional Domain
Humor; reflective of life experience (see responses under "Blind as a…")

Physical Domain
Fine motor control (if asking residents to select papers or cards)

Cognitive Domain
Listening; relationships (word linking); problem solving

Strengths
Delightfully creative and expressive interactive sessions. Limitless possibilities for self-expression. Unexpected surprise contributions from less verbal individuals. Given the opportunity and time, anyone can/will contribute.

Challenges
Complexity of language can reduce participation. Choose carefully and monitor response or lack thereof

Adaptations/Special Considerations
Use letters on bright colored cards. Ask what words people think of when they see a letter/phrase.

Notes/Ideas:

Food for Thought

"Don't forget, I'm inside this thing," he said,
and it turned out he was right.

—Ian Frazier (1994)

References

Angelou, M. (1994). *Wouldn't take nothing for my journey now*. New York, NY: Bantam Books.

Bowlby, C. (1991). *Therapeutic activities with persons disabled by Alzheimer's disease*. Gaithersburg, MD: Aspen Publishers.

Chödrön, P. (1994). *Start where you are: A guide to compassionate living*. Boston, MA: Shambala Publications.

Clemmer, W. M. (1993). *Victims of dementia: Services, support and care*. Binghamton, NY: Haworth Press.

Cousins, N. (1981). *Anatomy of an illiness: As perceived by the patient*. Toronto, ON: Bantam Books.

Dunne, R. (1995). The great discovery challenge. British Columbia Therapeutic Recreation Association Education Workshop, Vancouver, BC.

Dunne, R. (1997). Celebration of the self—The team quest. [Seminar] Vancouver, BC: Celebrations Unlimited Seminars & Press.

Dunne, R. (1999). *Sharing the magic: The caregivers' guide to quality dementia care in recreation and social programming*. Vancouver, BC: Celebrations Unlimited Seminars & Press.

Feil, N. (1993). *The validation breakthrough: Simple techniques for communicating with people with Alzheimer's-type dementia*. Baltimore, MD: Health Professionals Press.

Folstein, M., Folstein, S., and McHugh, P. (1975). Mini-mental state: A practical method for grading the cognitive state of patients for the clinician. *Journal of Psychiatric Research, 12,* 189–198.

Freeman, S. (1990). *Activities and approaches for Alzheimer's* (2nd ed.). St. Simons Island: Activities & Approaches.

Green, R. C. (2001). *Diagnosis and management of Alzheimer's disease and other dementias*. Caddo, OK: Professional Communications, Inc.

Gudykunst, W., Ting-Toomey, S., Sudweeks, S., and Stewart, L. (1995). *Building bridges: Interpersonal skills for a changing world*. Boston, MA: Houghton Mifflin Co.

Horn, D. (1991). *Comedy improvisation: Exercises and techniques for young actors*. Colorado Springs, CO: Meriwether Publishers.

Howe-Murphy, R. and Charbonneau, B.C. (1987). *Therapeutic recreation intervention: An ecological perspective*. Englewood Cliffs, NJ: Prentice Hall.

Jones, B. (1993). *Improve with improv*. Colorado Springs, CO: Meriwether Publishers.

Kitwood, T. (1997). *Dementia reconsidered: The person comes first*. Buckingham, England: Open University Press.

Kitwood, T. (1998, Spring). Toward a theory of dementia care: Ethics and interaction. *Journal of Clinical Ethics, 9*(1), 23–34.

Lucero, M. (1994). Presentation at the British Columbia Alzheimer's Association AGM/Conference. Delta River Inn, Richmond, BC.

Maddux, D. J. and Maddux, R. B. (1989). *Ethics in business: A guide for managers*. Menlo Park, CA Crisp Publications.

Milton, I. and MacPhail, J. (1995). Dolls and toy animals for hospitalized elders: Infantilizing or comforting? *Geriatric Nursing, 6,* 204–206.

Mitchell, G. J. (1990). Struggling in change: From the traditional approach to Parse's theory-based practice. *Nursing Science Quarterly, 3,*170–176.

Peterson, C. A. and Gunn, S. L. (1984). *Therapeutic recreation program design: Principles and procedures* (2nd ed). Englewood Cliffs, NJ: Prentice Hall.

Reisberg, B., Ferris, S. H., de Leon, M. J., and Crook, T. (1982). The global deterioration scale for assessment of primary degenerative dementia. *American Journal of Psychiatry, 139,* 1136–1139.

Reisberg, B., Ferris, S. H., de Leon, M. J., and Crook, T. (1988). The Global Deterioration Scale (GDS). *Psychopharmacology Bulletin, 24*(4), 661–663.

Reisberg, B. and Ferris, S. H. (1988). Brief Cognitive Rating Scale (BCRS). *Psychopharmacology Bulletin, 24*(4), 629–636.

Robbins, A. (1987). *Unlimited power*. New York, NY: Ballantine Books.

Sclan, S. G., and Reisberg, B. (1992). Functional Assessment Staging (FAST) in Alzheimer's disease: Reliability, validity, and ordinality. *International Psychogeriatrics, 4*(1), 55–69.

Thomas, W. H. (1996). *Life worth living: How someone you love can still enjoy life in a nursing home—The Eden Alternative*. Acton, MA: VanderWyk & Burnham.

Williams, M. (1983). *The velveteen rabbit*. New York, NY: Holt, Rinehart and Winston.

Willis Zoglio, S. (1997). *Teams at work: Seven keys to success*. Doylestown, PA: Tower Hill Press.

Wolfensberger, W. (1973). *The principle of normalization in human services*. Downsview, ON: National Institute on Mental Retardation.

Woods-Windle, J. (1993). *True women*. New York, NY: Putnam and Sons.

Additional Resources

Bennis, W. (1989). *On becoming a leader*. Reading, MA: Addison-Wesley.

Boyd, C. (1994, September). Residents First. *Health Progress*.

Buckwalter, K. C., Gerdner, L. A., Richards Hall, G., Stolley, J. M., Kudart, P., and Ridgeway, S. (1995, March). Shining through: The humor and individuality of persons with Alzheimer's disease. *Journal of Gerontological Nursing*, 11–15.

Chou, C., Jackson, L., Louie, V., and McAuley, M. (1996). *Geriatric nutrition in care facilities: A multidisciplinary approach* (2nd ed., pp. 7–22). Gerontology Practice Group, British Columbia Dieticians' and Nutritionists' Association.

Coons, D. H. (1987, September/October). Training staff to work in special Alzheimer's units. *The American Journal of Alzheimer's Care and Related Disorders & Research*, 6–12.

Coons, D. H. (1988, January/February). Wandering. *The American Journal of Alzheimer's Care and Related Disorders & Research*, 31–36.

Covey, S. R. (1990). *Principle-centered leadership*. New York, NY: Simon & Schuster.

Creasey, H. (1998). Brain and behavior [videotape]. Produced by the Alzheimer's Disease and Related Disorders Society in association with the University of Sydney, Australia.

Dunne R. (1998). *Discovering adventure in special care* (2nd ed.). Vancouver, BC: Celebrations Unlimited Seminars & Press.

Dunne R. (1999). *Sharing the magic: The caregiver's guide to quality dementia care recreation and social programming*. Vancouver, BC: Celebrations Unlimited Seminars & Press.

Fabiano, L. (1992). *The tactics of supportive therapy: A comprehensive intervention program for effective caring of the Alzheimer's victim* (2nd ed.). Seagrave, ON: Fabiano Consulting Services.

Feil, N. (1989). *Validation: The Feil method*. Cleveland, OH: Edward Feil Productions.

Hoffman, D. (Producer/Director). (1995). Complaints of a dutiful daughter [videotape]. Available from Women Make Movies, 462 Broadway, New York, NY 10013.

Larkin, M. (1995). *When someone you love has Alzheimer's*. New York, NY: Dell Publishing.

Lipovenko, D. (1996, Fall). Simple touches help dementia patients. *The Globe and Mail*.

Mace, N. L. and Rabins, P. V. *The 36-hour day.* New York, NY: Warner Books.

McCloskey, L. (1994). Applications in music therapy. BCACA Conference, Kelowna, BC.

McGregor, I. and Bell, J. (1993, September 8). Voyage of discovery. *Nursing Times, 89*(36).

Medina, J. (1999). *What you need to know about Alzheimer's.* Hong Kong: New Harbinger Publications.

Munson, P. (1991). *Designing facilities for people with dementia.* Ottawa, ON: Health Facilities Design Unit, Institutional and Professional Services Division, Health and Welfare Canada.

Nelson, D. (1996). *The power of touch in facility care* [videotape]. San Carlos, CA: AllenTouch Associates.

Parce, R. R. (1987). *Nursing science: Major paradigms, theories and critiques.* Philadelphia, PA: Saunders.

Pietrukowicz, M. E. and Johnson, M. (1991). Using life histories to individualize nursing home staff attitudes toward residents. *The Gerontologist, 31*(1), 102–106.

Providing dementia care: A teaching manual for educators. (1997). Alzheimer's Association, Western and Central Washington State Chapter.

Reisberg B. (1998). Functional Assessment Staging Test (FAST). *Psychopharmacology Bulletin, 24*(4), 653–659.

Reisberg, B. (1999). Alzheimer/EOS Conference: Dementia Stages & Caring. Victoria, British Columbia.

Reisberg B., Ferris, S. H., deLeon, M. J., and Crook, T. (1999) Toward a science of Alzheimer's disease management: A model based upon current knowledge of retrogenesis. *International Psychogeriatrics, 11*(1), 7–23.

Reisberg, B. and Ferris, S. H. (1988). Brief Cognitive Rating Scale (BCRS). *Psychopharmacology Bulletin, 24*(4), 629–636.

Robinson, A., Spencer, B., and White, L. (1989). *Understanding difficult behaviors.* Ypsilanti, MI: Eastern Michigan University.

Sabat, R. S. and Harre, R. (1992). The construction and deconstruction of self in Alzheimer's disease. *Aging and Society, 12,* 443–461.

Small, J. A., Geldart, K., Gutman, G., and Clarke-Scott, M. (1998). The discourse of self in dementia. *Aging and Society, 18,* 291–316.

Souren, L. E. M., Franssen, E. H., and Reisberg, B. (1997). Neuromotor changes in Alzheimer's disease: Implications for patient care. *Journal of Geriatric Psychiatry and Neurology, 10,* 93–98.

Zgola, J. M. (1987). *Doing things.* Baltimore, MD: Johns Hopkins University.

Zgola, J. M. (1999). *Care that works.* Baltimore, MD: Johns Hopkins University.

Zgola, J. M. and Coulter, L. G. (1988, July/August) I can tell you about that: A therapeutic group program for cognitively impaired persons. *The American Journal of Alzheimer's Care and Related Disorders & Research,* 17–22.

Zylstra R. (1999, May). *Preserving the art of dining when nutrition and mealtime abilities change.* Washington State Alzheimer Conference Seminar, 1–16.

Other Books by Venture Publishing, Inc.

The A•B•Cs of Behavior Change: Skills for Working With Behavior Problems in Nursing Homes
  by Margaret D. Cohn, Michael A. Smyer, and Ann L. Horgas

Activity Experiences and Programming within Long-Term Care
  by Ted Tedrick and Elaine R. Green

The Activity Gourmet
  by Peggy Powers

Advanced Concepts for Geriatric Nursing Assistants
  by Carolyn A. McDonald

Adventure Programming
  edited by John C. Miles and Simon Priest

Assessment: The Cornerstone of Activity Programs
  by Ruth Perschbacher

Behavior Modification in Therapeutic Recreation: An Introductory Manual
  by John Datillo and William D. Murphy

Benefits of Leisure
  edited by B. L. Driver, Perry J. Brown, and George L. Peterson

Benefits of Recreation Research Update
  by Judy M. Sefton and W. Kerry Mummery

Beyond Bingo: Innovative Programs for the New Senior
  by Sal Arrigo, Jr., Ann Lewis, and Hank Mattimore

Beyond Bingo 2: More Innovative Programs for the New Senior
  by Sal Arrigo, Jr.

Both Gains and Gaps: Feminist Perspectives on Women's Leisure
  by Karla Henderson, M. Deborah Bialeschki, Susan M. Shaw, and Valeria J. Freysinger

Client Assessment in Therapeutic Recreation Services
  by Norma J. Stumbo

Conceptual Foundations for Therapeutic Recreation
  by David R. Austin, John Datillo, and Bryan P. McCormick

Dimensions of Choice: A Qualitative Approach to Recreation, Parks, and Leisure Research
  by Karla A. Henderson

Diversity and the Recreation Profession: Organizational Perspectives
  edited by Maria T. Allison and Ingrid E. Schneider

Effective Management in Therapeutic Recreation Service
  by Gerald S. O'Morrow and Marcia Jean Carter

Evaluating Leisure Services: Making Enlightened Decisions, Second Edition
  by Karla A. Henderson and M. Deborah Bialeschki

Everything From A to Y: The Zest Is up to You! Older Adult Activities for Every Day of the Year
  by Nancy R. Cheshire and Martha L. Kenney

The Evolution of Leisure: Historical and Philosophical Perspectives
  by Thomas Goodale and Geoffrey Godbey

Experience Marketing: Strategies for the New Millennium
  by Ellen L. O'Sullivan and Kathy J. Spangler

Other Books by Venture Publishing, Inc.

Facilitation Techniques in Therapeutic Recreation
   by John Dattilo

File o' Fun: A Recreation Planner for Games & Activities, Third Edition
   by Jane Harris Ericson and Diane Ruth Albright

The Game and Play Leader's Handbook: Facilitating Fun and Positive Interaction
   by Bill Michaelis and John M. O'Connell

The Game Finder—A Leader's Guide to Great Activities
   by Annette C. Moore

Getting People Involved in Life and Activities: Effective Motivating Techniques
   by Jeanne Adams

Glossary of Recreation Therapy and Occupational Therapy
   by David R. Austin

Great Special Events and Activities
   by Annie Morton, Angie Prosser, and Sue Spangler

Group Games & Activity Leadership
   by Kenneth J. Bulik

Hands on! Children's Activities for Fairs, Festivals, and Special Events
   by Karen L. Ramey

Inclusion: Including People with Disabilities in Parks and Recreation Opportunities
   by Lynn Anderson and Carla Brown Kress

Inclusive Leisure Services: Responding to the Rights of People with Disabilities, Second Edition
   by John Dattilo

Innovations: A Recreation Therapy Approach to Restorative Programs
   by Dawn R. De Vries and Julie M. Lake

Internships in Recreation and Leisure Services: A Practical Guide for Students, Third Edition
   by Edward E. Seagle, Jr. and Ralph W. Smith

Interpretation of Cultural and Natural Resources
   by Douglas M. Knudson, Ted T. Cable, and Larry Beck

Intervention Activities for At-Risk Youth
   by Norma J. Stumbo

Introduction to Recreation and Leisure Services, Eighth Edition
   by Karla A. Henderson, M. Deborah Bialeschki, John L. Hemingway, Jan S. Hodges,
      Beth D. Kivel, and H. Douglas Sessoms

Introduction to Writing Goals and Objectives: A Manual for Recreation Therapy Students and Entry-Level Professionals
   by Suzanne Melcher

Leadership and Administration of Outdoor Pursuits, Second Edition
   by Phyllis Ford and James Blanchard

Leadership in Leisure Services: Making a Difference, Second Edition
   by Debra J. Jordan

Leisure and Leisure Services in the 21st Century
   by Geoffrey Godbey

The Leisure Diagnostic Battery: Users Manual and Sample Forms
   by Peter A. Witt and Gary Ellis

Leisure Education I: A Manual of Activities and Resources, Second Edition
by Norma J. Stumbo

Leisure Education II: More Activities and Resources, Second Edition
by Norma J. Stumbo

Leisure Education III: More Goal-Oriented Activities
by Norma J. Stumbo

Leisure Education IV: Activities for Individuals with Substance Addictions
by Norma J. Stumbo

Leisure Education Program Planning: A Systematic Approach, Second Edition
by John Dattilo

Leisure Education Specific Programs
by John Dattilo

Leisure in Your Life: An Exploration, Fifth Edition
by Geoffrey Godbey

Leisure Services in Canada: An Introduction, Second Edition
by Mark S. Searle and Russell E. Brayley

Leisure Studies: Prospects for the Twenty-First Century
edited by Edgar L. Jackson and Thomas L. Burton

The Lifestory Re-Play Circle: A Manual of Activities and Techniques
by Rosilyn Wilder

Models of Change in Municipal Parks and Recreation: A Book of Innovative Case Studies
edited by Mark E. Havitz

More Than a Game: A New Focus on Senior Activity Services
by Brenda Corbett

Nature and the Human Spirit: Toward an Expanded Land Management Ethic
edited by B. L. Driver, Daniel Dustin, Tony Baltic, Gary Elsner, and George Peterson

Outdoor Recreation Management: Theory and Application, Third Edition
by Alan Jubenville and Ben Twight

Planning Parks for People, Second Edition
by John Hultsman, Richard L. Cottrell, and Wendy Z. Hultsman

The Process of Recreation Programming Theory and Technique, Third Edition
by Patricia Farrell and Herberta M. Lundegren

Programming for Parks, Recreation, and Leisure Services: A Servant Leadership Approach
by Donald G. DeGraaf, Debra J. Jordan, and Kathy H. DeGraaf

Protocols for Recreation Therapy Programs
edited by Jill Kelland, along with the Recreation Therapy Staff at Alberta Hospital
Edmonton

Quality Management: Applications for Therapeutic Recreation
edited by Bob Riley

A Recovery Workbook: The Road Back from Substance Abuse
by April K. Neal and Michael J. Taleff

Recreation and Leisure: Issues in an Era of Change, Third Edition
edited by Thomas Goodale and Peter A. Witt

Recreation Economic Decisions: Comparing Benefits and Costs, Second Edition
by John B. Loomis and Richard G. Walsh

Recreation for Older Adults: Individual and Group Activities
by Judith A. Elliott and Jerold E. Elliott

Recreation Programming and Activities for Older Adults
by Jerold E. Elliott and Judith A. Sorg-Elliott

Reference Manual for Writing Rehabilitation Therapy Treatment Plans
by Penny Hogberg and Mary Johnson

Research in Therapeutic Recreation: Concepts and Methods
edited by Marjorie J. Malkin and Christine Z. Howe

Simple Expressions: Creative and Therapeutic Arts for the Elderly in Long-Term Care Facilities
by Vicki Parsons

A Social History of Leisure Since 1600
by Gary Cross

A Social Psychology of Leisure
by Roger C. Mannell and Douglas A. Kleiber

Steps to Successful Programming: A Student Handbook to Accompany Programming for Parks, Recreation, and Leisure Services
by Donald G. DeGraaf, Debra J. Jordan, and Kathy H. DeGraaf

Stretch Your Mind and Body: Tai Chi as an Adaptive Activity
by Duane A. Crider and William R. Klinger

Therapeutic Activity Intervention with the Elderly: Foundations and Practices
by Barbara A. Hawkins, Marti E. May, and Nancy Brattain Rogers

Therapeutic Recreation and the Nature of Disabilities
by Kenneth E. Mobily and Richard D. MacNeil

Therapeutic Recreation: Cases and Exercises, Second Edition
by Barbara C. Wilhite and M. Jean Keller

Therapeutic Recreation in Health Promotion and Rehabilitation
by John Shank and Catherine Coyle

Therapeutic Recreation in the Nursing Home
by Linda Buettner and Shelley L. Martin

Therapeutic Recreation Protocol for Treatment of Substance Addictions
by Rozanne W. Faulkner

Tourism and Society: A Guide to Problems and Issues
by Robert W. Wyllie

A Training Manual for Americans with Disabilities Act Compliance in Parks and Recreation Settings
by Carol Stensrud

 Venture Publishing, Inc.
1999 Cato Avenue
State College, PA 16801
Phone: (814) 234-4561
Fax: (814) 234-1651

"A beautiful and necessary work for all who are called to enter deeply into their own inner work and transformation."

—Sara Wiseman, author of *Messages from the Divine* and *The Intuitive Path*

"Donna DeNomme continues to amaze with new approaches in her already full understanding of healing."

—Tina Proctor, wildlife biologist, goddess storyteller, labyrinth facilitator, lover of trees

"Breakthrough self-limiting patterns and conditioned responses as you make your way through Donna DeNomme's discovery processes, guided contemplations and engaging stories."

—Melinda Carver, spiritual counselor, speaker, award-winning author of *Get Positive Live Positive*

As You Feel, So You Heal

A WRITE OF PASSAGE

Donna DeNomme

ILLUSTRATIONS BY SUSAN ANDRA LION

REDFeather

MIND | BODY | SPIRIT

4880 Lower Valley Road, Atglen, PA 19310

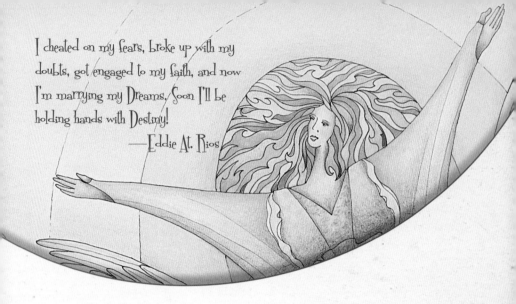

I cheated on my fears, broke up with my
doubts, got engaged to my faith, and now
I'm marrying my Dreams. Soon I'll be
holding hands with Destiny!
—Eddie M. Rios

Designed by Danielle D. Farmer
Cover design by Brenda McCallum
Type set in ITC Fenice, Raleway, and Fontdinerdotcom/Aperto
Closeup of painting palette, texture painting with old multi-colored crayons © Fotangel. Courtesy Bigstockphoto.com

ISBN: 978-0-7643-5810-4
Printed in China

Published by Red Feather Mind, Body, Spirit
An imprint of Schiffer Publishing, Ltd.
4880 Lower Valley Road
Atglen, PA 19310
Phone: (610) 593-1777; Fax: (610) 593-2002
E-mail: Info@schifferbooks.com
Web: www.redfeathermbs.com

For our complete selection of fine books on this and related subjects, please visit our website at www.schifferbooks.com. You may also write for a free catalog.

Schiffer Publishing's titles are available at special discounts for bulk purchases for sales promotions or premiums. Special editions, including personalized covers, corporate imprints, and excerpts, can be created in large quantities for special needs. For more information, contact the publisher.

We are always looking for people to write books on new and related subjects. If you have an idea for a book, please contact us at proposals@schifferbooks.com.

CONTENTS

INTRODUCTION   4

Chapter 1: SELF-DISCOVERY   11

The Awakening of Self-Discovery is an invitation to expand beyond the limitations of your present perspective. What's possible?

Chapter 2: TRANSFORMATION   35

With the Departure of Transformation, you consider leaving what is known, to journey into the vast unknown in search of greater meaning. Cultivate your emotions into more of what they can be.

Chapter 3: SACRED PATH   67

In this stage of your Write of Passage, you'll rise above Life's Tests and Trials to soar to new heights. Explore how human emotions help embody your divine experience; all you feel is a part of your Sacred Path.

Chapter 4: SOUL CREATIVITY   93

The beckoning of your soul voice inspires your personal contribution: by going into the darkness of an Inner Cave, you recognize your Divine Gifts and express them through your unique Soul Creativity.

Chapter 5: THE GREAT MYSTERY OF LIFE   121

While opening to life's infinite potential, you draw your new emotional insights forward in a way that benefits all. In this Returning phase of your Write of Passage, you come home and, at the same time, open wider to embrace the greater yet-to-be.

FINAL BLESSING   138

Your Write of Passage Home

ACKNOWLEDGMENTS   142

INTRODUCTION

Why do I feel like crying? There is an ache in my heart, and my eyes leak gentle tears without words. I'm weepy and acutely sensitive, with no clarity of thought or even questioning. Perhaps it's to purge a pain I no longer remember . . . or one I've somehow missed. It demands my face and washes me from the inside out. I let go and give myself to the river that calls my name, and the knowing current carries me downstream. It is a complete act. And so, I let it be.

My client, Denise, comes to see me in desperate need of relaxation and support. Pregnant for the first time in her early forties, this joyful transition has been complicated by the discovery of a mass growing in her left breast. Detailed research into her medical treatment options, followed by difficult conversation with her husband concerning the growth hormone that has been growing both their baby *and* the invader mass, culminates in a thoughtful decision to go ahead with the mastectomy and chemotherapy recommended by her doctor. This protocol will begin, right now, during her long-awaited pregnancy. As an alternative practitioner herself, she doesn't often feel the need to go to doctors, but now her life revolves around those visits. Normally cheerful and encouraging, Denise doesn't complain to anyone about this—not to her husband, not to her friends, and certainly not to her doctors—she just accepts the course they have chosen and moves forward.

As I focus my hands gently upon her head, the warm, sweet energy begins our Reiki session with a strong and clear focus, pulsing as it moves into deeper and deeper layers of nurturing and healing. Cradling her long, straight, brown hair, I think about how much this woman is going through, and my compassion naturally joins the life-force energy in an even-stronger flow of support.

Denise looks up at me through squinty eyes and with cheeks visibly flexing with the tension of clenched teeth. "May I speak freely?" she says, already sounding quite different than her usual self. "Of course," I respond firmly, sensing what will come next. She bursts forth with great emotion, blurting out, "I work very, very hard on my hair every day . . . and then, I come in here and *you* mess it up." I look at her natural head of straight, flat hair, and with gentle understanding simply offer, "I'm sorry." . . . Long deep sobs release, slowly at first, quickly building in momentum to find a necessary path. We both remain silent. No words are shared; what is important has already been conveyed.

    I stand impatiently listening to the phone ringing and ringing on the other end. It's the umpteenth time I've called in the past few days. Ryan and I have been working closely on a business project, and I really need to reach him because he holds the key to a significant piece that is holding up our collaborative progress. Literally, I am powerless to do anything else without him.

    We didn't quarrel or have some sort of falling out; yet, without warning, he has just disappeared. I've moved past concern into anger at being ignored. I know Ryan is okay and just choosing not to answer, because I've seen this kind of behavior before from him. John Gray calls it "going into the cave" as a way of processing emotionally. "Hello. Earth to Ryan, where are you?" I think to myself. I've already left several detailed messages.

    I wait. It's all I can do.

My dear friend Lucy is bursting with energy, and we enjoy many great adventures together. I truly love her. The thing is, we never talk about our feelings or how to move through any difficulty that comes between us. I've learned long ago the crazy frustration of going into that realm with her. Lucy would rather not explore difficult feelings or emotional nuances, and it's a stretch for her to hear or acknowledge my point of view. It's best that I don't expect her to understand what I'm experiencing. So, we limit our friendship to exploring mutually desirable activities and relaxing side by side on a sunny beach.

These stories show a vital emotional contrast. They're just a few of a myriad of possibilities when it comes to the deep and varied terrain of human emotions. As an intuitive empath, I've been able to easily pick up on other people's feelings. But that doesn't mean I've always been in touch with my own. And as a professional coach and shamanic healer, I've found that what we bury emotionally can, and often does, hurt us. And within those buried emotions, there are, in fact, at times, great treasures waiting to be mined: personal desires buried alive, qualities and characteristics left undeveloped, and sometimes sheer genius hiding in our own inner darkness.

You've been drawn to *As You Feel, So You Heal: A Write of Passage* for a reason. There is something within you that yearns to be seen, to be heard, and to be *felt*. An inner calling is beckoning you toward more of your precious authentic expression.

Together we'll explore well-traveled emotional pathways, as well as the uncharted emotional wilderness. In the depths of these woods, you might encounter an unexpected gem or two hidden within the natural richness of your own dark earth. There is infinite potential that lies within you, and our journey together may help you understand something with a new perspective or uncover something completely new. As a life coach and spiritual sherpa, I've learned how to help people with heavy emotional burdens rise to the challenge of their path and find their way over the proverbial mountain. My hope is that through these pages, you will discover your inner compass to guide your emotional path, and the most-effective strategies to navigate the clear, open trail, as well as the treacherous brambled brush. Through our Write of Passage, you'll release held emotions, so you can lighten the load in your emotional day pack. Choose to set off on a well-worn and familiar trail, finding new methods for being with what's been there all along, or be brave enough to embark upon the unfamiliar one that meanders this way and that with the delight of new self-discovery. A serene mountain pool holds the promise of self-reflection, as within the still water you see a crystal-clear image—and there you are looking right back at yourself with wise eyes and profound insight.

You'll give your emotions the time and space to find their true voice. Together we'll explore how to meet your disappointments, so you can release regret and sadness and move toward acceptance and understanding. As you openly connect with avoided or resisted emotions, your relationship with them shifts, and these pockets of trapped energy are pierced, losing their power *over* you. You join in a collaborative dance of information, feelings, and energy that points you in the direction of life unfolding—not with strained effort through struggle, but with a truly delightful inner collaboration. Build a conscious relationship with all your inner aspects, healing emotional rifts, so you can better allow the natural and divine expansion of your most authentic self.

When you appreciate and respect all your emotions as a natural human response, you elevate life to the place it deserves—recognizing it as the vessel through which you hone your spiritual character. When you develop your trust of self, of your experiences, and of the spiritual source that supports you, you unleash the beauty and the grace of the life you're living. Instead of struggling against "what is," you can embrace whatever happens, and through the process of finding precious meaning and divine purpose, you can consciously choose how to express in alignment with your innermost character, making clearer and more conscious choices that are right for you.

As you feel, so you heal . . . and by allowing yourself to feel, you can cultivate greater personal happiness and more grounded personal success. Glean the profound gifts of truth you find by following emotional guideposts as they lead to your personal healing and soul evolution.

WHAT IS A "WRITE OF PASSAGE"?

In the custom of the ancient cultures of the first peoples, there were rites of passage to introduce a new segment of life. Caring ancestors and loving mentors held energetic support, while providing tasks and challenges to usher one through a sacred portal. This process of solo discovery and transformation instilled great confidence; an assurance in one's ability to successfully move through changes in the outer reality, and a strong, resourceful belief in the innate relationship between woman and nature. Loving arms and knowing hands pointed the way to one's own sacred path and then, after a time, welcomed the initiate back—with sincere interest and appreciation for their unique soul creativity demonstrated in the form of visions, messages, and prophecy, not only for the individual, but for the whole tribe.

These "old ways," in many ways, have been lost. Yet, we still crave the self-discovery and deep meaning they provide. We long for a time of sweet mentoring and transition into a greater way of being. Some of us gravitate to the elders who still remember . . . and we recapture the language of the soul. Humbly and respectfully, we engage with the earth beneath us, the sky above us, and the whisperings of the allies from every direction, from the smallest creatures within the earth to the mighty wingeds above.

Within these pages you'll be given an opportunity to embark on your own Write of Passage. Wise ancestors and caring mentors energetically support you in this endeavor: As your hands move across the page, know they are blessed by your infinite and eternal connection with all-there-is and all-there-ever-will-be, and that life itself supports you in discovering more of the beautiful being you truly are, as well as the greater form of expression that you can truly be. These pages and the journal that accompanies them are your sacred place of unfolding.

FIVE ELEMENTS AND FIVE INITIATORY TRANSITIONS

This book was written with you in mind. There is something within you longing for your attention, sincere comfort, and deep healing. There is something wanting to be seen and heard. There's an inner push, an urging to expand and grow. What you are seeking outside yourself may be sitting in wait of you within the container of your very own skin.

> ➢ Do you believe you're in touch with your emotional self? All of it? Or have you avoided the depth of *some* of your emotions?

> ➢ Do you acknowledge and respect your emotions . . . or embrace only the ones you "like" and banish others?

> ➢ Are there times that you feel emotions welling up and spilling over, seeking a path of expression?

> Do you lash out at other people? Or turn your emotions inward toward yourself?

> Are you able to authentically show your emotions? Can you talk about your feelings in emotionally charged circumstances?

> Are there people who support you emotionally? Do you support others?

> Do you see your emotions as a strength? Or a weakness?

> Do your emotional reactions originate from a younger part of yourself? Or are they appropriate now?

> Is there a wisdom at times found within your emotions?

> Are you emotionally present? Or distant?

Let's approach our emotional selves with an honest curiosity about who we are and what we feel. When we let go of criticism and judgment, emotions feel safer. Then they are free to come out and let us get to know them better. Creating a safe space is key. We'll observe and explore the intricate contours, the various shades, the ins and outs, and the depths of our being. Together we'll do this by moving through five phases: **self-discovery, transformation, sacred path, soul creativity, and the great mystery.**

Initially, we'll look more closely at what is present within us, and then we'll expand beyond our limited perspective. As we set aside preconceived notions and allow ourselves to receptively observe, we can find what has not been seen before, exploring the light and the shadow of it. Self-reflection and Self-Discovery is essential . . . this is the Awakening stage of your Write of Passage initiation.

Once we've walked down the precious path into our own vast wilderness and uncovered our emotional essence with all its Earthy richness, we cultivate those emotions into more of what they might be. During **Transformation,** which is the Departure phase of your Write of Passage initiation, you'll be asked to nurture yourself in and through your own healing, letting go of what was previously known and opening your arms wide to receive the many gifts of expansion and growth.

Sacred path is where we explore how our human emotions help shape our divine experience in human form, acting as guideposts and portals to our unique personal path and bringing meaning and purpose to all we do. Denying our emotions can stunt our spiritual development as well as delay our human happiness. During the Tests and Trials phase of your Write of Passage initiation, you'll explore your sacred path with the understanding of the spiritual gifts you've been given by being embodied in your Earth suit, privileged to feel human emotions.

Soul Creativity is how we contribute to the outer world. *As You Feel, So You Heal* is an opportunity to understand that who you are and what you share is your gift to life itself. All you do and all you *feel* affect the collective consciousness and therefore impact all-there-is and all-there-will-ever-be. You not only impact the now, but the greater yet-to-be, so your feelings help shape our collective future. With the journey into your Inner Cave in this stage of your Write of Passage initiation, your personal reflection and the resulting illumination benefit us all.

And finally, the **Great Mystery** focuses on the vast infinite potential of life and how we can tap in and receive spiritual inspiration and guidance, how we can let go of "knowing" and, instead, enter the realm of infinite possibility. Understanding the great mystery enables us to trust our emotions, trust ourselves, and trust our life. In this Returning stage of your Write of Passage initiation, you "come home" to yourself.

Our five transitions relate to five initiatory steps, and like traditional rites of passage, our Write of Passage engages the presence and the power of the elements, cultivating them as treasured allies to assist in our emotional process: the Earth helps ground our discovery; by fiery illumination, we move in and through our transformation, forged anew; and currents of airy insight uplift us onto our sacred path as we learn to soar. Through the ebb and flow of water, the fluidity of our soul creativity is expressed through every aspect of our lives. These four core elements stretch backward and forward through eons of time, bringing an eternal continuity and depth of process; they are distinctively unique in their composition and qualities, and each one has value to our process. Yet, there's also a fifth element—the element of ether—and so, in our final chapter, we'll explore how the vast potential of ether can support us in embracing the great mystery, living from a sincere receptivity and acceptance for all our emotions.

As You Feel, So You Heal is for those who wish to live authentically and sincerely. It is also an important resource for coaches, body workers, and healers who help support others. It is an essential inquiry into what it is to be fully human . . . and from that authentic humanity to manifest what is essentially divine.

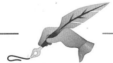

Choose a special notebook or a journal just for your Writes of Passage in As You Feel, So You Heal. You can jot a list of thoughts or write in paragraph form-whatever works best for you.

Dance
dance like the
lily, skipping,
slipping
against the wind
bobbing its white
pure face up to
the sun. As the
dance of life
erupts from the

damp fertile
earth and
continues its
life spiral
from corm to
bud to flower
to resting
corm.
Dance as
spring dances
as the lily
breathes the sun.

SELF-DISCOVERY

Chapter 1

GROUNDING IN: WHO ARE YOU?

Whenever we embark on a new adventure, exploring uncharted territory, it's helpful to first find our footing through a safe and solid grounding with the earth below us, to become fully present to our physical body and acutely aware of our inner character. So many things begin and end with who you are and the perspective you carry, and your emotions are certainly at the heart of your presence. Let's pause a moment and experience this awareness:

> Stand firmly where you are right now or imagine that you are outside standing on the solid ground. Connect to the earth beneath you and feel yourself fully present within your physical body. Notice what it feels like to be embodied in human form. Take a few breaths and just be in the moment of being fully present inside who you are physically.
>
> Now focus on how it feels emotionally inside you. What are your feelings in this very moment? You may notice one or two simple feelings . . . or you may notice a complex array of feelings within you. Just note what is honestly there.

There may be conflicting feelings, relating to different situations, all coexisting at the same time. Elise says she's overjoyed with her engagement, stressed and annoyed with her situation at work, and disappointed and challenged by how her mother is treating her right now. All those feelings are inhabiting her inner realm. Some days it's like a music fest with large crowds inside you playing various tunes!

> Take as much time as you need to openly observe your inner emotional reality.

Now list any observations. Write words or phrases to describe how you feel. People often don't listen to the cues and callings within themselves. Just pausing and doing a personal assessment of emotions and feelings can be quite informative.

Turn toward yourself, turn inward, and open with a curiosity to what is true for you.

I suggest you have a special notebook or a journal just for your Writes of Passage in *As You Feel, So You Heal*. Select one you really like to assist you in your discovery process. As you consider each of the following questions, take your time. Write honestly because this assessment is just for you! Sometimes people tell me they discover a piece or pieces they had no idea existed when we do this kind of inquiry together.

You can jot a list of thoughts or write in paragraph form—whatever works best for you. And if you don't have the time to fully focus on our first Write of Passage right now, then skip it and come back later. Find the best time and an appropriate place to effectively engage in this contemplation. Give it the time and attention *you* deserve.

We've found that this process of discovery sets the tone for everything that follows, as it clears the overgrown and brambled path: exposing a welcoming and creative channel for messages from your body, whispers of your heart, and callings from your soul. . . . To learn the full value that emotion brings, we open to the process of objective observation and curious inquiry by engaging in the following visualization.

Write of Passage: Mirror of Honest Reflection

Imagine you are looking in a mirror. This mirror can be simple or ornate, because its form is not of importance. Just pull up in your mind's eye a mirror of your choosing or be present with whatever kind of mirror appears to you when you call it forth. If it's easier for you, you can begin by looking in a physical mirror and then close your eyes and imagine drawing that outer mirror image into your mind, so you can look at it with your inner mind's eye.

What is special and unique about this inner mirror is that you easily and fully recognize it as one of honest and true reflection. Your image, outside and in, is reflected to you with crystal clarity; your reflection isn't in any way distorted, and there's no hiding the truth of what you see. It's an authentically real reflection. It's an image unaltered by thoughts or beliefs of "not good enough" or "unworthy"—self-defeating or self-sabotaging chatter cannot touch this place of open, receptive, and true reflection. This mirror is also limitless with your possible reflection, as it can see beyond the constraints of your current reality to the great potential beyond. In this mirror of self-reflection, you can catch glimpses of opportunities that await you.

Take a few moments to just sit in the energy of this inner realm and connect with the image of yourself. Sense it. Be with it. Feel into it.

> First observe your outer self as you know yourself to be . . . and open to seeing your reflection as you truly are.

> Then access your inner self and stay with your reflection for a little bit . . . as you open to see what is truly there.

> Soak in the presence of the energy you feel. This is you.

> You are safe here. You can find peace within this inner space. You can draw forward your personal wisdom and power from this inner connection.

> If it feels unwelcoming or difficult the first time you try, stay with it for a while . . . or come back again later. You are safe here and you *can find peace* here.

From this place of deep and sincere connection with yourself, contemplate and jot down any thoughts to the following questions. Every now and then, if you need to or when you want to, move back into your inner realm, connecting honestly with yourself and seeing with the *Mirror of Honest Reflection*. Take your time with this detailed assessment. The questions are presented for your honest inquiry, so answer the ones that speak to you or encourage you to explore in an area you haven't already. This personal assessment may be done at one time or over several sittings. Once you've focused on this inquiry, further insights often pop in later, so leave a little extra space in your journal, so you can come back and record later insights. Allow your process to unfold:

> Who are you? Record the first ideas that come to mind—whatever pops in. Don't censor yourself!

> What are the personas you show to the world? Persona literally means "mask" and is made up of the roles we play and the characteristics we share. What parts of yourself do you show your family? Your co-workers? Your friends? Are these parts the same or different in different situations?

> In what ways does the image you portray limit you? In what ways does it help shape you? In what ways does it allow you to grow and evolve in your identity?

> What are the most real or truest parts of you?

> Take a few minutes to assess your emotional "face."

* If you've been recording a list of words or ideas, you may want to take some time to write in paragraph form to explore these ideas. I suggest setting a timer for ten or fifteen minutes and writing whatever pops into your mind. This "stream of consciousness" writing has been found to pull forth information from our depths, enabling new insight and self-discovery.

I'll ask you to explore further by considering a list of questions. Approach this with a curiosity and realize that it's not a test and you can't do it wrong. You can't flunk "you." Just try grabbing the thoughts that surface as you allow yourself to answer honestly, without censorship, and you'll find that worthwhile information will make itself known. Look within and notice all your emotional nuances. Another way you could do this is to read the questions and then let them simmer on your mental and emotional back burner. You can choose to record your answers later after you've had time for contemplation.

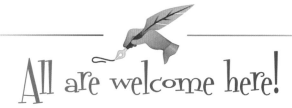

All are welcome here!

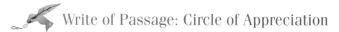

Write of Passage: Circle of Appreciation

We want to be sure *all* your emotions know they are welcome here, so let's pause a moment before you proceed to the questions, and create an energetically safe space to cradle your emotional assessment and all that follows. Each piece of information about every single emotion may be essential to your understanding. We invite them all into the circle with a sweet curiosity and a safe inclusivity. We observe and appreciate each one of them for what they are and how they contribute to our lives. . . . This mindset will encourage and optimize an honest and effective personal assessment. All are welcome here!

So now move even deeper into your inner wilderness by considering the following questions and remembering you can return to your *Inner Mirror of Honest Reflection* or your *Circle of Appreciation* whenever you need to or would like to for comfort and encouragement:

➢ What is your emotional status right now?

➢ What are the factors that are impacting you?

➢ What is your emotional identity? Do you think it's changing or static?

➢ Do you tend toward a doom-and-gloom, woe-is-me outlook or are you one who most often shows a positive face to the world?

➢ Are you emotionally reactive? Or are you even-tempered and somewhat measured in your emotional responses?

➢ Is there a variation in your emotional being depending on circumstances?

➢ Do you tend to be an emotional person? Or are you quite reserved in your expression of your feelings?

➢ How often do you express emotionally? And in what situations?

➢ Are your emotions pliable and changing? Or held stonelike stagnant, remaining the same over a period of years?

➢ What lens do you see the world through? Is it consistent or does it shift?

➢ What parts of your emotional self are you denying? What emotions do you shy away from? Which ones do you avoid at all costs? Which ones have been stuffed down or banished within you and never see the light of day?

➢ How do you react to disappointment? Loss? Success? Surprise? Stress? How do you process it?

➢ Do you feel Rage? Shame? Outrage? Depression? Do you feel Happiness? Joy? How do you express them? Just acknowledge whatever observations or insights you have here.

➢ What emotions are "good"? And what emotions do you consider "bad"? Which ones do you reject, and which ones do you embrace?

➢ What parts of you have been left emotionally undeveloped?

➢ What prevents you from feeling and expressing those feelings?

➢ What do you yearn to do? Experience? Be? And Feel?

WHY DO WE WRITE?

We write as a method to capture our thoughts—both conscious and unconscious. We may be aware of many of our thoughts, but often there is more beneath the surface, and writing with abandon opens us to ideas flowing off our pen onto the page . . . we literally discover ourselves through the act of writing. Our head with its mental gyrations may, at times, override and drown out sincere impulses from our heart, but engaging in stream-of-consciousness writing opens a pathway for the heart's strong voice to express what it thinks and feels. For that matter, all the parts of us are given the chance to make themselves known. We may even recognize a "higher self" finding her way to expression once we open the communicative channel. Writing, when it isn't forced, but simply allowed, can feel extraordinarily joyful and essentially productive to our healing and our growth. There is no one right way to do it; approach your writing in a way that works best for you.

Our Writes of Passage are not meant as assignments, but rather as an invitation. This is your time. Enjoy it! Answer each of my questions or just the ones that call to you. Be aware that the question that bothers you the most, the annoying question you don't like, may be the exact one you most need to consider. Watch for anything that has a strong energetic charge. If you need help getting motivated or you can't seem to find your traction, you might consider joining one of our online Write of Passage groups or forming one of your own with friends. Some of us like to trek solo, and others would rather enjoy a wilderness adventure with companion hikers.

> What are the defining moments that shaped your attitudes and beliefs about your emotions and feelings? Reflect on your past with honesty. What was your early programming about emotions? About expressing your feelings? Or were you taught to stunt that expression?

> How did you show emotions as a kid? How did you handle them? How did others receive or react to the way you processed emotionally? Were you allowed authentic expression? In what ways was your emotional evolution shaped by others' perceptions?

> What changed as you grew up? What were you told about your crying / your sadness / your anger? About your laughter/ excitement/joy? What were the messages you received? What experiences were pivotal for you? What specific events shaped you emotionally? And how? How do these still influence you? Who's perpetuating that now? Do you think you have jurisdiction over your emotional realm? Part of what we'll be doing is to encourage you to claim that power.

> What was your most intense emotional experience? Why?

> When did you feel the most nurtured? The least?

➢ Do you have any emotional role models? In what way? Movies? Media? World?

➢ How do you meet your emotions? How do you avoid them? In what ways are you open emotionally? In what ways are you shut down?

➢ What do you do to avoid your emotions? For example: binge eating, shopping, drinking or doing drugs, excessive TV watching.

➢ When are you most emotionally real? Why?

➢ When do you feel stirred up emotionally? When are you at peace?

➢ On a scale of 1–10, how open are you emotionally? How closed are you emotionally? How pliable and evolving are you? Or are you set in your ways?

➢ Do you process emotions in the moment? Or stew?

➢ When you are upset emotionally, how do you process? By venting somehow? By talking? By doing?

➢ Do you typically process with someone? Do you want your hand held? Or would you rather be left alone? Are you a solo processor?

➢ Do you think/feel you came into this world with an emotional burden or emotional karma? In what way?

➢ How do you feel when a family member cries / gets angry / is sad?

➢ How do you feel when a friend is being emotional?

➢ How do you relate to your partner or mate emotionally? Do you have similar modes of expression or do your ways of sharing emotions differ?

➢ What makes you uncomfortable emotionally?

➢ What is the most difficult to deal with emotionally? Why?

➢ What would you need to feel emotionally safe?

➢ What do you consider emotionally healthy? Unhealthy? How would you like to change emotionally?

When we claim our emotions as useful gateways taking us through necessary transitions for our evolution and growth, we can accept their great value. If we're denying or cutting off this essential channel, we may miss important input that can enrich our self-discovery, our experience with others, and our experience with the outer world. Emotions are valuable treasures that can be mined to excavate their brightest gems. They are a very real part of being human. Let's learn from and understand our unique ways of feeling or *not feeling* so we can enhance the quality of our lives.

THERE'S SO MUCH MORE TO YOU

Although it's helpful as a point of grounding to explore where you've been up until now, each day is a fresh new canvas waiting for your most beautiful creation. If you can reflect on the past and look honestly at what's in the present, you can actively choose not to be limited by either what's been or what is, but rather choose to shape the future according to what you'd really like it to be. Wherever you've been and whatever life experience you've had, there is so much more to you.

Thomas Edison said, "If we did all the things we are capable of, we would literally astound ourselves." Wherever you have been, whatever your life experience, wherever you are right now, believe in your ability to move forward, into the potential of what lies ahead. I *believe* in you. And if for some reason you don't believe in yourself—if you're living in reaction to some wounding or traumatic life experience, if you're stuck in a limited reality, if you've lost faith in yourself or life itself—know that I can hold the vision for you, until you can hold it for yourself. Even if we've never met, I believe in you . . . because I've seen human resiliency and know human potential. It's there—within you—even if you can't see it or feel it . . . yet.

The most significant message my inner guidance ever gave me came in the form of the gentlest comforting voice that whispered, "The point is not in the wounding . . . the point is in the healing." That message helped me continue moving, dragging myself through even the most-difficult times; that sentiment became a mantra that has shaped my life and, through me, others. Wherever you are, in times of success and times of challenge, please remember to keep moving because there is so much more to you than even you know.

And this is especially true when it comes to your emotions. We are evolving emotional beings, right? Who you are now, emotionally, is not the same person you were at two. Or twelve. Or even twenty. Thank goodness!

When people have a safe space, a listening ear, and time for honest reflection, we're able to "break through" to a place of emotional sincerity, one in which we can feel our true feelings and express them in ways that open a portal to healing. When we learn what an emotion is about, and explore what is behind or beneath our feelings, we gain valuable information and insight into ourselves, and we can shape and reshape or repattern those emotions to

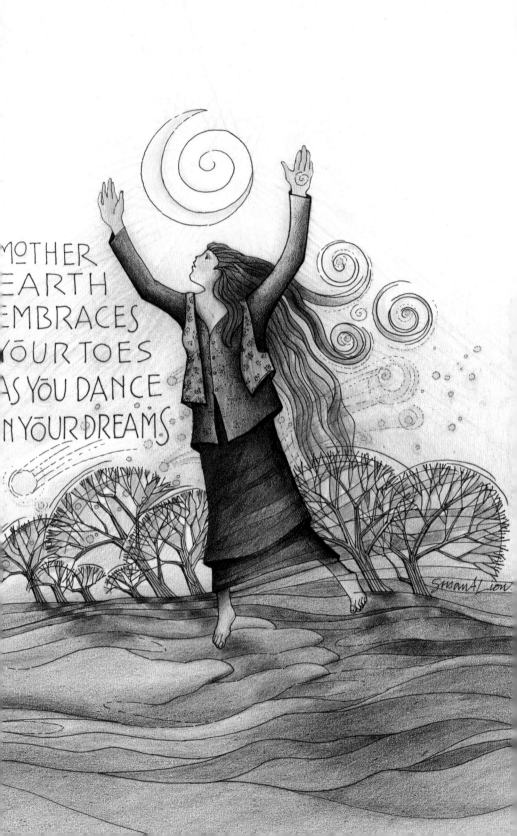

MOTHER
EARTH
EMBRACES
YOUR TOES
AS YOU DANCE
IN YOUR DREAMS

be more in alignment with what we desire them to be. We can enrich our lives by focusing less on any resistance or doubts we hold about the value of who we are, and instead feed our heart's desires and soul's longings.

Becoming and expressing who you're meant to be is life's eternal promise! Trust in your ability to find solid ground, the strength and know-how to navigate life's twists and turns. Learn to trust your true character and stand with assurance as the root of all you do, so you may cultivate an unshakable trust in self, partnered with an enthusiastic zest for life. This attitude will enable you to wade through the mundane and surmount difficulties, as you triumph as an individual. Don't settle for mediocrity. Be more, have more, express more. Why? Because you can.

WHAT'S STUCK?

Just as your physical body digests food and eliminates waste, emotional digestion is a necessary part of your healthy balance. If you don't process or digest your feelings, you can become emotionally constipated. Pretending that emotions aren't there doesn't make them go away; holding them back or stuffing them down doesn't keep them from expressing. It just leaves them untapped and raw, aching to be consoled.

Sometimes an emotional backup can look like someone *void of emotion*—one appearing distant, cold, or unmoved by what's happening around them. One time I was at a particularly disturbing movie—one that had a strongly personal emotional charge. It portrayed stories similar to my own harsh childhood wounding. My friend sat next to me, seemingly unaware while I cried my way through scenes that ripped to the core of my heart. At several points, I openly sobbed, highly unusual because I'm not a person who cries easily. She didn't reach out to me or even acknowledge my pain. Perhaps she was uncomfortable with the force of my emotion, or what I suspect is that she has her own unacknowledged and unresolved pain.

We may intellectualize why we shouldn't be feeling our feelings, and in doing so we push them away, denying them. Talking ourselves out of our feelings is not the same as dealing with them, and honestly, it's offensive. "Suck it up, buttercup," is what one woman who was raised in the South says when she encounters an uncomfortable or distasteful emotion; it's a common saying she learned as a child. "No, no, no," I said, "don't suck it up—that's the opposite of what it's asking of you." When we ignore or bury emotions, they continue to live on and then we have a backup or stockpile of "old" emotions to clear before we can reach emotional authenticity and sincere expression. Surely you know what it's like not to get what you need. You may not be able to have influence over how others treat you, but you can give *yourself* (and your emotions) the attention you deserve. What would it be like to provide the nurturing you need? To do that for the parts of yourself you honestly like and even for those you don't: for the good, the "bad," and the ugly. Clean your cupboards, clear your closets, and open the gate to the dungeon. Let the prisoners run free . . .

    ★ *note:* If you come from a harsh background of abuse or trauma, seek a professional to support you through this process.

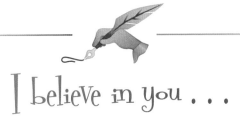

I believe in you . . .

there is so much more to you than even you know.

Process: Let's Unplug the Channel

Dr. Bernie Siegel suggests watching classic comedies and laughing to raise patients' immune systems when confronted with a physical-healing crisis. I recognize movies as effective fiber to help clear emotional constipation; when you're all stopped up, a good movie can unplug the blockage. I remember crying with abandon at a particularly moving moment during a TV program many years ago—of course, the *Wheel of Fortune* contestant *had* won a car! Seriously, this was during a very challenging and hurtful time in my life, and as I've already mentioned, I was a tough cookie when it came to tears . . . and yet, there it was, this magical moment that popped through my resistance and allowed my emotions to freely spill. If something feels stuck or stifled, you can pull out a comedy and laugh, or view a drama and cry, or watch a story of courage and resiliency and tap into your own well of hope. Watching someone else's pure emotional expression can trigger your own, and it's interesting to note what makes you laugh or what makes you cry (or brings up any other feeling, for that matter). I notice my tears flow from seemingly "ordinary" everyday people living heroically by overcoming adversity and blossoming beautifully in some inspiring way.

ANXIETY IS THE OTHER SIDE OF NUMB

I wake up with my heart pounding and a strong sense that I might jump out of my skin. Extreme hypersensitivity coupled with a need to escape where I'm at . . . and I don't even know what triggered it. Was it a dream? Or some stuffed emotion demanding expression? Is this the basis for something truly threatening me, or is it an underlying, undefined anxiety? Sometimes we learn the meaning beneath a feeling that comes in, and at other times, it simply comes and goes without definition. How can we learn to navigate through or manage it, without being sucked mercilessly into its grasp?

First, focus on your breath. Consciously slow down and elongate your breath. This is not the time to contemplate why you're anxious or to try to figure anything out, but rather to bring your entire focus to your breath. Breathe in slowly and purposefully.

Then, release the breath slowly, too. With the outbreath, you imagine letting go of the feeling of anxiety. . . . Then the inbreath feeds you with nurturing and calming energy. . . . Outbreath again releases more of the jittery feeling. Inbreath supports you. . . . Outbreath clears you.

You surrender to your own breath. Let go of needing to put forth effort; let go of any struggle and instead relax into the natural and dependable movement of your breath. You don't have to think about breathing for it to happen; you don't have to force it to be. Your breath is most often just there for you. When you let go of an outbreath, the next inbreath is there waiting for you to pull it in. And when you breathe it in, your breath feeds you with oxygen and vital life-force energy.

So, in this conscious focus on the breath, relax into the natural and dependable flow of your breath. Let go of any need to concentrate or effort to breathe. Relax into the inbreath and relax with the outbreath. . . . Out with anything that is upsetting you. And in with all that supports you.

Take as long as you need to focus on the simple act of breathing, easily and fully, until you feel calmer.

You are not alone. All of life supports you through the life-connecting and life-sustaining inbreath . . . and the releasing outbreath . . . in and out . . . out with anxiety . . . in with peace. . . . Out with anxiety . . . in with peace. . . . Out with anxiety; in with peace.

Write of Passage: Leaky Emotions

We can gain great insight, energy, and personal dominion over our lives when we face the feelings we've been trying to avoid. The truth is, they find us anyway! No matter how hard we try to stuff down our ignored, rejected, or disowned emotions, they'll somehow find a way to "leak" out—those are the times that you have a sudden outburst, raising your voice way too loud for the situation, or perhaps, bursting unexpectedly into tears.

Leaky emotions are sneaky, too, impacting our happiness in subtle, self-sabotaging ways, like causing us to run in the other direction every time a dating relationship gets close, threatening true intimacy. Pushing another away with our inner or outer criticism may initially appear to offer relief, but it only prolongs our self-discovery process, as we replicate intimacy-challenging scenarios as catalysts for our growth.

Emotional backup, emotional numbness, or persistent anxiety are all toxic. Left untreated, over time, they erode our emotional health and can even cause somewhat of an emotional death—one in which you are in a constant state of fight-or-flight anxiety or perpetual numbness to natural human senses. What can you do?

> Meditate with our simple breath meditation, outlined above.

> Watch your thoughts and emotions as they float by, naturally—let them pass like clouds in the sky. Some may be puffy and white, others dark and ominous. Let them pass through your mind's eye regardless of their content, as if you're observing a beautiful spring day or a dark winter's storm. You notice them, neutrally, without analytical judgment or "charged" engagement. Just see them. Just be with them. This is the first step to acceptance!

> Practice mindfulness techniques: Simply observe what's around you. I like choosing something in the natural world like a tree, a bird, or an animal in the yard or a city park.

> Take a pause: Stop moving in the hyperactivity—and sometimes chaotic outer world—and get still with yourself, even for a moment. Just stop your body and sit or lie down. Remember to relax into the breath. Then ask yourself, "What emotion is here for me? What am I feeling?" Describe its nuances in as much detail as possible. Connect with its essence.

> And ask, "What am I not feeling in this moment? What wants my attention?" Once something surfaces, you may choose to follow the thread to a deeper understanding. We can, at appropriate times and in a safe place, consider what is underneath our emotions at the root. What are you afraid of? Angry about? What keeps you caught in a churning sea of confusion? Or stuck in overwhelming sadness?

What takes you to the depths of despair or chronic depression? If you choose to do an in-depth exploration, you may want to draw in a trained professional to help you with this task. No one can give you answers, but they can offer support as you find your own. Having an objective and nurturing guide can help you navigate through even harsh emotions.

> Ask another clarifying question: "How old am I?" Identifying the age of the part of you that is feeling the emotion can be quite helpful. If the answer is "I feel sixteen . . . or twelve . . . or seven," that information may bring insight into the roots of the cause of the feeling. And even if it isn't true for you today, "old" feelings can be projected into "new" circumstances, perpetuating old patterns. Identifying that reality may be enough to help you find your way out of the emotional maze . . . or you can choose to reshape or repattern the old script. This remarkable process of rebirthing yourself is not necessarily simple or easy, but it's quite doable. One of my greatest passions is to witness others as I midwife them through this dynamic process of rebirthing.

* Learn more about this in the "8 Essential Keys: Tools for Hope-Filled Healing and Expansive Evolutionary Growth" online program.

WHO CAN JOIN YOU AT THE TABLE?

Let's invite doubt to breakfast . . . anger to lunch . . . and have fear over for tea . . . engage disappointment in conversation at dinner. Commune with all of them—but don't encourage any of them to spend the night! This is a Write of Passage to meet and accept difficult aspects of your emotional self. What if you stopped trying to avoid or run from your emotions, and instead, you invite them in. Remember, "all are welcome here."

My friend's children are taught to accept and learn how to appropriately express their emotions, but many of us weren't given this skill as children. We may have been told (or shown) that certain emotions were not to be expressed. Anger is a common example. Resisted or denied emotions, no matter how deeply buried, have a way of digging themselves out as they seek the light of day. Once you take responsibility for your own emotions, you can look at them, learn from them, grow to understand and appreciate them, and ultimately work in partnership with them.

The opposite of denial is a type of emotional hoarding. Have you ever known someone who stockpiles anger? They collect injustices and replay them over and over in their head, sharing them with anyone who will listen. What do you think happens when your focus is on injustice? You become a magnet for it. You see it everywhere . . . and you expect and even project injustice into your private world.

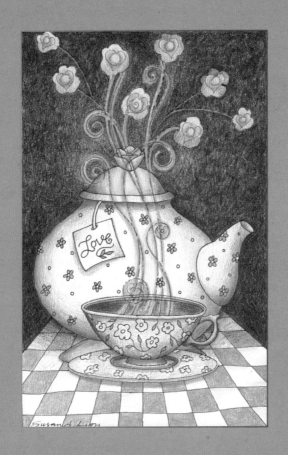

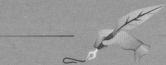

LET'S INVITE DOUBT TO
BREAKFAST . . . ANGER TO LUNCH
. . . AND HAVE FEAR OVER FOR
TEA . . . ENGAGE
DISAPPOINTMENT IN
CONVERSATION AT DINNER

This principle works for whatever we hold our focus on. So, what would it be like to stockpile peace . . . appreciation . . . joy? If these qualities seem too unfamiliar or out of your reach, begin with gathering moments of quiet . . . contentment . . . and little pings of happiness. What you turn your attention and intention to receives energy to grow.

Wherever you've been, whatever you've experienced, and however you're showing up right now contribute to the shaping of who you are and how you live your life. At any given moment, you can make different choices and take conscious action to shift your reality. I suggest that no matter what the raw material is and regardless of the emotions connected to it, in the vein of open objectivity, we look at the color of its life blood and the value it holds, without embarrassment or regret. That which is not pretty may have the greatest value, ultimately, for our life's lessons.

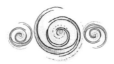

I was introduced to the striking courage of resilient individuals when I presented a program in the county jail for incarcerated women. Every day they're forced to face the repercussion of their past actions, with the only choice within their control being to either remain caught in the quicksand of those consequences or put forth the effort to extract themselves and find freedom in a new pattern of being. Many of these women speak with such conviction, recognizing that even being imprisoned has value in their overall scheme of life. How many of us create our own "jails" every day without regard for how we might escape to a higher path of expression?

Yet, as a collective, we've made great strides toward becoming more conscious in the creation of our destiny. Many of us recognize that we have "choice points," and what we do with them makes a difference in our ultimate reality. It's never too late to be who you might have been if you embrace your core potential, your spiritual essence, and your uniquely blessed blueprint, pushing you toward all you can be. Thomas Holdcroft said, "Life is a grindstone. Whether it grinds us down or polishes us up depends on us." May we consciously use every experience, and all our emotions, to enhance our personal and collective growth.

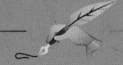

WHEREVER YOU'VE BEEN,
WHATEVER YOU'VE EXPERIENCED,
AND HOWEVER YOU'RE
SHOWING UP RIGHT NOW
CONTRIBUTE TO SHAPING
WHO YOU ARE . . .

LOOK AT THE COLOR OF ITS LIFE
BLOOD AND THE VALUE IT HOLDS,
WITHOUT EMBARRASSMENT
OR REGRET.

I came from a tightly knit French American family with loving parents, grandparents, aunts, and uncles. Little did they know that I was being terrorized and sexually abused by people responsible for my daily care. Years later, as a rebellious fourteen-year-old kidnapped by dangerous gang members, I unexpectedly found myself in an outlaw society that was the perfect container for venting and healing my huge emotional baggage. Emotions pushed down (and kept secret) for so many years found their righteous expression. Whenever I was physically pinned with the weight of a body on top of me, I literally blacked out and one way or another found escape. I had so much rage that even at eighty-nine pounds I could make a lasting impression. "She's loco," they said. I was crazy and bold from deep wounding, choosing empowerment by saying, "No more." As a young adult I faced my not-so-hidden demons and terrifying fears to get to the root of the problem, and life became lighter and brighter.

No matter what a person's outer reality appears to be, you never know what's going on beneath the surface. My rebellious years were terrifying to my concerned family, who thought I literally went off the deep end, but that time was essential to my healing path. People are never broken, never lost, and at times, life may take a strange detour to self-correct. Through my wild and crazy years, I reclaimed my sense of power and dominion over my own life . . . and once I knew the pathway through that darkly dense forest, I chose to become a guide for others making their way through their own dark wilderness. I celebrate life's great adventure, knowing the importance of every part of my journey . . . and yours.

It's important to note here that I understand some of us deal with enormous emotions, unbelievably trying situations, ongoing chronic stress, and unbalanced personal biochemistry. As an intervention specialist, I've seen a range of mental and emotional challenges, including agoraphobia, obsessive/compulsive tendencies, bipolar disorder, disassociation identity disorder, and various forms of anxiety disorders. A growing number of individuals suffer from debilitating anxiety, living in a cycle of emotional battering, where even the simplest task can throw them into overwhelm and life is a perpetual struggle. One woman I know manages her professionally diagnosed, previously medicated anxiety attacks by loving them into submission. She "grabs ahold of them" and purposefully beams loving energy and bright light to them. She, in the moment of extreme panic or apprehension, just loves the feeling despite its intense discomfort. So far, this approach has had dramatic results. Once ruling her life, these anxiety episodes are now merely a slight inconvenience, a blip in the overall scheme of things, and the side benefit is that periodically, throughout her day, Julie is literally sending love and light *to herself* through the portal of these anxiety attacks. Julie is an example of someone who meets her emotions straight on by acknowledging them, learning from them, nurturing them, and, in some cases, choosing to simply accept and manage them.

Write of Passage: Make Room at Your Table

> Pause here. Make a cup of tea or grab your favorite (nonalcoholic) beverage! Consider what emotion you would like to "sit" with for a little bit of time . . . and invite it in. Approach it with respect and all the curiosity you would show a new acquaintance you hoped would become a friend.

> Open to hear whatever your feeling has to say. . . . Record what comes up through freestyle writing or by creating a list of points. You can also use a mind map to connect your ideas or sketch a picture to capture what's being communicated to you. Take your time with this process.

> You could take a situational approach in which you unpack its meaning by taking out pieces and looking at all the facets of that situation, including your feelings. Acknowledge all its parts and see them from as many angles as possible; thoroughly examine its content. Be real about the pain or injustice if there is any, without pinning the blame on anyone (including yourself). Be open and receptive during this discovery phase.

> *Listen* to your feelings at every point along the way. It's an evolving dialogue, with the emotion doing most of the talking! *As You Feel, So You Heal* is not about wallowing in our feelings but rather giving those natural expressions their due. Opening yourself to this type of contemplation and consideration is a courageous act. Listen to your pain, your sadness, your confusion; truly see and acknowledge your own joy as you come emotionally home to yourself.

> With the greatest empathy you possess, feel the feeling that's being shared with you . . . be attentive. Sometimes the simple act of being seen is enough to heal a lingering emotion. It's about having your eyes wide open.

> There may be appropriate times to invite the emotion to begin to loosen or let go. Offer it something to soothe or comfort, helping it move through that demanding transition. Unburdening the heaviness of bitterness, anger, and grief is a great catalyst for healing. The same is true for repatterning a subtle, but undeniable, ongoing sadness or underlying discontentment with life.

> Our attempt is to meet our feelings without judgment; instead, with curiosity and acceptance. This attitude creates a freedom on so many levels and allows our emotions to be bold enough to speak to us, sometimes in their own language, which may be one of the symbols arising in our mind's eye, or more feelings coming forward

in ripples or waves. Realization (and healing) is not a "quick fix" but unfolds like a flower in the rising sun. You cannot rip the petals open but must be patient, allowing the beauty its natural growth. Each stage has merit; each opening reveals a precious truth. Honor and allow the process.

> Know that life is not doing something to you but, rather, is conspiring to help shape your truest form. No matter what the situations or experiences that have challenged or hurt you, you never know what is percolating, since there are lessons in every experience, and meaning in all our days. You are never broken, never lost. Despite the way the outer picture looked or looks, what have you learned? What have you gained? What was in its rightful process?

I've observed thousands of times through the years that this kind of open sharing with parts and pieces enables people to learn things about themselves they've never known. Locked within these buried emotions are precious gems of understanding . . . and those insights and realizations are as close as your own heart.

If you have a lot of fear or have other intense unresolved emotions, please seek out a professional support person. I work with people by phone and Skype, as well as in person. There are many qualified professionals who can mentor you through this process; know you are not alone, and reach out for help if you need it. Your pain and your healing impacts all of us. Take good care of yourself and be brave enough to begin. Once you do, you'll be encouraged by those forgotten or banished pieces from within, and you'll find the stamina to continue. When you look at, are open to, and learn from what presents itself with an approach of compassionate understanding, you are the one that, ultimately, benefits from this attentive process. You are emotionally rebirthing yourself.

EMOTIONS = FEELINGS?

There are entire disciplines of psychology dedicated to researching, categorizing, and defining human emotions, and helpful lists of words to draw on when you're considering or describing your emotions. Exploring those avenues may be helpful to you, but they are beyond the scope of this book. What I'm sharing is not a comprehensive study of emotions. I'm interested in what you are feeling . . . and am suggesting a way to evolve those emotions so you can heal and grow.

So, is an emotion the same as a feeling? Not necessarily. An emotion describes a physiological state generated unconsciously and felt physically—the feeling is the result of that emotion. For the context of *As You Feel, So You Heal*, we'll use these ideas somewhat interchangeably, but it's important to understand that, at times, you might experience emotions because of external or internal events, without feeling the feelings related to them. Watch for that happening and record the details. It may be interesting to explore. At other times, you may act out unconsciously or express your feelings reactively without being aware you're doing so. Typically, those around you will reflect this back to you or in some way acknowledge its occurrence. Learning to give your inner realm, with all its emotional content, the attention it needs is a necessary rite of passage for all of us.

 ## Write of Passage: Emotions Are Precious Gems

Consider developing a list of words to describe your feelings or an emotional state.

> ➢ Start with those you know by naming them. Write as many as you can think of without censoring yourself. You can Mind Map them for a visual of how they interrelate. Consider them further, looking at their nuances. Your emotional list or map will be helpful as we proceed.

> ➢ Don't expect your list to be comprehensive. There are 3,000 words in the English language alone for describing emotions!

> ➢ Add to your list as new words arise . . . and be open to adding words used by people around you.

> ➢ You may experience emotions that are difficult to name or describe. We are expansive and complex emotional beings!

Once you have your list, consider each emotion as invaluable. Examine them as you would a fine piece of art or a precious gemstone. Inspect its contours carefully as you gaze into its enticing depths. Observe its uniquely distinct sparkle (or lack thereof). Marvel at the precious treasure found within yourself.

AN ADVENTURE OF SELF-DISCOVERY

Of all the paths you take in life, make sure a few of them are dirt.

—John Muir

As we engage the earth beneath us and the natural world all around us, we can find our personal grounding by appreciating what's naturally within us, too. Just as we accept the value in the variation of a dense, dark, redwood forest; an open meadow speckled in multicolored wildflowers; and a majestic mountain range with crested peaks and deep valleys, so too we learn to appreciate the varied landscape of our own rich inner wilderness. We discover the highs and the lows, the open and the dense, and the light and dark within, moving through the Awakening Phase of delightful Self-Discovery as the first step of our initiation.

A wise teacher, Mary Antin, once said: "We are not born all at once, but by bits. . . . Our mothers are racked with the pains of our physical birth; we ourselves suffer the longer pains of our spiritual growth." We are faced, again and again, with the physical, mental, emotional, and spiritual pain of birthing into the fullness of our truest self. I offer to serve as a midwife to assist with the birth of your most authentic self through the labor of your emotions. Connect deeply with the element of earth below you . . . think of yourself as "earthy" and ground into your body, claiming it as the little mobile home that moves you from place to place. Anchor yourself within your naturally unique and complex personal character. Look with wide eyes of wonderment as you gaze upon where you are right now in your life, seeing and accepting all that is, so you might clear away the debris of what no longer serves you. Open your vision to the path ahead, knowing it leads to the great beyond.

Here are a few additional practices to help further ground and anchor you before we move through the sacred portal of self-discovery and onto the fiery adventure of transformation:

1. A "GOOD MORNING" CENTERING

We rest and rejuvenate during our nightly sleep, having the potential to travel far and wide in our dreams. As you notice your awareness coming back to your daytime world, take a couple of minutes to fully land in your body and sense how it feels to be inside your human form. Be grateful for your physical container and notice if anything on a physical level needs your attention today. As you get out of bed, consciously connect with the earth beneath you and spend a couple of minutes in gratitude, before you rush into your day.

2. PRACTICE A DAILY ASSESSMENT

How are you feeling? Are you happy or are you sad? Tense or relaxed? Hopeful or discouraged? If no one is asking how you're feeling, ask yourself; acknowledge and be accountable to yourself for the emotions you're feeling. Do this once daily or several times a day. Observe what feelings arise from images, situations, or experiences. Checking in is important because it encourages your emotional awareness to become heightened to what's going on with you.

3. CEREMONIAL RITUAL

Create a Gathering Place of Stones symbolizing each of your emotions to "ground them in" as a viable part of you. These are not rocky burdens, but rather foundational stones or stepping stones for your success. Choose regular yard rocks or gather stones from a special place. You can leave them unmarked and note in your journal the emotions they symbolize . . . or you can mark, draw, or paint on your stones. You could also purchase stones with words on them to season your evolving sacred space. Know there are emotional "gems" among your stones—even if they appear as one of those common rocks. You are acknowledging the value and the sacred hidden within the mundane.

Another way to symbolically work with stones is to bury them in a ceremonial manner to cleanse or release a destructive emotional pattern. After the earth cradles the stone for a time, you may choose to dig it up again and reclaim it as fresh and new, accepting the emotion's evolved state as a part of your personal wholeness.

4. CREATE A HEALING SANCTUARY

Forget not that the earth delights to feel your bare feet, and the winds long to play with your hair.

—Kahlil Gibran

Tina Proctor and I, years ago, facilitated a special girls' group at an alternative school for kids with learning challenges, and one autistic girl shared that her way of dealing with a teasing brother and other frustrations was to go to her "safe space." She had created a little hideaway under a favorite bush that shielded her from the world. I, too, remember finding solace as an abused child under my grandparents weeping willow tree; the long branches hung down all around me, holding me hidden and safe within the arms of my beloved tree.

This approach is energetically sound: Connect with the Earth and nature when life gets overwhelming to release, ground, and recharge. "Go for a long walk on a dirt path," I tell clients, or "Sit under a tree and just relax." One of my favorite recharges is to walk by the river, connecting with the large granite rocks surrounding the banks as the glistening crystal water flows by. Then I have Earth and Water to help clear and recenter me.

Where is your healing sanctuary? Do you have one? Write about it in your journal as you honor this special place. If you don't have one, where would you like your safe space to be? Describe it in as much detail as possible. Look around you and try to find or create your own safe and nurturing space. I've fashioned a lovely contemplative meditation garden with an arbor entry, sitting benches, water features, and special rocks in my own backyard. A variety of plants, bushes, and trees provide texture and shade. On my wish list for this year is to visit a gentle, natural waterfall and stand underneath for a cleansing shower.

➢ What can you imagine as a cleansing natural space?

> A comforting one?

> A regenerative or recharging one?

Have you ever gone somewhere in a natural setting and had a sense of being nurtured in some way? Perhaps even a feeling of coming home? Some places just seem to surround you with a caring embrace.

5. CONTEMPLATION/MEDITATION

Think of a tree—it may be one you know well, or it may be one you simply imagine. Now think about the changes that tree goes through and the many faces she shows you: naked, spring buds, bursting forth with leaves, which eventually turn colors, and in the fall becoming naked again. There are many types of trees and various life cycles, but all trees, from the time they're planted until the time they are no more, go through physical changes, and yet, they stand firm (and some stand tall). Even when a tree has lived out its lifetime, its essence remains, blending back with the totality of the natural world.

Trees can be an inspiration to us. One may experience an injury or need to be trimmed of dead or disruptive branches; yet, it continues. Trees blossom with delight and let go without resistance. Trees honor their cycles and have faith in the next

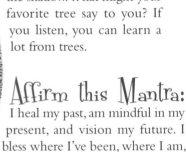

phase of their unfolding. They reach for the sun and cast shade upon the Earth, embracing both the light and the shadow. What might your favorite tree say to you? If you listen, you can learn a lot from trees.

Affirm this Mantra:
I heal my past, am mindful in my present, and vision my future. I bless where I've been, where I am, and where I'm going. Life is good!

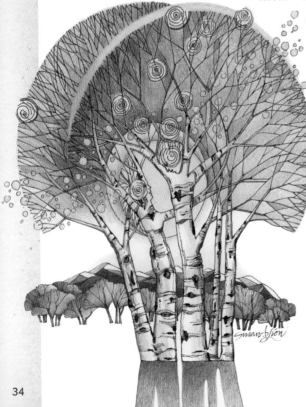

Chapter 2

TRANSFORMATION

Now **that** we've "come home" by being fully in our bodies and present to our ourselves and taken the time to anchor a grounding cord into the Earth; now that we've sat with our emotions and practiced feeling the feelings that are evoked by those emotions; now that we've discovered there are bountiful treasures hidden in our own rich, dark earth, we are ready to go deeper. Our emotional health is greatly enhanced by movement—which is why expressing emotions is so important. When we get stuck or hold onto old emotional paradigms or when we only allow ourselves to express certain emotions while rejecting others, we can become emotionally toxic. Learning to deal with our emotions as soon as possible after they come up is an ability that will serve us well.

As we journey through the portal of Self-Discovery into Transformation, we gain a confidence in our ability to work *with* our feelings and emotionally thrive. Observational and coping skills enable us to understand the reasons for our emotions and to navigate through the emotional arc faster. No longer simply "at the mercy" of our most difficult emotions, in the Transformation phase we learn how to best examine all our emotions in order to better understand ourselves. Emotions contribute to actualizing our greater humanity as they feed our overall evolution of life.

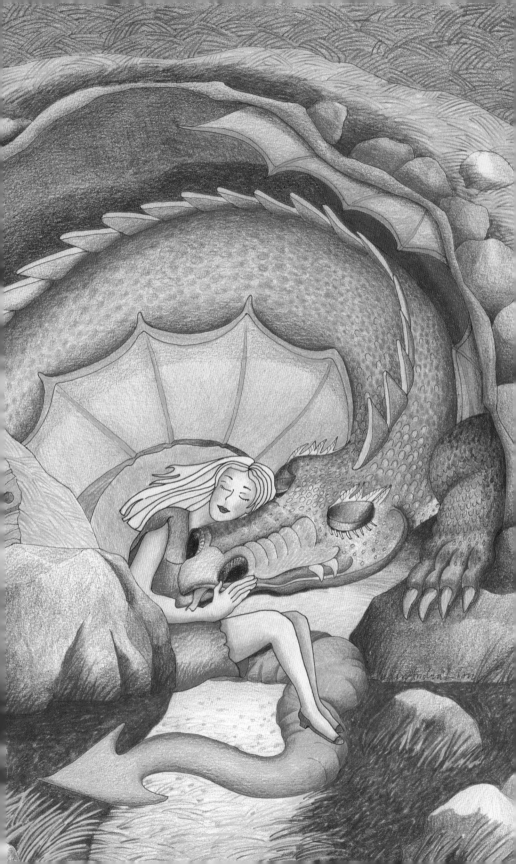

DRAGONS INTO PRINCESSES—
THE POWER OF TRANSFORMATION

In the Departure Phase of Initiation, we leave what is already known to journey into the unknown in search of greater meaning. Although we may traverse treacherous terrain and encounter terrifying turmoil, the richness of the gain outweighs the risk. No one says it better than Rainer Maria Rilke in his *Letters to a Young Poet*:

> How should we be able to forget those ancient myths that are at the beginning of all peoples, the myths about dragons that at the last moment turn into princesses; perhaps all the dragons of our lives are princesses who are only waiting to see us once beautiful and brave. Perhaps everything terrible is in its deepest being something helpless that wants help from us.
>
> So you must not be frightened if a sadness rises up before you larger than any you have ever seen; if a restiveness, like light and cloud shadows, passes over your hands and over all you do. You must think that something is happening with you, that life has not forgotten you, that it holds you in its hand; it will not let you fall.
>
> Why do you want to shut out of your life any uneasiness, any miseries, or any depressions? For after all, you do not know what work these conditions are doing inside of you. . . . just bear in mind that sickness is the means by which an organism frees itself from what is alien; so one must simply help it to be sick, to have its whole sickness and to break out with it, since that is the way it gets better. (Translated and foreword by Stephen Mitchell, 1986)

What a perfect image to hold in mind when dealing with the enormity and sometimes harshness of our emotional process—dragons! And the idea of turning those dragons into princesses by befriending them, recognizing that they're not as scary as they seem but, rather, are just waiting for our curiosity and our caring . . . and to know that they are at work within us, doing something productive, rather than destructive. It is through our acceptance and partnership with our emotional self that we transform our difficult feelings from dragons to princesses.

WANTING TO BE RESCUED

My little self came in as one who was independent, proficient, and capable. I come from a large family of nine kids, and I'm the oldest. My mother says that unlike the others I never needed help from her since I could walk, which was early, at about nine months. And my father remembers me climbing stairs on my own at six months. He says that I never really struggled to walk but just wanted to climb those stairs over and over . . . and then I ran!

Even though I consider myself strong, capable, and independent, I sometimes still recognize an inner desire to be rescued. I've handled things on my own ever since I can remember; yet, underneath was often a tired, discouraged part of me wanting to be saved and, frankly, taken care of—so, for once, I wouldn't have to do it on my own. Is it just me? Or like the princesses in fairy tales, do you, too, have a part of you that wants to be rescued? Honestly, the idea of an external something or someone who can come in and dramatically shift reality presents itself as a common theme with those who come to sit with me in sessions:

> "If only I'd meet him, my perfect mate, then I would be loved and supported. Then I could take on the world."

> "I'm wanting my mother to really see me for who I am, to accept and love me in the way I've always wanted her to appreciate and love me."

> "I handle everything that comes across my desk at work, but at home, I want someone to take care of *me*."

> "I'm just waiting, hoping, and praying that *someone* will rescue me from all of this."

Are you having similar thoughts or feelings? Do you recognize a wish that someone or something could somehow make it all better? Does your satisfaction and happiness hinge on this magical thinking? Instead of running on a scenario that longs for something outside you to create change, pause and look at your own internal dialogue and consider its content. Feel the feelings that lie below face value. What insecurities are motivating this wish? What fears are showing up as what appears to be a desire? And how can you reckon with them?

As demonstrated by Abraham Maslow's well-known and widely accepted "Hierarchy of Needs," our motivation toward self-actualization as humans is dependent on our more basic needs being first met. Once our physiological needs for food, water, and shelter are satisfied, as well as our basic safety needs, then a sense of belonging and connection is of next importance. As humans, we *need* to be accepted and loved: to connect with others, love them and have them love us, and have a sense of belonging. We weren't born to exist completely alone. Finding the balance between autonomy and intimacy is a universal core issue, a significant issue that each one of us is encouraged by life events to explore in various ways, work through, and resolve for ourselves.

Write of Passage: A Human Need for Giving and Receiving

> Consider in your journal: How do you need to be cared for? And how are you being cared for now? Who supports you? In what ways do you still wish to be supported or loved?

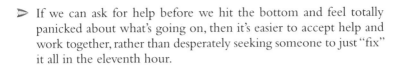

> If we can ask for help before we hit the bottom and feel totally panicked about what's going on, then it's easier to accept help and work together, rather than desperately seeking someone to just "fix" it all in the eleventh hour.

> It's not a sign of weakness to ask for help, but rather one of great strength and interconnection. We learn to stand strong and *still* ask for help.

> Do you recognize and "feel" when someone supports you? Sometimes we can be numb to it.

> Whom do you care for? How else might you show up in support of others? In what ways do you wish to care for someone else?

> Are these two facets of your character in balance—giving and receiving? Are you most often the giver supporting those around you? Or are you most often the receiver, having others care for you? What adjustments or shifts would you like to make? At first glance, we might see givers as contributing and receivers as taking, but, if you only give, you deny those around you the experience of giving to you. You block their human need to give.

> How can you open to give if your natural pattern is to reach out a hand to receive? And if your typical pattern is to give, how can you sit back and open to receive?

The truth is, YOU are the one you've been waiting for: See her, hear her needs, and learn about her weaknesses and strengths. Draw toward you those who can support you, and, at the same time, learn how to best support yourself. It's too much to expect a friend or a lover to never hurt you, because they're human, after all. No one will ever rescue you, and if it appears he does, he'll only later disappoint. Or she'll hurt or leave you in one way or another. No one or no "thing" can be your foundation. We must each rescue ourselves . . . and support each other through healthy interconnection.

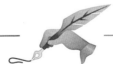

The truth is, YOU are the one you've been waiting for: see her, hear her needs, and learn about her weaknesses and strengths.

THE DANCE OF THE FLAME

In our quest for transformation, let's engage with the alchemical element of Fire. When I was a Girl Scout, I used to love to stare into the fire and watch the images that seemed to come alive within the heat, transforming shape in the dance of the flame. Sometimes I would try to guess what the flame would become next.

Within the alchemical fire, we can see and transform aspects of ourselves:

Take a pure white candle and light its flame. Observe the fiery essence for a few moments . . . and when you're ready, gently close your eyes.

Breathe easily and fully into the awareness of your own body and ground yourself with a taproot you imagine going into the Earth. As you continue to breathe, easily and fully, relax into the sanctuary of your own inner realm, as you remember the image of the flame.

Use that image to light a campfire in a safe and contained space, in a beautiful and serene spot, away from the hustle and demands of everyday life. Watch as your fire begins to grow in brilliance and intensity, as you savor the warmth of its welcoming heat. Sit here for a time . . . just soaking in the nurturing warmth of this fire.

When you're ready, begin to allow your thoughts to wander, as you call forth the parts of you needing attention. They may be situations of the past or present—they may be aspects of yourself—or certain emotions may ask for help. Whatever pops in is right and perfect—don't question it. Trust yourself and trust the wisdom of the fire; know what shows itself is meant to be here with you around this welcoming campfire. Know that all is well and in divine-right order as you sit with yourself and you sit with the fire.

Observe what happens naturally with these parts and pieces. Are they sitting next to you or do they seek the comfort of the hot flame? If they enter the fiery dance, in what way are they changed or transformed? Do they continue to exist in another form or are they reduced to a dark, peaceful ash? Whatever happens within this safe space is good. Don't force or manipulate it: Simply see it, observe it, follow the movement, and then record it once you bring yourself gently out of your contemplative state. Take as much time with this visualization as you need.

Know that whatever is being worked on by the fire is the death of the false self or the death of the false sense of self. Because often who we think we are is much more limited than who we really are at core essence. Working within the transformative quality of the images frees your soul to express, as you release inauthentic or outgrown parts of yourself.

Thank the parts of you that presented themselves. Thank the fire. Offer your gratitude as if offering a gift to all involved with sincere appreciation.

You may need to return again and again to your candle and your transformational fire, working piece by piece with the layers that arise for clearing and release, cradling the one that asks for understanding and integration and letting go of the one that inspires you to birth anew.

* If you need help with this process, you can access my extended guided meditation at WriteofPassage4me.com. This meditation is useful to unravel aspects of yourself, see what parts are ready to shift, observe what old behaviors can change, let go of any remnants of an "I am the Victim" story, and create new pathways for success.

AS YOU FEEL, SO YOU HEAL

Transformation is like taking a road trip from point A to point B—you need to allow time for the journey. Sure, you could push the gas pedal to the floor with the hopes of getting there faster, but it might not be the easiest, most efficient, or safest way. Better to have an idea where you want to go and a map to get you there, keep your focus on the piece of road you're on, pay attention to the traffic pattern, notice the scenery, and enjoy the ride. Then when you arrive at point B you can fully BE there, too! Being present with your emotions is like that road trip: if you have your eye on the destination and rush to get through it, you miss the experience and value of the journey.

Emotions want to be seen and heard. When feelings summon you, the most powerful thing you can do is validate them. When you're brave enough to stop avoiding your feelings and, instead, stand and face them full on, you'll find they easily lose power over you. Staring fear in the face, for example, will show you that it can't hurt you anymore. Sharp, undesirable emotions such as sadness, anger, rage, and jealously need your attention too. These "dragons" might want to stir something within you or alert you to a looming danger. Once you learn the language of these so-called negative emotions, their intensity softens, helping them become manageable. Being attentive typically helps resolve them faster and more effectively.

Acknowledging your emotions and tending to your feelings will allow you to rest in the assurance that your emotional needs *will* get met. Instead of running away, move *toward* and embrace your feelings to interrupt any sort of downward emotional spiral. Look at difficult patterns that perpetuate themselves, and find a way to beat the heat by shifting those patterns. YOU have the power to activate a change, so let go of any nagging sense that it's your lot in life to suffer (release any victim story). Make choices to stop the pain. No matter what has happened in your life or what may be happening now, there is nothing about you that's broken, and you don't need to be "fixed." There is a part of you that always remains intact and unscathed; true healing is uncovering, revealing, or bringing forth the part of you that is always well. The place is right here; the time is now.

★ We focus on this deep work in the "8 Essential Keys" online program.

 ## Write of Passage: "What Am I Feeling"?

Choose one or two emotions you're experiencing, and record anything and everything that appears to be connected to those emotions and feelings. Give them a way to express through you onto the page. Then sit back and be present with the feeling and the words that present themselves; be with your emotional reality, without expecting anything specific. See what opens inside you as you meet each piece and experience its contours and sensations. Get to know your feelings intimately—it's from this place of awareness that you can truly awaken.

> ➤ Our first step is to get curious and acutely aware, so you can aptly describe the emotion. We practiced this technique in our Self-Discovery section.

> ➤ Observe and put words to the feeling. Some feelings may be subtle, but you know they're there; others may "smack you in the face."

> ➤ Once you acknowledge them, then be open to their most intimate story.

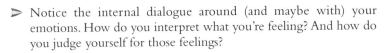

> Notice the internal dialogue around (and maybe with) your emotions. How do you interpret what you're feeling? And how do you judge yourself for those feelings?

> How do you build your emotions? How do you disperse them? Are your coping mechanisms appropriate or inappropriate?

> Are your feelings expressed in alignment with your truest integrity? Or do you have a tenancy to lash out or be destructive in some way?

> Can you be present with what you're feeling and simply "be" there for a bit, or do you feel inclined to push it away or deny it in some way?

> Writing about a problem or difficulty you're having, and detailing the emotions connected with it, may be another approach. Through written exploration, you may see aspects you've previously missed.

Confusion lifts like smoke clearing from a stifled flame when you allow the sensitivity of your emotions to burn freely in the fire of transformation. Be conscious of these little writing prompts in your Write of Passage. Shape them in alignment with who you are and what you desire, because they hold long-reaching potential. When you record your feelings and your thoughts about those feelings, it's as if you're creating a physical altar, a grounding space to see, acknowledge, honor, and respect those emotions. Perhaps you did this with a physical altar of stones in our Self-Discovery phase. Now it's as if you create an altar of words—and your words are fiery potent. As you work through these transformational processes, it's as if you're physically changing or moving sacred items on your altar with the power of your honest reflection and the words you use. When you shift your written expression, your writing cultivates a shift inside you. And once that shift stirs embers, the sacred fire ignites and burns with a steady light that illuminates far beyond where you now sit.

You know stuff happens in life. We do the best we can. Don't become stuck in the appearance of any past challenge, outer circumstance, or what seems to be true about you in any one individual moment. You are a beautiful soul evolving . . . snuggle up to your true reality in the dark of the night; let its enormous radiance warm you against a harsh winter's chill. Honor your process and allow yourself whatever time you need to see it through. Trust you're in the right time and place to heal, to grow, and to stretch into the greater yet-to-be.

NOTICE WHAT YOU TRY TO AVOID

Whatever is overflowing within you will spill out when you are bumped.
—Indian proverb

We can sometimes be sneaky when it comes to our emotions, nudging aside, hiding, or burying one that is difficult to feel, and pushing another one forward in its place. That emotional decoy becomes our focus, and our time is absorbed in intellectualizing and understanding the imposter. All the while the real root is beneath the surface, smoldering with unexpressed heat.

Alexandra, a self-proclaimed "Daddy's girl," was extremely close to her father, and she enjoyed helping to take care of him almost as much as being spoiled by him in the way only a special father can. They adored each other! When Alex's father became terminally ill, she continued to care for him with an emotional weight that shouldn't fall on a young girl's shoulders. And that little girl had to withstand an even-greater hardship when her beloved dad passed away.

Years later, Alexandra found there were still more than a few triggers that mercilessly poked at still-sore places when it came to the loss of her father; a magnitude of grief remained within her. "Why?" she would ponder. "I wish I could flip a magic switch and be in another place." Grief does not have an expiration date—people grieve in their own time and in their own way.

As I listened further, it became apparent that Alex was resisting the huge emotions of her grief and nudging forward feelings of "not good enough" or somehow being "bad." Her words clearly demonstrated that she was blaming and even shaming herself for current situations, perceiving herself as somehow "messed up" by the way she was handling her current challenges. While she was sacrificing herself to the fire of "what's not good enough with me," what was staying untouched in the ground below? The grief.

Alexandra thought she was sabotaging her life. While closely listening to her transparent words, it appeared that seeing herself as one stuck in sabotaging behaviors was, in fact, the real saboteur. The busier she was feeling sad or frustrated or even confused, the more she could avoid her grief. It was easier to cope with "I'm bad or I'm wrong" than it was to fully feel that her father was gone. It was a tried-and-true pattern for avoiding the enormity of her emotion . . . one that had been a familiar pathway over the years.

What do you do when you suspect a decoy emotion? Once you become aware of it, you can meet it with a sincere desire to move past its distractive surface and discover what lies beneath.

In this case, it was important for Alex to know and accept, "There is nothing wrong with me." And her grown-up self understood why the little girl might feel responsible for somehow not stopping the death of her father, and why, because of that failure, she might not believe that life could ever be good. "It's hard and it hurts so much." But Alex was ready to move past that old reality. She knew she had to confront her old feelings, and even though so much time had passed, they were still so raw and burned to the touch. She had the courage to be with them in their fiery intensity because she was wise enough to know that something better waited for her on the other side.

The most effective solution is to meet the feelings and let them run their course. Certainly, to take care of yourself along the way and draw in trusted support. But there is no escaping it; you need to take the time necessary for healing. As we feel, so we heal. When I checked in with Alex days later to see how she was doing, this was her response:

Much better. I took most of Wednesday and made myself sit in the grief, cried, slept, cried, cried some more, and did meditation. I feel stronger and lighter today (funny that even the number on my scale is lighter this morning). . . . Grieving is really super hard work.

Feelings are magnificent keys to doorways leading to your innermost self. Instead of tossing them carelessly aside and leaving those rich inner chambers locked away . . . instead of leaving parts of you held captive in the dark, innermost dungeon . . . go ahead, pick up the keys. Open those locked doors to expose more of who you truly are.

> What would happen if you could look right in the face of that scary grief and really *see* it? What if you felt its feeling—the enormity of it? How can you honor your loss without continuing to be immersed in it? Captive to it? Defined by it?

> And what about fear? What would it be like to admit to your fear? To examine it for what it holds? To see what is rationally based and what is simply an "old fear" carried forward without current relevance or merit?

> What would it be like to feel your anger, even your rage?

> What would it be like to savor the feelings of joy and happiness? To take time to pause with them before rushing on to the next thing on your to-do list?

Like the complete transformation the little worm makes in the solitary chrysalis, take time to explore your emotions with curiosity for the beauty that will emerge. Explore one or more further in your Write of Passage journal. "I love the voice you are putting to this experience. Powerful work" was my response to Alexandra. Find *your* voice! Emotions warmed by the fire of transformation become friendly. Cultivate the courage to walk hand in hand with your feelings and see where they might lead.

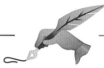

Feelings are magnificent keys to doorways leading to your innermost self.

WHAT'S HELD TIGHTLY BETWEEN GRIPPED FINGERS

It's not the daily increase but daily decrease; hack away at the unessential.
—Bruce Lee

What about an underlying sadness or a deep sense of hopelessness? Some of us are subject to a complex weaving of repetitive feelings that never seem to leave or find resolution. Perhaps you've felt something heavy and overshadowing, or a frustration or anxiety that comes and goes but remains under the surface of whatever else is happening, never really disappearing. Clinical depression affects countless Americans every year—some say as many as 16 million. Even more suffer from feeling discouraged or unable to cope with the challenges of daily life. And we're all confronted with natural disasters, unthinkable acts, and a world that struggles with intense growing pains.

Watch for perpetuating cycles of regret, bitterness, resentment, or any other emotional state that spins round and round. Notice repeating themes that show up again and again in various settings with different people. Directing negative thoughts toward people with bitterness or resentment keeps you chained to the past. If you're still in reaction mode, playing the scene over and over in a repetitive manner, you're stuck in a destructive groove of a limited, unresolved perspective. Don't hold yourself captive in the pain of the past.

Even a little movement to create a new pattern could be healing; the quickest way to find the path of resolution is to move in and through the difficulty. In *8 Keys to Wholeness: Tools for Hope-Filled Healing* (2014), I suggest that traumatic situations often hold unforeseen opportunity to tap into our own wisdom through the resilient act of rising to meet and move through adversity, gaining the momentum to thrive. I believe our experiences—all of them—are rich in effective motivation to catapult us toward growth and soul evolution.

What do you cling to? What are you holding tightly between gripped fingers? What emotions are eating you from the inside out? How many things do you harbor that serve no useful purpose but, rather, continually erode your self-confidence, strain your ability to act, and block your true happiness? How can you let those pieces go?

➤ Admit your pain when you feel hurt—at least to yourself.

➤ Remember to be kind. Don't take your frustrations out on those around you, and don't take them out on yourself. Your kindness contributes positively to the energetic field, actively moving you toward successful resolution.

➤ Struggle is painful and exhausting. Once you learn to sustain the heat of the transformational fire within, you can reprogram and repattern, letting go of what's toxic and retaining what sustains you.

➤ When someone can't appropriately express their feelings, it may result in passive-aggressive behavior. She says nothing's wrong, but her actions demonstrate something else. The antidote? Giving her permission to speak her truth. Is this you? Give *yourself* permission to speak.

➤ Let yourself "off the hook" for any decision or choice that had painful results. Allow the past to be past—and send a blessing to the person you were from the person you are now. Notice and celebrate the growth you've made and be grateful for your life's path, complete with all your life's lessons. It doesn't have to become "baggage" unless you choose to carry it with you!

➤ What can you do to nurture yourself? A little tender caring can be a boost that lifts you up and catapults you forward. I've found even fifteen to thirty minutes of doing something you love can offset difficult emotional processing.

➤ If there's a small voice within you begging for help, listen, before it turns into a bloodcurdling scream . . . or worse, goes silent.

Don't go it alone. Reach out. Ask for help, and be open to receive support from those you trust. If you believe you're chronically sad or clinically depressed, please seek professional help.

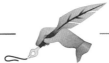

If there's a small voice within you begging for help, listen, before it turns into a bloodcurdling scream . . . or worse, goes silent.

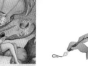

Write of Passage: What Have I Missed?

Are you able to express your sadness? Your anger? Happiness? Joy? What emotions are still missing in action? Like a spark to flame, giving them an invitation to find their voice and way of expression is a powerful catalyst—one that can have far-reaching repercussions:

> ➢ Distinguish the nuances of your feelings: For example, what are the variations of guilt? Of shame? And how do those feelings feel when attached to various scenarios? Are they always the same or are there different ways of feeling guilty? Shameful?

> ➢ Observe when you become emotional and whether you feel those emotions as a part of you? Or *all* of you?

> ➢ Do your emotions take over and define you? In what ways does this happen? Are there times that you feel a specific emotion *is* you? Are you perpetually held captive to any one emotion?

> ➢ Can you give voice to persistent feelings that no longer serve you, and explore how they've served a purpose in the past . . . and notice if that purpose is no longer relevant today: describe what it still has to say. Record this in your journal.

I've said it before—this is all a process. We can't just jump into the raging fire and expect to be healed. Whenever there's a magnitude of emotion, a surge of anger, or a river of tears, something's either in process or not fully healed. Please take care of yourself—like a lovingly tended marshmallow dangling on the end of a stick over a crackling campfire, easy does it, with great attention and care, slowly turning and turning, until it's a sweet golden brown.

COMFORT ≠ GROWTH
(But Growth Can Still Be Comfortable!)

I'm surprised how many times the idea of being "comfortable" comes up during times of transformation. Growth is not necessarily comfortable, and our discomfort does not mean we're on the wrong trail; the most arduous uphill climb can bring us to the most beautifully astounding view. Sometimes repatterning old ways of coping, or stretching into a new area, can be downright *uncomfortable*! Just keep moving . . . don't stop and get stuck or wallow in it. On the other hand, entertain the idea that you can grow without excruciating pain and agony. Sometimes you can painlessly accept your next evolution! So, comfortable or not, the question is this: Are you headed in the right direction? Are you growing toward the person you want to be? Are you evolving into the very best you? If so, then follow these wise words from an old Buddhist saying: "If you're pointed in the right direction, keep moving."

SO GOOD IT HURTS

Sometimes what we've buried alive is our ability to know feelings of happiness or joy. I've met more than a few clients who initially experienced aversion when good came their way. For some, being given a compliment or shown gratitude is difficult to take; it's not only uncomfortable but actually causes pain because it feels so overwhelming. It's unfamiliar . . . or perhaps, they've been taught not to believe or trust praise. "So good it hurts" is an unfortunate reality for some people.

Does this ring true to you? Can you receive and accept positive comments and compliments? Do they penetrate your outer core; can you let them into your heart? Or are you somehow guarded? Does "good" hurt? Somewhere, somehow, you may have learned not to trust when people sent goodness your way. Like a child who's offered a piece of candy and then harmed, you were given sweetness with one hand and slapped with the other. So, you'll have to desensitize yourself from the natural, perhaps learned, reaction of avoiding what hurts. Practice opening just a little to receive a compliment or a kindness. Little by little, stretch yourself into being able to receive. Build trust. Over time you'll learn that good can really *be* good!

DISAPPOINTED IN YOURSELF?

Mistakes. Yikes! We all make them. And every mistake or "failure," it is hoped, gives us helpful information that moves us closer toward our success. That's how Thomas Edison looked at it, anyway. He said, "I have not failed. I've just found 10,000 ways that won't work." When you make an honest assessment of disappointments or regrets with you as the common denominator, look at them as chapters to your entire story and recognize them for the value they bring. You wouldn't expect the heroine to show up victorious in chapter 1, now, would you? Life is a great adventure, predictably one with its twists and turns.

Be patient with yourself. Edison suggests, "Just because something doesn't do what you planned it to do doesn't mean it's useless." And my belief is that everything we experience has meaning and purpose, including our challenges or disappointments. Be forgiving of what you perceive you've done wrong. If there's someone who warrants your apology, then offer it sincerely; believe in the power of your words to at least open the door for healing. Admitting regrets and mistakes can cultivate empathy for others who might stumble on their path too. Keep trying. Our friend Edison says, "When you have exhausted all possibilities, remember this—you haven't."

Strive to align with your core values and act in accordance with your authentic self. Stand on the strength of your true character, not on what might appear to be defined by one or more individual occurrences. You can make different choices and take actions to shift your reality– it's never too late to be who you might have been.

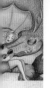

In times of doubting or being disappointed in yourself, try this:

> Take a safe and objective step away from the drama of what's occurring and hear the story you're telling yourself. Notice the words you're saying internally.

> Practice following where your thoughts go, and observe how your mind behaves when you're hurt, or angry, or fearful. This is a proactive stance that can be invaluable in repatterning ineffective ways of dealing with your emotions.

> Don't believe the "ick" of harsh, critical, or destructive thoughts.

> Acknowledge when it's a difficult or painful place, and know that no matter what, you are never broken, never lost.

> Instead of getting caught up in the storyline, gently bring yourself back, again and again, to observing your emotions and allowing the depths of your feelings to find their voice. Be open to your own emotional wisdom.

Be kind and considerate to yourself, comforting and encouraging in this transformative process. "This feels terrible. It's tough to be me right now!" is a useful thing to admit. Ultimately, know you came into this world as a precious and worthwhile person, uniquely blessed. Matthew Fox calls it your "Original Blessing."

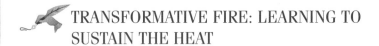

TRANSFORMATIVE FIRE: LEARNING TO SUSTAIN THE HEAT

The Phoenix must burn to emerge.

—Janet Fitch

The process of transformation can be an arduous one, producing an alchemical heat. At times, it may feel warm and comforting, and at others, quite uncomfortable. Our natural inclination may be to avoid our most difficult feelings. Practice being with what's difficult and may even burn to the touch. Discover appropriate methods for venting your "hot" emotions and temper them, instead of dismissing them. What you do contributes to your character, your attitude about life, and whether, or not, you perpetuate those emotions (and the experiences that evoked them) or learn to effectively defuse them.

Life has challenges. As a part of our human experience, there are, most certainly, painful times. Everyone experiences some degree of challenge: a physical pain or illness, an emotional heartbreak, confusing times, doubts, or insecurities. You may carry emotional baggage from your past. Yet, challenges can

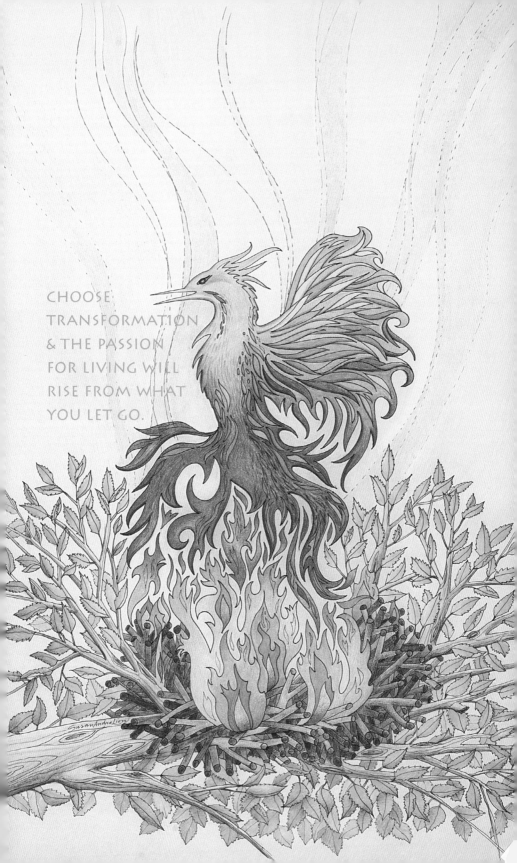

CHOOSE
TRANSFORMATION
& THE PASSION
FOR LIVING WILL
RISE FROM WHAT
YOU LET GO.

be the spice of life, drawing out richer flavors. All your experiences contribute to your highest evolution; difficulties you've encountered add to who you are in the present and who you might become in the future. Know that how you show up and work through adversity is what matters most. The character you discover through hardship is what remains long after the challenge has passed. It is most helpful to come to terms with whatever happened, and its emotional aftermath, because it is a meaningful part of your story. Listen to whatever feelings are there; they'll lead you in the direction of healing yourself.

> Notice the story you're telling: Who's listening to that rendition? Are you repeating it over and over to yourself? Are you inflaming what's upsetting?

> Are you like someone a friend described in this way? "She'll pick a hard emotion and she'll live in it without venturing outside." Do you perpetuate your pain?

> Or are you bound to it like one who said, "Fear is a recurring nuisance in my life."

> Are you utilizing your feeling's transformational potential? . . . and when appropriate, letting its embers die out.

> Recognize the fallacy of any fleeting thoughts that someone or life itself is doing something bad *to* you. Look for the personal significance of what is happening to you.

> Assess where you are right now and where you'd like to be. Discover what's in your power to shift and then move forward toward the change you desire.

> Regardless of how difficult, complex, or overwhelming the darkness of your emotions might seem, there is a way—and the quickest way out is through!

Alchemy

Alchemy is a seemingly magical process of taking something ordinary and transforming it into something extraordinary in a way that is unexplainable. With medieval roots, alchemy pertained to the task of converting metals into gold or discovering the magical elixir of life. Modern-day alchemists (like you) understand that they can take their own heavy material and spin it into gold by utilizing the heat of the fire of transformation. Being in touch with yourself by consciously acknowledging, reshaping, and integrating the influence of your past enables you to sip from life's sweet elixir, bringing forward acceptance, a renewed vitality, and enthusiasm for what lies ahead.

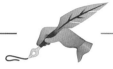

Combine five parts of the present with two parts of the past, mix with understanding and insight, and season with a dash of inspiration.

—Turtle Wisdom:
Coming Home to Yourself

While immersed in problems, it may be difficult to see them as productive. You might wonder, "What's the point?" There is one, I promise you—every experience, every challenge has one. You may not realize it or learn from it, but it's there. Nothing in life is worthless. Tending the sacred fire of your pain transforms pain into something useful, as you take that dense, heavy emotional energy and spin it into gold. As you realize the value in the obstacles on your path, you won't shrink from them or cower in fear. You'll meet them full on and move right through even the most complex difficulty once you've learned the way through the dark and scary forest. There's an amazing resilience within the human spirit that helps us rest in the comfort that we can do this— whatever "this" may be. Every moment has significance. Every contribution affects the whole.

I heal my past, am mindful in my present, and vision my future. I bless where I've been, where I am, and where I'm going. Life is good!

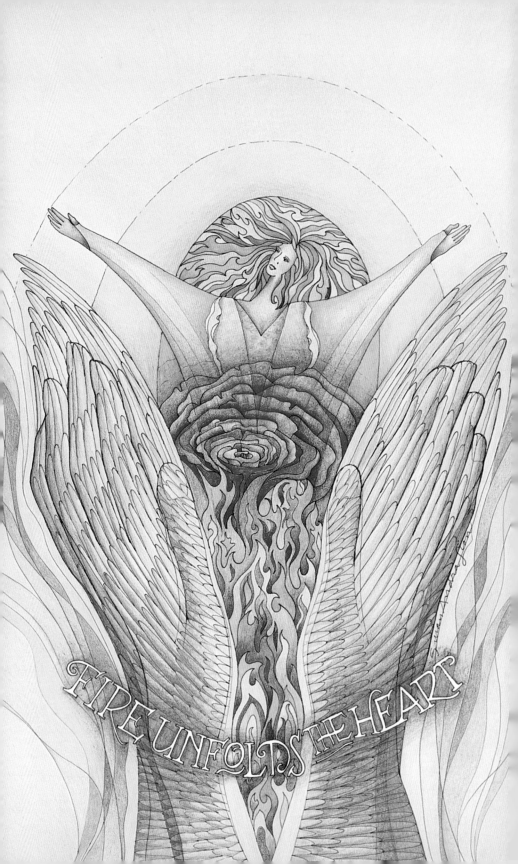

FIRE UNFOLDS THE HEART

Write of Passage: What Is within Your Control?

Yesterday I was clever, so I wanted to change the world. Today I am wise, so I am changing myself.

—Rumi

Believe that you aren't stuck with your old patterns but, at any time, can move toward emotional and experiential change. Even minute movements matter when they're heading in the direction you desire. Explore these questions:

➢ How useful is this emotion?

➢ And how detrimental?

- -

➢ How has this shaped me?

➢ How has this limited me?

➢ How has this empowered me?

➢ What can I release about the old conditioning?

➢ What can I embrace or further develop?

- -

➢ What is within my ability to control? Or effect in some way?

➢ What is outside my control?

➢ What new story can emerge on the shoulders of the old one?

Emotions can be incredibly intense, but typically we know we're going to be okay even when we're immersed in heavy or hurtful emotions. What about when you feel you have no control over your situation or your emotions? Understandably, you may try to claim sovereignty by striving for the very thing you don't have—control. It's a normal part of our natural defense mechanisms to try to grab ahold and attempt to *make* something happen, to push our personal agenda, which only creates an internal, and often external, tug-of-war. It's counterintuitive, but often very effective, to relax into the process, surrendering to what we cannot change, and putting our efforts into effecting what is within our reach.

➢ Ask for divine guidance from your higher self or your angels, guides, and helper beings.

➢ Find a healthy and safe outlet.

- ➤ Reach out to a trusted friend or trained professional.

- ➤ Explore ideas beyond the limitations of what has triggered your feelings. Explore what else is there.

- ➤ Be kind to yourself. Draw in what comforts you.

- ➤ Believe there is something on the other side of where you are right now.

- ➤ Studies have shown that doing something to serve others often is the best medicine for short-circuiting the repeat cycle of hurtful emotions: for example, volunteering has been shown to help shift chronic depression. In what way can you help others?

Human beings are so resilient! We tap into that innate knowing rather than just to be battered by life's twists and turns.

affirm

I let go of any resistance and move into and through whatever challenges face me. I learn my lessons with ease and grace.

EMOTIONS ARE SUBJECTIVE

When I was in my early thirties and my son was a teen, I became a nanny, as a solution to my motherly instinct craving another baby. My little guy, Weston, was blessed with a nurturing and supportive, close-knit family, including an aunt and grandparents within walking distance to his spacious house nestled among the red rocks of Morrison, Colorado. We spent delightful days exploring outside, and in, with plenty of enriching activities to occupy our time. Anything we needed or wanted, the family provided for us, and what especially impressed me was how loving and attentive his parents were toward Weston. So, I was completely shocked to hear this toddler's sad little voice from the back seat of my car one morning, "My mother hates me." I pulled over. "What do you mean?" I asked, looking deeply into those wide eyes—as round as a full moon. "My mother hates me," he repeated. . . . Yikes! We sat on the side of the road for quite some time, as I listened to what happened over breakfast that morning. I can't remember the exact content, but honestly, whatever the transgression, it was obviously not meant to be mean or hurtful. But there you have it; this four-year-old was crushed.

That's the thing about emotions—they're quite subjective and not necessarily an indication of what is the honest reality of any given situation. Yet, they could still be truthful for us: they are *our reality.*

Our perpetrators may be real or imagined, but our pain is significant either way. And so, we heal our feelings by acknowledging and respecting them for what they are and valuing the understanding they may carry about who we are and how our character has been shaped by them. Many of us have sustained very real difficulties and sometimes outright horrific trauma. *As You Feel, So You Heal* is about honoring the emotional content that lingers and helping those feelings grow and evolve into an integrated part of who you are. Kahlil Gibran says, "Out of suffering have emerged the strongest souls."

IS IT REAL OR IS IT TRUE?

Is it real or is it true? Sometimes it's both. Even if it isn't true, a feeling is still real if you're feeling it (and remember, dismissing it or talking it away is offensive). This is the case with anxiety, right? You may think an anxiety is unjustified or it might seem unwarranted through another person's eyes, but if you're feeling it, it's real for you. True for grief too. Anger. Sadness . . . ecstatic joy. Our emotions are real, whether they seem true, or untrue, for the situation at hand. For the times when you resist your honest expression of emotion, it's helpful to notice when and how these situations arise, and to explore how you might dance with both the resistance and the emotional expression in a way that brings forth a healthy balance for honoring yourself. Regardless of what it is you're feeling, and whether or not you consider it true, in the moment you're feeling it, it's very real.

Write of Passage: Body Speak

The mind has intricate ways of communicating, but sometimes our emotions are speaking a foreign language. We can turn to the body for understanding: pain, imbalances, or diseases are often a symptom of deeper emotional pain. Migraines, digestive problems, chronic pain such as arthritis, back issues— literally, pain or illness in any part of the body may indicate emotional distress. And when you learn the body's language, you can discern what emotion is held there, the content of that emotion, and how to deal with it directly.

Physical symptoms or body imbalances can be a gift that alerts us to something that needs our attention. There is a partnership between our bodies, our hearts, and our minds; the body will provide us with strong messages when we aren't hearing our emotions. It's as if they're saying, "Help! Help! You're missing something here." Or "Enough. I can't take it anymore. I'm carrying such a burden."

> Are you at home in your own skin?

> Do you know the language of the body and how it communicates with you?

➢ Write about how your body is currently responding to your emotion(s). What is your body trying to tell you?

➢ What have been your patterns in your past? What "old" wounding still manifests through physical symptoms? You may forget a trauma, but it can still be stored in the body.

➢ We may also carry emotional pain in our bodies that comes down through the generations in our DNA. Epigenetics is a fascinating study of this phenomenon.

➢ What can you learn from this? Listening to the body, in and of itself, is a powerful act.

Have you ever needed to make a decision, and your gut tells you not to go a certain way, letting you know you're headed in the wrong direction? Or you have a full-body feeling you're on the right track—you "feel it in your bones"? This kind of intuitive sensing has an emotional base. Our bodies are intelligent and wise: they'll let us know when we need something such as food or sleep, and they'll also let us know when something isn't right. Our palms sweat when we're nervous, our stomach aches when we're apprehensive, or our chest may feel heavy when we're burdened . . . listen to your body and its sensations. There's a piece of your story there.

Where in the Body Do You Feel Emotions?

➢ What physical symptoms are speaking to you? Is there pain involved? How painful is it on a scale of 1–10?

➢ Where in your body do emotions reside? Do you bury them in your tummy or choke them off in your throat? Do you have a heart that's heavy with all the feelings it carries? Do you literally sit on them in your buttocks? Or walk all over them in your feet? Discover where they are hiding or resting in full view.

➢ Draw attention to an area that is symptomatic or houses an emotional charge. Describe it as specifically as you can with as much detail as possible.

➢ Describe the images you see as you pay attention to that space. And any activity that happens as a result of your presence in that area.

➢ If there's pain, make note of any tension or other sensation below the pain. Again, describe it as completely as possible.

➢ Now f-e-e-l into everything further. As you feel, allow the body to physically move if it wants or needs to . . . notice what kind of movements emerge.

- Speak words out loud if there are any, even if there's no one but you to listen.

- Observe any thoughts and new feelings that arise as you stay present to the symptom or the emotion in this part of your physical body, your little mobile home.

- Write until you feel done.

- Now check in again. What does it feel like now in the place the emotion lives? How would you now assess the symptom on the pain scale?

Power of Emotions on the Body

I worked with a woman for a few years as she went through a cancer journey. Actively involved with her healing, Constance is extremely bright and analytical, coming from a successful career as a financial advisor. Although she was well grounded in extensive research to physically support her healing in practical ways, Connie was open to exploring in a new direction. Through intuitive visualizations and guided journeys, we explored her body: what was balanced and working in harmony and what was not. We observed how particular areas presented themselves, and we listened when they communicated in their language with us. And then, this highly motivated and responsible woman optimized the ways in which she met those needs. At times it was something physical—such as a change in diet or supplementation. Other times it involved an emotional exploration or release. Connie worked it through piece by piece with remarkable results. She reflected to me a journey from fear to trust. "When you came in, I was in a place of great fear. Now I'm in a place of trust!" As she worked with the process as opposed to "fighting it," she came into partnership with her body and even the cancer. As she saw the impact of talking with her various parts, her confidence grew, and even though it was slow and meticulous, she felt it was invaluable. She possessed an ability to affect her physical health in a profound way. When fear shifts into trust, it can contribute to a very different physical reality. Trust can be very healing.

Head to Heart (You Have More Than One Brain)

Native cultures speak about the longest journey being the one from our heads to our hearts. And science has shown that the intelligence housed in your cranium isn't your only brain; according to research done by the HeartMath team, there is a distinct, measurable intelligence found in your heart. More than an essential pump circulating your life blood, the heart is now believed to also synchronize your heartbeat with the natural world, being a vehicle for your universal connection.

> Drop down into your heart. What do you feel there? What do you "see" there?

> Does your head typically run the show? Or do you allow your heart to chime in?

> Are your head and your heart in alignment? Do they communicate with each other? How can you encourage both parts to share with you?

> And in what ways can you draw forward your authentic heart essence and live from that perspective in your daily life?

A woman with bouts of anxiety visualizes a bright light around her heart and then encourages its warm radiance to spread throughout her entire physical form. She rests in the comfort of this beautiful heart essence. Terri also visualizes bright light emerging from her partner's heart and traveling through his body; so, when they hug or kiss, their heart lights merge. Anxiety no longer has the same power over her; she's free of its tormenting grasp, as she gives way to the brilliance of her own heart.

COLLABORATE

We've been talking about listening to our emotions and being receptive to the wisdom they carry, and by doing so, acknowledging them as guideposts. Emotions show up to give us a vital pulse about where we are and at times to alert us to something we're missing. They help us reinforce our trajectory or regroup and refocus in another direction. As we cultivate a healthy emotional intelligence, we accept our emotions—all of them—as an integral and beneficial part of us. They help us clear reactive energy and find balance through life's experiences.

 Write of Passage: Negotiating with Your Emotions

You are in this together! Take this idea further by exploring how to negotiate with your emotional parts:

> Let's say that you are both excited and scared about a new opportunity.

> Remember when we had our emotions over for tea? Negotiating with them can begin like that. You first connect with your feelings of

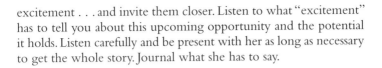

excitement . . . and invite them closer. Listen to what "excitement" has to tell you about this upcoming opportunity and the potential it holds. Listen carefully and be present with her as long as necessary to get the whole story. Journal what she has to say.

- -

> Thank your "excitement" for sharing . . . and ask her to remain present as you connect with your feelings of being scared. This is an important piece because now "excitement" can listen to what "scared" has to say.

> Be present and attentive as "scared" conveys the picture from her point of view. Take your time and journal about this piece too. Thank her for sharing.

- -

> Now ask "scared" if she has anything to say to "excitement." . . . This may sound strange, yet it's remarkable what surfaces when you ask the question!

> Ask "excitement" if there's anything she needs to say to "scared."

> Depending on what arises, you may be complete . . . or if you find these two feelings are in conflict, you can be a mediator between them, helping them come to a place of partnership, not necessarily in agreement, but at least agreeing to work together. So, for example, "excitement" may need "scared" to not be such a downer when she's feeling great about the new potential. And "scared" may need to have her fears heard and considered. If you can get them to work together to meet each other's needs, there will be harmony in the home. And where is that? Inside you!

I hope this gives you some idea of how effective these techniques can be. Every situation is unique, so your approach may differ, but I have found what I've described as a great starting point. Your open curiosity is what matters the most.

affirm

Today I choose to accept, respect, love,
and honor all my emotions!

Write of Passage: Live in the Question

Have patience with everything that remains unsolved in your heart . . . live in the question.

—Rainer Maria Rilke, *Letters to a Young Poet*

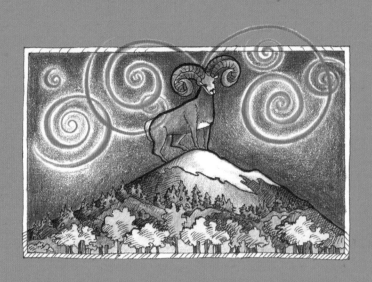

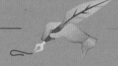

LEARN MORE ABOUT YOUR OWN
PATTERNS . . . AND TRY
SHIFTING A DOWNWARD
SPIRAL TO AN UPWARD ONE.

JOURNAL ABOUT YOUR
OBSERVATIONS AND INSIGHTS.

Do you think you need to know the answer to understand or find resolution? The truth is that when you ask a question, the Universe rallies to answer it . . . and your own wisdom and insight step forward too.

> Be curious and launch into inquiry mode.

> Is there something you'd like to know about your emotions? Would you like to gain insight about how you feel?

> Create a running list of cosmic questions in your journal. They'll sit on the "back burner," simmering on the transformational fire.

> Expect to receive clarity . . . be poised for it.

> Observe what bubbles forth within you and what shows up in your outer world. Life will demonstrate your "answers" in a variety of ways.

THE ADVENTURE OF HEALING AND TRANSFORMATION

Transformation is vast and deep; its parameters cannot be contained or defined. Like the element of Fire that's supported us through this phase, transformation can be small and simmering, or massive and raging out of control. Developing strategies for coping with even the most intense transformation leads to a masterful life—one infused with trust and belief in your ability to navigate through, regardless of the intensity of the challenge that presents itself.

Having come from your initial Awakening in Self-Discovery, you've stepped right into the initiation of the Great Departure held within our Transformation piece. Releasing the grip of attachment on what exists allows you to venture into the great unknown, which holds unforeseen treasures and golden opportunities. Learning to sustain the heat of the alchemical fire enables you to spin gold from even your most difficult and heavy emotions. And being present, befriending, negotiating, and collaborating with your emotions shifts them from the status of a strange outsider to an integrated aspect of the wholeness of you. There is so much more to your journey of transformation; return again and again to explore more deeply and venture further into your own wilderness and the great beyond.

1. CREATE A LIST OF WAYS TO BLOW OFF EMOTIONAL STEAM

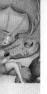

2. ASSESSMENT: NOTICE WHEN YOU'RE IN AN UPWARD EMOTIONAL SPIRAL OR A DOWNWARD ONE

The physical sensations of fear and excitement are very similar. We spoke about honoring both of these feelings by inviting them to negotiate with each other. Once they work collaboratively, forming an alliance, are there times when you can shift a fear to curiosity and even excitement?

3. A LITTLE BIT ABOUT "CORD CUTTING"

This is an important and complex topic. When undergoing our transformation, at times it's important to cut the cords that bind us to the past or to individuals who stunt our forward thinking and development. If you are unfamiliar with this concept or strategies for accomplishing this form of release, visit my website to find out how you can access my video about cord cutting.

4. CEREMONIAL RITUAL: BURNING-BOWL RELEASE

Partake in a Burning Bowl ceremony by burning a piece of paper or papers with a few words to describe the emotion (or emotions) you are ready to release. Be sure you have a physically safe container or fire pit to create this ceremonial ritual.

➢ Bless your space in a way that's meaningful for you.

➢ Record your emotion (or emotions) on one or more slips of paper.

➢ Bless them for the ways in which they've served you. We often find our greatest strength in our weakest moments. Look for that strength and then acknowledge it. A lens of gratitude helps you see their value.

➢ You most likely will not be releasing the entire emotion, but perhaps a manner in which you've expressed that emotion or a nuance of it that you wish to grow or develop into a more effective expression. For example, lashing out in rage . . . you might release that with the intention of embracing healthier ways of expressing your intense anger.

➢ As you see that which no longer serves you go up in flames, let it go.

➢ Give thanks for this sacred process.

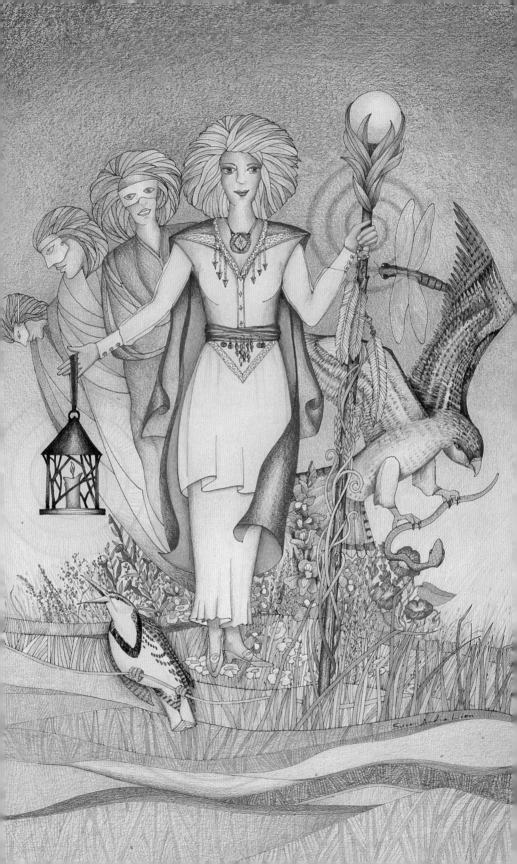

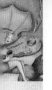

Proceed slowly if you want to release a multitude of pesky issues and sticky emotions. By taking your time with this process, your flame will be strong and steady, rather than tossing everything in at once and causing a raging fire to erupt.

5. CEREMONIAL RITUAL: BY THE LIGHT OF THE MOON

Follow the moon cycle by observing its beauty in each stage of its appearance. Write about an emotion in the dark void of the New Moon, recording your hopes and intentions for the emotion you've chosen. In whatever way is right for you, show appreciation and gratitude to Grandmother Moon for being present in her returning light as you receive inspiration for staying present to your own cycles of unfolding.

Take time throughout this moon cycle to reflect on the emotion you chose to focus on . . . and be open to your understanding coming into the light with the expanding belly of the moon. In the brightness of the ripe Full Moon, reflect once again, being grateful for whatever you've received. Thank yourself. Thank the moon—you may want to offer her a prayer or a song of gratitude.

Our powerful connection with the natural world clearly demonstrates cycles of life that move in and through all things, including us. Cyclical movement doesn't go backward but progresses in an upward spiral. The moon is constantly changing her appearance right before our eyes; that same moon has been seen in our night sky since the beginning of time . . . and it will be there long after we are gone. That same moon is seen across the globe as well as in your own backyard.

6. CONTEMPLATION/MEDITATION: DRAGONS TO PRINCESSES

Consider how your "dragons" are transforming. Your body knows how to heal, your feelings are keys to the dungeon, you've been asked to step up by being brave enough to realize you are your own knight, your own prince, and you're here to rescue yourself. You can do this . . . you're discovering your adventurous, warrioress self, and she is fiercely able to walk through the alchemical fire to transform what no longer works for her.

Honor your journey, realizing it's the steps along the way, not just the destination, that matters. As you recognize and let go of what no longer serves you, you create fertile and receptive space for what can come forth, revealing new layers of your authentic self and your greater yet-to-be.

Chapter 3
SACRED PATH

You absolutely belong here. It was no mistake that you were born. There is something so uniquely precious about you; no one else is exactly like you.

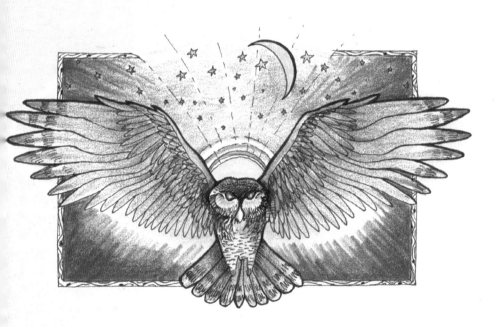

You are a meaningful part of the Divine Plan. You have the ability to contribute to this world in a way no one else can, and without you, that piece would be lost. It's your birthright to create through your life's expression and by acknowledging the magnificent gift of life; every moment becomes precious, every experience valued for its significance. Accepting your special reserved spot in the "circle of life" points out your responsibility to care for yourself and enhances your appreciation of the seemingly mundane found in everyday pursuits—even going to the grocery store can become a wonderful adventure. You never know what you might see or who you might meet or where it could lead. Your path, every day, in every way, is sacred. The choices you make are sacred. Your emotions, and the feelings you feel, are sacred. Your *entire life* is your sacred path.

 Write of Passage: The Wheel of Life

On a fresh page in your journal, create a Wheel of Life.

> ➢ Choose a photo or take a picture out of a magazine to represent you, and glue it in the center of your page. Or you could draw one (even a stick figure).

> ➢ Write your name in the center, too, as you bless the center sacred space. That center represents the center of your life's wheel.

> ➢ Draw spokes that radiate out from the center. Each spoke on this wheel represents an aspect of your life. Draw as many as you need, and label them. Since they originate from the center, they are energetically intertwined and interconnected through their connection with you; you are the center of your wheel of life. With this visual image it's easy to see clearly that no matter how seemingly separate, one aspect of your life affects the others as they each impact the overall balance through you. If one spoke is too heavy, it'll throw the entire wheel off-kilter. Your work life affects your home life. Your friendships affect your marriage. Your motherhood entwines with work, even if you attempt to keep them in their separate compartments.

> ➢ Observe and interact with your feelings related to all aspects and every role in a respectful and productive manner.

BREATH OF LIFE

In the Sacred Path component, we engage with the element of Air. When you entertain thoughts of "Air," you might think of air to fan your transformational fire or to cool you in your transformational heat; you might draw in an image of wind beneath your wings to lift you up to a higher vantage point . . . drawing in a winged ally like the graceful owl is helpful when working with the element of Air. And we also know that air is essential for being alive and is expressed in and through every breath of life. And that breath may be powerfully utilized as a vehicle to bring us home to ourselves when we breathe deeply to our center and get in touch with what we're feeling inside. That essential breath can be used to manifest our desires when we choose our words wisely and create affirmative statements to inspire and motivate ourselves. Our ever-present breath can be used purposefully when we shape and reshape how we show up in the world, through potent words that focus our thoughts and escape our mouths even when no one else is around.

> Know you are embodied in this human form to experience and to feel.

> Connect with the air around you, the Earth beneath you, and the Cosmos above you every morning.

> Keenly observe what you see. Keenly observe what you feel. Marvel at its expansiveness. This seemingly simple act connects you with all-there-is in our grand, creative universe . . . and subtly opens you to the greatness wanting to express through you.

> Take several long and deep, conscious breaths. Allow your breath to clear, and release anything that hangs heavily upon you. Allow your breath to feed you with vital life-force energy. Allow your breath to bring you fully present within yourself.

> Light a candle to give thanks for your light in the world. Then, speak (out loud) your prayers or your mala blessings—for love, for joy, for peace, for happiness . . . for whatever you choose.

> Speak words of gratitude for people, situations, and lessons you've learned or are learning.

> Speak affirmations for how you will show up today as the gift you are in this world.

> Record and speak aloud any intentions for your day. Infuse them with confidence and assurance in your ability to bring them forth. Commit to step forward with purposeful steps.

> Smile with delightful anticipation for what lies ahead.

> If you need an extra boost, listen to Karen Drucker's "Thank You for This Day" or Scott Kalechstein's "Say YES to Your Dreams" or Jana Stanfield's "If I Were Brave," or a similar upbeat song.

> Reflect and repeat one or more of these practices as your day ends. Infuse the morning and evening with what is sacred as you honor your own sacred path through morning and nighttime rituals.

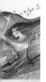

DIVINE TIMING

When you're confident with your ability to process emotionally, you are better equipped to handle anything that comes along, and you can relax into trusting life unfolding. Recognize and believe that you're in the right place, and the right time NOW. You are in sacred divine timing for your highest and your best, in spite of any appearance to the contrary. Believe that you are in sync with what serves you now. Celebrate your successes . . . and be open to the wisdom held in your challenges.

 ## Write of Passage: Traumatic Timeline

In the midst of pain and trauma, we can bless the thing that's cracking us open, exposing our most raw inner core. I've seen time and time again when we ask, "What needs to be revealed?" valuable information surfaces. Emotions can take us to a mountaintop or send us plummeting into a swamp; either way, there's something we can learn from the terrain. As we navigate through difficulties, moving, in spite of our vulnerability, becomes one of our strengths.

> Create a timeline of your life.

> Mark points of injury, loss, pain, and traumatic situations.

> Connect two points when there's something that spanned over a time period, so it'll be easy to follow.

> Label your marks.

> Sit back and reflect on your timeline and how your life has evolved. When you do so, you'll see things from this perspective that you might not realize when you're living through it.

When I did this process many years ago, I realized how reactive I'd been during my younger years, acting out from my place of childhood wounding. Having my baby at twenty and then later becoming a single mother shifted my rebellious, downward spiral into a positive upswing. I was "getting it together" for my son, and recognizing that fact enabled me to treasure him even more!

The power of imagination has long been utilized for healing trauma. Through visualization techniques, difficult parts of our life's story can be resculpted into something useful—or, at the very least, tolerable. We can also explore ways of taking care of the inner child or the wounded adult who went through harsh experiences. We discover the path of acceptance for what has already happened by shaping its contours in a way that pulls forth the meaning it contains. Instead of resisting the harsh content, when we go to the heart of the matter and see it for what it is, we neutralize its power over us. The "traumatic timeline" can be an effective tool, and journaling on various

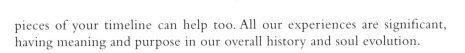

pieces of your timeline can help too. All our experiences are significant, having meaning and purpose in our overall history and soul evolution.

* If there is a major difficulty or a persistent pain you're dealing with, please know that your feelings matter; your pain matters. Your process may not be a simple or easy one, and I suggest you seek support from someone trained in trauma resolution and healing. I care about you and the burden you carry. And I'm knowing you are led to the right people and the most-beneficial support systems to help you through it. As you work with the overwhelming feelings that confront you, you'll build both a tolerance for them and a confidence in your ability to navigate through them. It takes time. It takes attention. But trust me when I say, it's doable.

IT'S *ALL* DIVINE TIMING

I'd planned to get together with a dear friend on Friday, and he, being a thoughtful planner, called early in the week to finalize our arrangements. Since I was in the midst of a demanding writing project and couldn't really think four days ahead, I suggested we reconnect later in the week. I blinked, and it was already Friday morning. I started to text to finalize our plans when I realized that it would be best to call and maybe apologize for leaving our plans for the last minute.

"Hello!" An unfamiliar and hurried voice answered the phone. She sounded a bit desperate. "Oh, I'm sorry, I think I have the wrong number." "No you DON'T!" she said. "Who are you calling?" "My friend Randy." "Yes, this is him . . . I mean this is his phone . . . I found a phone in the snow. Cars have run over it, but it appears that it's still working. His driver's license and credit cards are here too." "Thank goodness someone like you found it," I said. "When I lost my phone someone used it until I shut it off." I thanked her for being an angel today. When I called my friend on his business landline, he had no idea that his phone, his credit cards, and his driver's license were even missing! I had been concerned about needing to apologize for not contacting him sooner . . . and instead, my last-minute call was obviously Divine Timing!

Synchronicities and mini-miracles happen every day. When disasters happen, we often hear stories of how individuals' typical timing patterns were altered, reshaping their day, so they were not in their usual place, avoiding the disaster that occurred. We're on our sacred path with each part of our day: the good, the challenging, and the mundane. Completing a project, being recognized with an award, or having a perfect date night—part of your sacred path. Working through a difficult situation, struggling with an addiction or getting dumped—yep, part of your sacred path. And

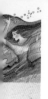

getting up in the morning, cooking or sharing a meal, sitting in a chair reading this book, or even cleaning the toilet are all a part of your sacred path. From the time you begin by opening your eyes, greeting the new day, until you rest your head on your pillow, every part of each day is you on your sacred path. For that matter, when you shut your eyes at night and go into the dreamtime, you've got it—you are still on your sacred path.

ABOUT PERSPECTIVE

I saw a Facebook meme that caused me to laugh out loud: There's a rose that's wilting on the vine, saying, "Oh, dear . . . oh, my. The pH of this soil isn't right . . . I'm d-y-i-n-g." And then there's a dandelion, stretching through a crack, screaming, "Yahoo!!! Cement!" It's all about perspective.

> I was thinking about dandelions recently. I couldn't help it. There's a portion of our fence down right now, and my next-door neighbor is growing dandelions—hundreds of them! I've gone over and picked bagfuls of those white-headed sprouts to avoid them coming my way. I even tried using a hand vac to capture those pesky white heads. Then, I picked yellow ones in an attempt to keep them from turning to seed. The more I picked, the more that grew. And my neighbor was not participating in slowing or halting the repetitive cycle I was so invested in stopping.
>
> Finally, one day I looked at the white seeds wafting over into my meditation garden, and fondly remembered how we'd blown the full, round puffballs with delight while making a wish as children. I started seeing the white wispy seeds as "wishes" landing in my garden. They seemed to fit perfectly in my sacred meditation garden. Now don't get me wrong, I'll still dig out those plants to avoid dandelions taking over my yard, but first, I'll envision that they're wishes, energetically finding their ground and coming to fruition before my eyes.

Perspective. I'm sure you've heard the story of people blindfolded and stationed at various points around an elephant and how they each described that animal quite differently. When we shift our perspective, our reality often shifts too. One of my friends who's had a longtime happy marriage speaks about her younger years of criticizing the differences she saw in her husband. and thinking, "this can't possibly work. How can I be married to someone who _____." Then she realized all his fine points and ever since has focused her eyes on what's precious. Decades later, they're still in love and launching into new paths of discovery together.

Look at a situation you're in or an emotion you're experiencing. Would it be helpful to shift your perspective? Write a paragraph or two from one vantage point. Now shift and look at it from another angle. Continue as long as you have additional possible perspectives to explore.

Your perspective colors your experience and leads to your suffering or your sense of success. One person's challenge is another's opportunity. There's an amusing story about two shoe salesman who go to a remote village where no one wears shoes. One sends a disappointing message: "Leaving today. No market here." The other one pens an urgent plea: "Send cases of shoes immediately. Wide-open field. Unlimited possibilities!"
(www.forbes.com/sites/ronashkenas/2011/04/13/do-you-have-a-mindset-for-growth/#24fadbca2e30.)

RELEASE THE IDEA OF "NOT ENOUGH"

When I was growing up in a large family with a lot of kids, there never seemed to be enough bananas. We had an incredibly frustrating banana shortage. Mom would buy a bunch, and, as if they fell into a great void, they'd disappear almost as soon as she walked through the door. It was one of many messages around me that said, "There is not enough for you"—not enough time, not enough space, not enough treats, not enough attention . . .

And then, of course, there were experiences that seemed to say that I, too, was "not enough." No matter how skillful or how gifted one is, there will be others who are achieving in a more visible or greater way or are a few steps ahead of you. We'll focus on trusting yourself in our fifth chapter as a part of life's great mystery. The only way to shake this paralyzing perspective is to take steps to rise above it. The antidote to this source of suffering is to focus on what you *do* have, what you are achieving, and what wonderful strength of character you possess. Move through any sense of lack or limitation and recognize the infinite potential of the Universe. If all possibilities are available to you, which ones will you choose? The Mayan elder Angel Chiquan says: "You are a star that shines in your own Universe . . . you don't need to search anywhere else. You have it in you" (September 2017, For Heaven's Sale Books).

YOU ARE THE ONE

It's been said many times, but it bears repeating: You are the one you've been waiting for. There's no other person or situation that will bring it all together for you—no perfect job or great love that will bring you what you desire. That task, that adventure, falls onto your shoulders. Joseph Campbell said it best when he talked about the hero's journey with all its challenges and pitfalls leading to each of us carrying home the gold. And in our transformation section, we explored the idea of alchemically creating gold from the heavy, dense emotional material within us. When we recognize that the gold is truly within us, perhaps still in its

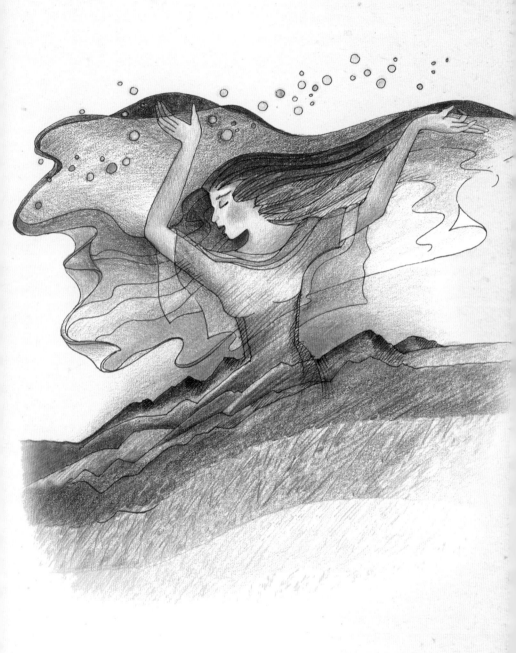

raw form, life becomes about the weaving of those golden threads in and through all we are and all we do. Somewhere in the midst of our grand adventures and within the intricacies of our many valuable lessons, we navigate our way home to who we really are and who we were meant to be. There is so much more to us than what we've known up to this point; there's a wealth of indescribably lavish treasure within us to find and share.

 Write of Passage: Creating the Space

My dear friend Jana Stanfield, a well-known motivational speaker and singer, wrote a call-to-action song, "All the Good" (2014), with powerful words, suggesting:

"I cannot do all the good the world needs. But the world needs all the good that I can do!"

www.janastanfield.com

Look inside yourself and explore through your writing.

> What is yours to do?

> What wants to birth through you?

Hint: Notice what is hovering around you, asking to be given the breath of life.

> What is it that only you can do?

> Yes, there is something, and probably more than one thing, that only you can do.

> Own yourself as unique; you are not a copy of anyone else. You were put in this world to be yourself. How can you show up more authentically?

> Believing—even when something seems too large or far, far away— feeds its possibility. What you believe becomes.

> Give your ideas and inspirations life expression by speaking their names, unapologetically, out loud.

> One shamanic practice is to bless something sacred with your breath. Bless your ideas and inspiration with your breath by speaking them alive!

You may not be the very best at something; perhaps you're even stumbling or struggling along the way, but if you're willing to show up and put in the effort, you may be the exact right person to manifest that idea into form. When my son was young, I started a children's theater. Having grown up in Stratford, Connecticut, at a time when it was home to the American Shakespeare Theatre and a thriving children's theater, I'd had precious times in that world of imagination. I wanted my bright, intellectually gifted son to have similar memories. And at almost four, he memorized our scripts word for word long before anyone else did, by listening to our actors reading them, so Michael became our official prompter. I wasn't the most experienced in theater; there were a few Broadway actors and a director who lived in our small town. When the inspiration came to me, I acted upon it and gained quite a following. Our small troupe was eventually sponsored by the county Arts Council and received a grant to tour several counties; a reality way beyond my original vision.

Your true nature has infinite potential. You are designed for greatness and can program yourself for success. Look to the horizon and catch a glimmer of what's possible—as grand as the cosmos, as grounded as the earth—that is your spiritual inheritance. Recognize your innate wholeness and reach inside to touch the root of your truest character residing in your most evolved self. Everything you do is your sacred path home. How can you express your true Essential Self? How can you develop and realize your unique awesomeness, bringing it into form?

Can you hear the sweet and sacred sound of your own breath? That's life breathing through you. That's you breathing life. Bless each breath and make your moments worthwhile.

> Try writing a personal fairy tale. Written in the form of a myth, our stories take on a different cadence, a different style. You can begin with "once upon a time" or "there once was a girl" to set the mood.

> Then just let your thoughts spill out on the page. You'll find that you may access a deeper part of yourself; one that speaks metaphorically and describes symbolically.

> This personal myth is geared toward the unique shape and contour of your personality and your life's adventure. Through the act of writing, you may reach parts that are still hurting and have not yet healed.

> Weave a tale of hope. Be your own healer, putting a potent salve on old wounds still tender, as well as new ones still raw with injury.

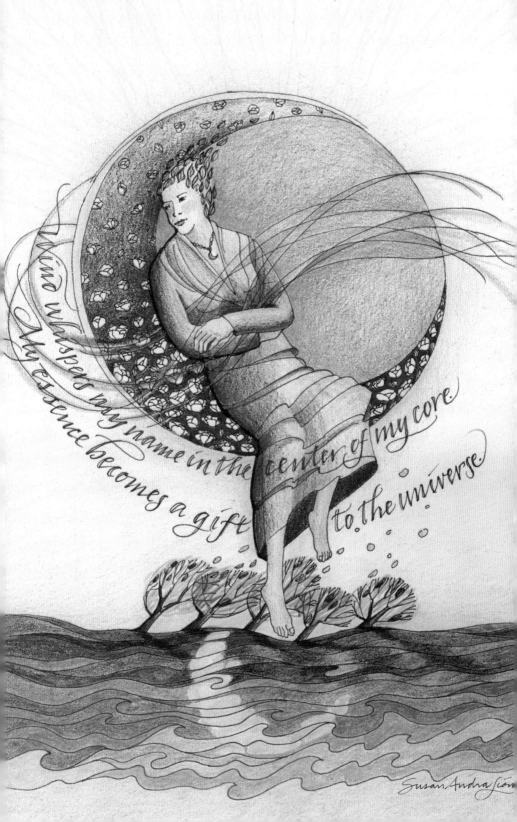

I whisper my name in the center of my core.

My essence becomes a gift to the universe.

Susan Andra Lion

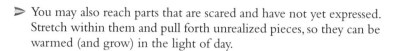

> You may also reach parts that are scared and have not yet expressed. Stretch within them and pull forth unrealized pieces, so they can be warmed (and grow) in the light of day.

> You may access characteristics you never dreamed existed; they've been waiting for you to discover them. Your personal myth can tell you the most-insightful truths.

> Every part of your journey has meaning and purpose; every piece of your learning is significant.

WHAT'S IN THE AIR?

The Universe responds to who you believe you are, what you believe is happening, and what you imagine is possible. Yes, there are outside factors that contribute to your reality, but the single most important piece within your control is your attitudes and beliefs. What can you do to positively influence the reality you experience? Examine the content connected to each emotion you feel, and let go of any thought that someone (or the Universe) is doing something to you—that you're at the mercy of what life brings you. Instead, observe and praise all that is being done for your good, and notice the ways in which life, Itself, is conspiring for your growth. Be careful how you "spin" the truth—the story you tell reflects how you think and feel, and your words blow life-giving air on a seed that plants itself in fertile soil that creates anew. Believe that anything is possible, and you'll bring forth more than what you think *might be* possible!

 Write of Passage: "I Believe in Me" Letter to Self

> Begin with *Dearest Woman* or *My Dearest* or whatever you choose as an endearment. Make it super loving and accepting!

> You may want to acknowledge where you are emotionally. So, if it's been a difficult day or week, don't sugar coat it, but don't stay stuck in it either. Then shift into appreciation and gratitude: for who you are, for how you're showing up, for what you bring to the situation, and affirm that you'll get through it.

> Explore the possibilities available to you. How are you inspired to move forward?

- - - - - - - - - - - - - - - - - - - -

> Writing a "love letter" to yourself when things are going well reinforces the goodness of the Universe (and yourself). It invites in more of the same . . . and helps you imagine receiving it. Praise what's working in your life. Include clear, encouraging statements such as "You are incredibly beautiful" or "I am so proud of you."

➤ If you're rushed for time you can make it short and sweet, try this: Dear _____, You are doing the best you can and I'm proud of you. Keep moving . . . Love, me

Or simply:

Dear *(me)*,

I love you.

Practice giving and receiving love from yourself. And take care of yourself in nurturing ways; protect yourself from destructive people. Albert Einstein said, "Stay away from negative people. They have a problem for every solution." Don't you just love that? Of course, sometimes having a solution for every problem isn't helpful either. But finding something positive in every challenge can be encouraging and inspirational. Draw toward you the people who support you in the way you need, and return the favor to your dear ones in the best ways you can.

Trust and know you are worthy to receive the goodness of life. Affirm that awareness, in different ways, every day. Raise your consciousness level and your manifestation will be more successful. Emma Curtis Hopkins says, "There is Good for me and I ought to have it."

GUIDEPOSTS ON YOUR SACRED PATH

Our outer reality often reflects to us what we need to know—not only about other people or situations, but also about where we are developmentally, where we are in our life's evolution, and the characteristics we possess at our core. Our emotions can act as pointers to understanding ourselves and our true feelings, so we can make better choices that lead us in our desired direction.

How many of us were taught to embrace our emotions and learn how to effectively deal with them? You lived through the terrible twos with the typical outbursts, but were you told, "Yes, sweetie, you're really feeling now. Good girl. Keep it up. Keep on feeling those feelings!" Probably not. Yet, stuffing emotional content doesn't work either. Repressed emotions typically pop out when you least expect them to or when it's most inconvenient—in the midst of an important meeting or when you're entertaining your in-laws for dinner, suddenly you blurt out something in a fit of rage or become a puddle in the middle of the conference table. All that bottled-up energy has its way with you, my dear.

Become more present to yourself—your real self—all of you. That which looks pretty and all composed, and that which is messy and raw, with a runny nose. Honor the shades and nuances of your colorful self and you'll learn to appropriately and effectively vent all those parts of you. You literally stretch into every nook and cranny of who you are as a human being, and you love her. YOU love her. You LOVE her. By accepting your emotions, you love yourself. For she's a sacred being in a human suit on the path of life; at essence, she's a divine being. And she's doing the best she can. So cut her some slack, okay?

If we get stuck in the harsh dichotomy of right and wrong, black and white, good and bad, we miss the point. Life is rarely that simple. Having a big, fat, ugly emotion does not mean that you made the wrong choice or a bad decision. *As You Feel, So You Heal* enables you the time and the space to take an objective look at what's coming up within you, so you can listen to what it has to say and learn how to best handle that emotion. Your feelings give you the opportunity to repattern old patterns of reaction or past-programmed patterns of behavior to be more in alignment with who you hope to be. Again, they're guideposts, showing you the way down the next trail on your sacred path.

Feel your feelings in the time and the space in which they're meant to be. When you do, you bypass the need to heal later. You do it, right here and right now. You move in and through with a confidence of knowing you can do this. True emotions serve you in even the most challenging situation: we're wired that way as humans for a reason.

It's time to revisit these ideas:

> Is your heart open or closed?

> Is your mind receptive or set in its ways?

> How deeply do you feel? Are you in touch? Or detached?

> Do you dramatically feel? Are you overly sensitive? And how do you manage that extreme sensitivity?

> Life is a potent schoolhouse enabling us to feel and to grow. Being present—whether or not it feels "good"—ensures that we make the most of its potential.

> Are you stuck rigidly within parameters of what is acceptable and true, or are you open to new discovery?

> Life is a glorious adventure: How much of it are you allowing yourself to experience?

 Write of Passage: The Emotional Me

Continue to objectively observe and chronicle your emotions. This can be free-form writing in paragraphs, or it can also be a list. Here's another idea of a way to look at your feelings:

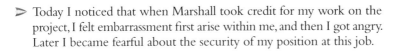

> Today I noticed that when Marshall took credit for my work on the project, I felt embarrassment first arise within me, and then I got angry. Later I became fearful about the security of my position at this job.

Or:

Marshall—credit for my work
   # 1 embarrassed
   # 2 angry
   # 3 fearful

_ _

> Next, you'll want to think about what you observed, and record your understanding about what happened to you.

When he first spoke about my work as if it were his own, I was embarrassed because it appeared like I hadn't done anything to contribute to this project. Then I was angry that he put me in that position. Much later I felt fear rise. What if they don't think I'm doing a good job?

This longer process is helpful because sometimes through the longhand writing we discover insights about what happened or our reaction to it. Your contemplation may be much longer than this example and include details about the environment, conversation, and a more in-depth description of your feelings

> or the short-list version:
   #1 embarrassed: for how I looked.
   #2 angry: that he didn't give me any credit.
   #3 fearful: for my job security.

This can be beneficial when your time to write is short or if you don't want to take a lot of time with it. Sometimes a very brief written reflection may stir and surface great insights. And you might also think about it a lot but record just the highlights.

Choose which method works best for you. Learning to do this type of self-reflection can inspire us to turn our faces right into the wind and be confident that any storm that comes our way will, in its proper time, pass. Consider brainstorming possible actions you might have taken or can take right now in support of what you're feeling, and also what you might do moving forward.

BE CONSCIOUS OF YOUR WORDS

A new client was referred to me for a thyroid imbalance. Emily had never been to an energy practitioner before and spoke to me at length about what she was (and was not) comfortable with pursuing during our bodywork treatment. "No meditation . . . or relaxation techniques," she said; "if I totally relax, that's when the devil will get me!" I looked at her intently, assessing her statement and realized she was serious. "Okay, no meditation or relaxation techniques," I said matter-of-factly. My role is to support a client in the best way possible, as long as it's within the natural parameter of my personal and professional integrity.

Continuing with our intake, I explained that the energy I utilized worked on all levels, simultaneously, and that I, the practitioner, did not control or manipulate that energy. My role was not to diagnose or prescribe anything specific. My place was to support and assist the partnership between the energy and the person I was serving. As an experienced "bridge," I was blessed to have witnessed many wondrous and even-miraculous occurrences.

Emily was ready. Her thyroid had been surgically removed, and initially she said she wanted it to grow back. After some questioning, we identified her desire more specifically: "I'd like my thyroid to function at full capacity as a healthy thyroid." She believed this was the best course for her—and she was under a doctor's care. In fact, Emily had an appointment with blood work later this week, the day after our three sessions were complete. And so, we began.

Typically, I would talk a person into a more relaxed state, but since Emily had already made her wish known in this regard, I simply sat still. I didn't even ask her to focus on her breath. As I moved through a couple of positions with my hands on her head, I could feel her body relax ever so slightly. When I cradled my hands above her throat, she inhaled deeply with an audible sound. "My husband is literally choking the life force right out of me!" she said. I shuddered with an eerie wave of energy moving through my entire body and up through the top of my head. An intuitive sense of the power of this moment struck me.

"What?"

"My husband—he sucks the living life right out of me."

When Emily returned for her second session the next day, her face looked very, very pale, and her eyes were red and puffy. "When I got home yesterday, there was a suitcase in the hallway at the front door . . . my husband . . . he left me last night . . . he says for good."

Choose your words wisely! And think about what you're saying:

➤ "I'm sick and tired."

➤ "She's a pain in the neck" or "he's a pain in the ass."

- "It scares me to death."

- "He's killing me."

- "I hate her."

- "Kill two birds with one stone." Louise Hay spoke pointedly about this one, saying, "Why would you want to kill two birds?"

Emily went to the doctor the day after our third session, and he cut her thyroid medication in half. She took an energy class from me a couple of weeks later, and her medication was cut in half again. After a couple of months, she was taken off all medication, and her doctor said, "The small piece of your thyroid is functioning at full thyroid capacity." His words matched what Emily had spoken as her desire.

Emily's husband never returned, and eventually they divorced. She went on to pursue a master's degree in social work, something she'd always wanted to do but hadn't because her husband didn't approve. Years later I bumped into her and was pleased to hear she was very happy. I don't believe Emily's words caused her husband to leave . . . but I do think they aptly described a situation that was contributing to her emotional and physical health problems.

Words have power and meaning; they have energy and a vibration that ripples on beyond the moment you let them go. Don't let confusing or counterproductive words cultivate realities you wouldn't choose. Language has power and holds great potential to help or to harm, to build or to destroy, to cut right to the inner soft core of a person or encourage one with a heavy heart. Practice neutralizing or clearing anything you say that you don't really mean. Reshape and repattern words that aimlessly fall from your mouth, and be mindful when you start to say something that isn't going to be easy to "take back." Each word is an entity unto itself—is it really what you want to put out into the world?

- Observe the words you use to describe how you feel.

- How do others receive them?

- Notice how others describe how they feel—and how you react to any of their words. What kind of "charge" is there?

- When words just spill over, coming out without much thought or consideration, do they portray what you really want to say? Or do you need to filter?

- You may use words learned a long time ago; perhaps even in childhood. Are they true to your present way of being? Have you evolved past them? What outgrown words or phrases do you still speak?

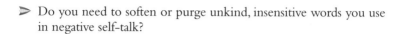

> Do you need to soften or purge unkind, insensitive words you use in negative self-talk?

Words have much more of an impact than only in the time they're spoken. People may hold onto our words for decades, and their impact ripples forward in consequences long after we've let go of them. Consideration and thought will help evolve your words to be less of an emotional venting and more apt emotional communication. Develop an emotional intelligence and an emotional maturity by learning how to acknowledge and convey your emotions in appropriate, effective ways. You have power in your words. Use that power wisely.

My accountant spoke to me proudly about her niece. Both Jan and I have been licensed spiritual coaches for decades, so we know a little bit about being positive and supportive. Still we had to marvel at Suzie's way of handling young children in her care. When one child wants a toy that the other one has, or gets frustrated over something that comes up naturally in their daily play, words sometimes get mean and biting. Suzie looks them deeply in their little eyes and gently asks, "Is that an encouraging word?"

Don't you love it? When you speak to others, ask yourself: "Is that an encouraging word?"

When you speak to yourself with your internal chatter, ask yourself: "Is that an encouraging word?"

Affirmations

One remarkably helpful use of our life's breath is to speak positive and affirming thoughts. Powerful declarations can color our inner and outer world. When we think and speak ideas of possibility, they help us accept the idea, and our outer reality often begins to shift toward our success.

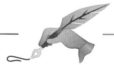

When you speak to others, ask yourself: "Is that an encouraging word?" When you speak to yourself with your internal chatter, ask yourself: "Is that an encouraging word?"

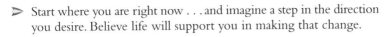
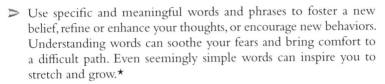

➢ Start where you are right now . . . and imagine a step in the direction you desire. Believe life will support you in making that change.

➢ Use specific and meaningful words and phrases to foster a new belief, refine or enhance your thoughts, or encourage new behaviors. Understanding words can soothe your fears and bring comfort to a difficult path. Even seemingly simple words can inspire you to stretch and grow.★

➢ Make strong, clear statements to those around you and to yourself, being careful to catch and neutralize any defeating ones, so as not to confuse the energetic field of creation.

- -

➢ One technique I learned years ago that really helps get past the part of the brain that doubts, or resists change, is to say, "In the past this was true, but what I know now is _____."

➢ Don't perpetuate old stories of disaster or defeat, but embrace new and uplifted ones and feed them daily. By acknowledging your earlier days and honoring your lessons, you can build on your past as you move forward.

- -

➢ As you guide yourself to develop in a desired direction, sometimes your experience still mirrors the old belief with patterns of the old behavior. By noticing your thoughts, and the words you use to describe your thoughts, you can refine what you say to reflect the new you. By changing what you think and say, you reinforce your evolving self, propelling you forward. Momentum builds with the power to continue moving in ever-widening circles of success.

★ I outline, in detail, creating and using affirmations effectively in *Turtle Wisdom: Coming Home to Yourself* (2007) and the *Turtle Wisdom Playbook: A Motivational Coloring Adventure* (2016).

In the poignant memoir, *A Stolen Life* (2012), Jaycee Duggard chronicles being kidnapped at eleven and held captive in the backyard of a twisted and perverted couple for eighteen years. She drew on everything she could just to survive almost two decades of sexual abuse and torture with complete loss of control. Even her most basic needs weren't met—it was months before her perpetrators gave her a toothbrush, she was kept in a dark shed with no light, and for years she was at the mercy of a dangerously demented sexual offender. Jaycee attributes her love of reading, and the self-help books this man had from when he was in jail, for enabling her to cultivate an attitude that not only helped her survive but, once she gained her freedom, has led her to do the meticulous

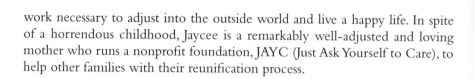

work necessary to adjust into the outside world and live a happy life. In spite of a horrendous childhood, Jaycee is a remarkably well-adjusted and loving mother who runs a nonprofit foundation, JAYC (Just Ask Yourself to Care), to help other families with their reunification process.

GRATEFUL FOR THE ABILITY TO FEEL

Faith is an oasis in the heart which can never be reached by the caravan of thinking.

—Kahlil Gibran

We are gifted with our human capacity to feel. Even our most basic animal instincts bring a valuable aspect of feeling that contributes to our overall emotional repertoire.

Continue to affirm this mantra:

I appreciate my ability to feel. By opening to, acknowledging, and honoring my feelings, I can heal the past, be mindful in the present, and vision my future. I bless where I've been, where I am, and where I'm going. Life is good!

GUARDIANSHIP

What do you think it means to be a guardian? It *doesn't* mean ownership. When we try to possess, dominate, or control, we block the ability to expand and grow; we impede development. When you're a guardian, your influence is one of support, reinforcing the human right-to-be. Your protection comes from a soul-level respect and appreciation, motivating you to allow people their natural evolution. Guardianship is a cooperative effort between the guardian and what is being guarded.

If we imagine being the guardians, rather than owners, of our emotions, it affects how we relate to them. Instead of trying to dominate or control them, we support their natural evolution—one that can contribute to our overall growth. As we move through our emotional processes, developing emotional intelligence and emotional maturity, the face of our emotions naturally changes. It develops deep wisdom lines and playful, happiness crow's-feet!

 Write of Passage: Revisiting the Sacred Circle

Many sacred practices utilize the universal dynamic of a circle. A circle is symbolic of no one person being in charge: A circle is collaborative. We created a *Circle of Appreciation* to welcome all our emotions in chapter 1, the self-discovery phase, because a circle is inclusive and connected, with all parts helping to set the containment and all being contained within its embrace.

Let's set another sacred circle. This one will create a natural boundary and a natural shield (or protection) so that when you move inside the circle, you move inside your Whole Self. The circle gives your feelings another safe container, a place to interact and get to know one another even better. Because they exist separate of each other, they don't necessarily know about each other, or if they do, they don't necessary care about the other. In this circle, they can learn from each other and perhaps find ways to work together. Your various emotions can call upon one another in times of need for your greater benefit. The circle supports you from a universal perspective; it carries the seed of your personal right-to-be and it sets an electromagnetic field that is conducive to healing and growth.

The following Write of Passage brings your emotional parts into an arena prime to cultivate alliances. No one is viewed as good or bad; none avoided or banished, but rather all meeting together. Once again, all are welcome here.

> Physically draw a large circle in your journal or notebook.

> Draw a broken line through the edges—pointing from inside to outside—to indicate that the boundaries are permeable. Or draw the boundary of your circle as a broken line. You aren't holding your emotions *in* the circle; you're just giving them a safe place to land.

> Connect with the circle physically by touching your paper. What do you observe? Note anything that stirs within you.

> Connect with the circle emotionally. How does that feel? Is it comforting? Grounding? A feeling of safety? Security? Or does it feel constrictive in any way?

> Connect with it mentally. What thoughts come in? Now, I know this kind of thing may be new to some of you . . . but be honest. What do you think about this process? There's no one here but you. Speak freely.

> What's coming up on a psychic or an "energetic vibe" level?

> When you're ready, place one or more emotions inside this circle. Again, move through the observational process. How does it feel? What thoughts arise? What else can you sense here?

> What emotions protect or shield you? Which ones cover or hide other emotions? And how do YOU shield your feelings? In what situations? Is it appropriate?

➣ What do you perceive within this circle? Does the circle have anything to teach you? Anything else it wishes to say? Anything else you wish to reflect on?

➣ Ask the circle how you can work with your emotions in a way that's constructive. How can you dispel or vent energy when needed? How can you boost your emotional energy? How can you refine your energy?

- -

➣ When confronted with something overwhelming, take a moment to step back and step out of the emotional setting and the emotional ride . . . just pause. Then breathe. Connect with your sacred circle (no matter where you are, you can psychically connect with this circle even if it isn't with you). Observe your feelings in all their characteristics, all their nuances. Just f-e-e-l.

➣ You can draw a circle wherever you are in a time of need, and put your feelings within it to symbolize their safety. Remember to include the lines crossing outward as the way the emotion still expresses in the outer world. The line is permeable; your emotions are not held captive but instead can cross the boundary.

➣ When times are emotionally confusing, invite all your emotions into the sacred circle. Corral the wild horses so you can observe and support them. You can always open the gate and let them run free again.

- -

➣ When you are complete, each time you use this circle technique, remember to thank the circle. Thank the emotions and feelings that have participated. Thank yourself for engaging with this discovery and transformative process.

Within this sacred circle and within your sacred writing, there is great safety. You can return to this part of your journal again and again to deepen your connection and strengthen your alliances; as you cultivate your relationship with this technique, the power and the presence of your circle is enhanced. Like any relationship, it deepens over time.

PARTNER WITH YOUR EMOTIONS

The visual image of the circle and the energetics connected with it encourage you to partner with your emotions. On your sacred path, which is every part of your life's journey, emotions are key. You've been connecting with your emotions and learning from their wisdom. If you encounter one that seems harmful or even destructive, you can work with it in a way that helps it evolve into something more beneficial. Based on a true story, the movie *Chasing Mavericks* (2012) follows surfing icon Jay Moriarity as a young man learning to surf Northern California's most dangerous waves. "Frosty," a local surfing legend, mentors Jay, and the two form an unlikely bond as they push the limits of the sport. As a significant part of his training, Frosty told Jay, "Fear and panic are not the same thing. Fear is healthy; panic is deadly. Identify what you're afraid of to avoid panic."

THE ADVENTURE OF THE SACRED PATH

Your sacred path stretches before you and cradles every aspect from the simplicity of the mundane to what you might think of as your wildest dream. Your sacred path is not one chosen direction or one preferred way of being: Life with all its twists and turns is your sacred path. Like the element of Air that's supported us through this phase, your Sacred Path is lofty, seemingly without boundaries. It stretches far and wide, offering you limitless potential. In addition, recognizing and honoring life as your sacred path is as essential as breath itself.

We've shared our initial Awakening through Self-Discovery, ventured into the Great Departure of our Transformation phase, and now have encountered the many Tests and Trials that life presents as we move along our Sacred Path. Those challenges, coupled with our joys and successes, are what help us step through this portal of initiation, stretching onward and upward as we move toward our uniquely precious Soul Creativity.

Here are a few more ideas for your Sacred Path consideration:

1. MENTORS FOR FEELINGS

Whom do you know that you see as emotionally balanced and emotionally healthy? Observe them to learn how they deal with emotions. Like two tuning forks placed near one another, one fork struck can enable the other one to sing. Spend time with positive role models to be energetically fine tuned. When appropriate, you might consider asking them to witness your Writes of Passage and mentor you.

 ## 2. WRITE OF PASSAGE: SACRED CONTRACT

We are in a sacred circle as I write these words to you. The Source connects us through time and space . . . and I feel you right here, right now. Many blessings to you as you read my words and do our next Write of Passage: negotiating a sacred contract with your emotions. Ask. Explore. Record.

> What do they need?

> What do you need from them?

> How can you cooperate?

➤ What will be your signal that you need space to vent? When you need time alone? When you need to reach out for support?

➤ Draw up an official contract, recording what you are asking of your emotions and what they can expect from you. Be specific. And sign your name as you commit to your emotional health.

3. WATCH WHAT YOU IMAGINE

Scientists studying brain waves have found that when you visually imagine eating an apple with all its sweetness and its crunchy juiciness, the brain registers in the same manner as it does when you are really eating that apple. So, what do you think happens in your brain and in your body when you summon up feelings that aren't there? Yes. It "thinks" that is your reality. Of course, this can work for you if you're conjuring feelings of happiness or wellness. It's how we can sometimes shift out of a rut.

But if you're pretending to be disappointed, confused, or sad, well, you're contributing to the reality of those feelings too. When I was a teen and wanted to skip school, I let my mouth droop, summoned up a pained expression on my face, and watered my eyes. The false outer façade successfully released me from my day's activities. Just like the teen me, for one reason or another, people sometimes "fake" emotions—pretending to be happy or sad, disappointed or perplexed. The answer to why you might do this is complex and often situational; to do so on an ongoing basis not only confuses those around you but has confusing repercussions within you as well.

HMT: What is the one physical expression of a feeling you can't fake? Those little bumps that rise from the skin when you hear something that particularly moves you or resonates with you. Sometimes it happens when someone speaks, and other times it happens when you hear a meaningful poem or see a moving performance. I call them Truth Bumps!

LIFTING YOURSELF TO SOAR

Wisdom is found in doing the next thing you have to do, doing it with your whole heart, and finding delight in it.

—Meister Eckhart

What might you do differently if you trusted your ability to soar, knowing that you have proverbial "wings?" What is it you DREAM of doing? Who is it you long to be? Consider how fear, disbelief, or a sense of unworthiness

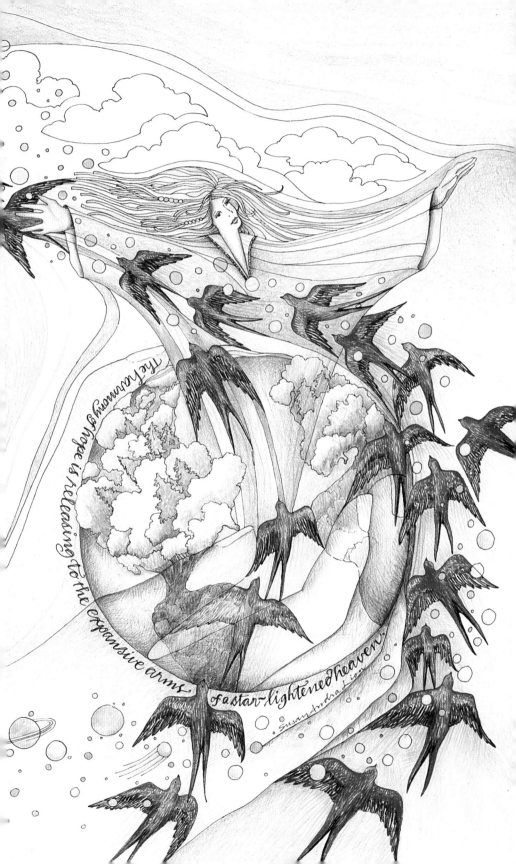

The harmony of hope is releasing to the expansive arms of a star~lightened heaven.

Susan Andra Lion

might be limiting your ability to catch or keep your dreams. Are you trying to cling to a limiting space you've already outgrown just because it's known and feels safe?

Choose life and be fully present. Embrace your humanity by knowing that in spite of your imperfections, you are, at core, quite perfect—and a brilliant work in progress. Enhance and expand your outer reality by allowing the time and the space to evolve in a chosen direction. Be gentle with yourself and honor the process. Every step has value, every stage merit. Build trust as you move forward. Like birth, our growth may, at times, be painful, but a new expanded life awaits. So, comfortable or not, if you see your next chosen move, take it. Ready or not, here you come. Lao Tzu says, "The journey of a thousand miles begins with a single step." And Victor Hugo says, "Be like the bird who, pausing in her flight awhile on boughs too slight, feels them give way beneath her and yet sings, knowing she hath wings."

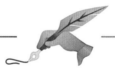

Every stage merit . . . so, comfortable or not, if you see your next chosen move, take it. Ready or not, here you come.

Chapter 4

SOUL CREATIVITY

We've awakened into the grounding of self-discovery, explored what was unknown through fiery transformation, and soared to new heights as we've risen above our trials and tribulations on our sacred path. Now, we open to receive the insights and gifts possible through our personal soul evolution. Do you question who you are or what you want to be? Perhaps you feel solidly centered in the strength of your character but long for more and aren't quite sure how to find it? Are you hoping to better navigate through life's intricate maze? The answers, my friend, lie in your soul essence. In the depths of your soul, you'll find a voice; one that whispers with an undeniable beckoning that draws you closer to where you really want to be. At times, it will call your name, asking you to wake up, and bring forward a part of you that is yet unexpressed. Within your soul is the secret that will set you free—helping you embrace your greatest potential by living life authentically with your most sincere personal expression.

The ultimate truth of the health, wealth, and happiness formula is that you, yourself, are precious beyond measure: You are *the most precious treasure*. You have something to do, and a way of being, that's not like anyone else. Your contribution to life, through how you live that life, absolutely matters and is essential to all of us. Your innate uniqueness is your gift from life itself . . . and what you do with it, your Soul Creativity is *your gift* back to life. You have the capacity within you to do more than you can imagine. So, open to receive many blessings that come from the inside out. You are the most precious treasure.

WHAT IS "SOUL CREATIVITY"?

Soul Creativity encompasses those aligned endeavors that best express who you are at soul level; they lie in your soul imprint or soul code. As authentic expressions of your innermost and highest self, soul creativity wells up from your most essential self, pushing and stretching into form. Sometimes you may need to coax your soul creativity forward, especially if you were told "you can't" (paint, dance, write, etc.). There may be mental, emotional, and energetic sludge that needs to be cleared to allow your most playful creativity to find its rightful pathway.

Soul Creativity is not limited to what you may think of as "creative." In addition to artistic pursuits, Soul Creativity is your unique expression in a myriad of ways: how you offer help to a friend in need, the way in which you arrange your home to welcome people in, your creative methods of problem solving. You express your Soul Creativity in the way you treat family, how you interact with friends, and the person you choose to be. It encompasses the activities you seek, the type of work you do, and how you make your way in the world. Honest soul creativity through right-livelihood (doing the work you came here to do) is a sincere sharing from the depths of your being, and like artistic inspiration, this type of creation is divinely inspired.

Coleen serves many people as a human resource manager. She brings an insight and compassion to her work that elevates even the most difficult piece, like problem-solving employee conflicts or telling someone they are being fired. But Coleen has a deep desire to connect on a different level—she wants to feed people with a welcoming inn that can provide for their physical needs and, at the same time, touch their hearts. She is listening to her inner beckoning and opened to possibilities.

Although she's had the glimmer of the idea for many years, she'd given up hope of ever seeing it come to fruition, since it seemed impossible to ask her husband to leave his childhood home, especially when their daughter, who lives a mile away, just had their first grandchild. Yet, once she propped open that metaphoric door, options began popping in: One house was in poor shape, another sold to someone else, another had beautiful views but an oddly arranged physical structures. And then it happened: Coleen walked into an old Victorian and felt immediately that it was hers. The rooms were nicely sized, and the caretaker suite would provide a cozy spot for her and her husband, Steve.

Now you'd think that'd be the end of my story, right? But it's not necessarily always that easy! Feeling "right" about something doesn't mean it comes together seamlessly. Coleen had to wade through difficult blackout periods where the owner went completely silent, not returning emails or phone calls. She was often left unaware and confused as to where buying this house stood and if they were even moving forward. Each step of the way she trusted . . . and she knew if it didn't work out, there'd be another place to call her new home. Despite dealing with uncertainty, Coleen didn't make the owners wrong for being inconsistent and unpredictable. At one point, she wrote a compassionate letter, empathizing that this home might be hard to let go. In the end, it became evident that this was poor timing, compounded with mounting complications. She let go as gracefully as she navigated through this challenge.

Still, my friend's patience and persistence paid off. Steve is now fully in with the plan, and they are moving forward, together, with an adventurous search to find their perfect spot. They look forward to welcoming friends and tourists alike with the special touches only someone as sweet and caring as Coleen can provide. Even now, she is living and expressing her deepest longing, her brightest soul creativity, as this story continues to unfold. It is not the destination that determines our character. It's how we show up during the journey that matters the most.

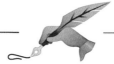

Soul Creativity recognizes that how you live your life is your greatest masterpiece.

How can you realize your fullest potential? By opening to your natural flow and listening to the musings of your soul. You'll never be given a soul's longing that is wrong for you. That inner voice knows and wants only the best for you, so honor what speaks to you and calls your name. Be brave enough to let go of the known so you might express more of your inner self. You don't need to know exactly how to make all the pieces come together; you need only accept the next assignment and begin by taking a step in the right direction. Then take another step. And another. You'll be shown the way and given the power to create this inspired reality.

Sue is a gifted graphic designer with small- and large-scale clients; she assists solopreneurs and provides service to large corporations. When I met Sue many, many years ago, she saw herself as a graphic designer and not necessarily as an artist. Yet, not only was she artistically gifted, but she has a mind that often sees things from interesting angles, providing uniquely inspired perspectives in her art.

I approached Sue to illustrate my books, as did others who recognized her talent, and after a bit, she began creating her own books too. Her list of titles is growing, and she has a line of prints, journals, and other products displaying her delightfully inspired images. As a matter of fact, it's Sue Lion's illustrations that grace the pages of this book! I include her story because it's a sound example that even when you're doing what you think is your work, there may be more that wants to come through you—another gift or talent wanting to express more fully.

Soul Creativity recognizes that how we live our lives is our greatest masterpiece. One way to shape-shift into our authentic soul creativity is by acknowledging and expressing our emotions. By its nature, a "feeling" evokes us to feel. So, when we deny that feeling, we set ourselves up for that feeling having to push stronger to get our attention. When the gentle spring rains come, the water seeps into the earth, bringing nurturing and new growth. But when torrential rain falls in massive amounts all at once, it causes destruction and devastation. Seen and attended emotions are like the spring rain, gentle or wild but in manageable doses. Pushed-away or suppressed emotions can bring forth an uncontrollable storm.

Natashia was a competent professional, yet she had one repetitive problem that followed her from job to job. No matter how many times she changed positions or companies, this problem persisted. Someone in some way would "push her buttons" over something real or imagined, and Natashia would explode. She would yell and spurt nasty words, cutting the person who triggered her off at the knees. Do you know what happened? Even when Natashia had a valid complaint, she was the one who appeared at fault because of her explosive behavior. In fact, once this pattern surfaced at any job, she would then be set up as the scapegoat, blamed for things she had nothing to do with, because her anger made Natashia an easy target.

There's a difference between feeling anger and being immersed in that anger. When some part of us is being pushed on or something we live by is threatened, we may naturally become angry. I've heard that one minute of anger weakens the immune system for five hours, and that one minute of laughter strengthens the immune system for twenty-four hours. I can't swear to that, but as a body worker, I've observed the power of laughter and the destructive quality of anger with no proper release. When we stew in anger, it takes a destructive toll on our bodies; yet, properly vented and addressed anger can be motivating and empowering. Ask yourself: What is this situation or these specific words triggering? What is threatening about it? What within me is being violated? Answers to these questions can help begin to shift our part in the equation. Feelings are not meant to destroy or compromise our success. They are a blessed aspect of the divine soul creativity that is one of our most valuable human birthrights.

Have you ever been at a store or business and watched a customer explode with frustration and anger, berating the stunned salesperson behind the counter? Perhaps, on a difficult day, you've been that person.

Recently I was concerned with a tire that kept losing air, so I went back to the store where I'd purchased it. They checked and repaired the tire for free. A day later my TPS light came on, which sent me to the dealer, and $75 later I was told that the tire store had put the wrong valve on my tire, causing the tire pressure system to malfunction. It would be $250 to replace the "new" stem for the proper one. The dealer also pointed out a different tire that had a cut in it, telling me I was at high risk for a blowout. It would be another couple hundred dollars to replace two of the tires as suggested. The news was disappointing because my tires weren't very old and hardly worn.

I returned to the tire store and explained the situation. It was obvious when you looked at the other three tire stems and the newly installed one that they were not the same, and I wondered why a skilled technician would have missed that they appeared so distinctly different. I voiced my surprise and disappointment to one of the managers. He promptly apologized and offered to change the stem personally. Okay, problem solved. Except that I also had this $75 charge for going to the dealer about that warning light, so I presented that fact calmly, without blame. The manager credited my card for the charge.

"Thank you," I said, "and I wonder while I'm here if you could check your price on my back tire because the dealer told me it should be replaced. He looked at my car again, researched the tire price, and came over to let me know that the tire would be free because they were still under warranty.

"Oh, but it happened when I was in the mountains, backing up a steep drive. I ran right into the side of a large rock. I damaged it. The slash isn't due to a faulty tire."

"Doesn't matter, ma'am, the tire is still under warranty. Let me order it for you."

It's not the "what" of our experiences that matters as much as the "how." It's about "how" we show up to deal with "what" happens that contributes the most to how we evolve as human beings. Our unique abilities, in all their nuances, are the gifts we receive when we come into this human form, and what we do with them is our gift back to life and to everyone we touch. Create your greatest masterpiece by living with bold strokes of honest authenticity, seasoned with a bit of awareness for those around you and their feelings too.

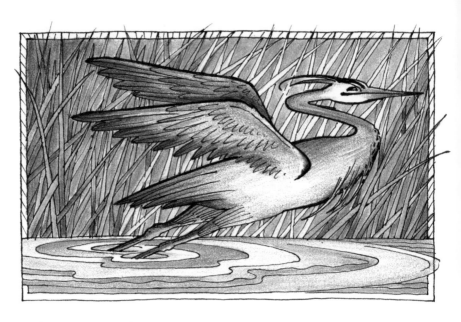

THE ELEMENT OF WATER

In many traditional philosophies, emotions have been compared to water. It's helpful to imagine an ally when engaging with Water, like this beautiful heron who is a symbol of self-reliance and self-realization, the perfect one for strengthening our Soul Creativity. An extra bonus is that the heron can fly above, giving us a bird's-eye view that can see far and wide as we look at our overall emotional perspective. There is a fluidity to emotions. Soul Creativity, too, is like Water: it may express in little spurts or a giant wave. There are powerful emotional analogies and symbolism found within the element of Water, so let's engage with it as we explore our emotional fluidity.

I had just enough time to get there if everything fell perfectly into place: The traffic lights were on my side, and I-70 didn't have any unforeseen congestion. Because it was Sunday, I had a good chance of making it. At least I thought so. As I was heading down 54th Ave., the little connecting road between Easley and McIntyre, my focus wandered to the day at hand. I had a lot ahead of me.

I loved this little street with its mix of architecture, from the spacious southwestern sprawling stucco with its grandparents' residence in the back, to the warmly familiar two-story with the wraparound front porch complete with rockers, the sprawling white-picket-fence horse property, and even the oddly modern two-story new building down the end of the road. But today, I wasn't looking at the houses in this patchwork community while driving down this short little road, or being aware of the road itself; instead, my mind was miles away.

Until I saw it. The face of it loomed ominously when my mind snapped back to attention. And even though I couldn't see the markings, I knew what it was immediately. There was a certain strong energy coming from the large SUV on the left side of the road. Or perhaps it was coming from the radar gun. Of course, I braked, way too late, and rolled on by. Glancing in my mirror, I saw the unfriendly but unavoidable flash of lights and the determined pull of a swift U-turn of a vehicle on a mission.

"You were going 45 in a 30-mile-per-hour zone," he said, in what sounded like his purposely gruffest voice. His words blasted in through the open window, smacking me into the gravity of the moment.

In my haste to provide my driver's license, my arm nervously vibrated as it reached toward him. My insurance card was front and center, ready to be seen, but the credit card in my outstretched hand only served to lesson my credibility, as he asked again for my driver's license. I stumbled to give it to him, and he hunkered off to the dark giant behind me.

As I sat there, I felt so many emotions. To be honest, the first one was frustration at having my down-to-the-wire trip interrupted midstream. I had a full day of back-to-back appointments, and now my schedule was already running behind. I called ahead so they could warn my first client that I'd be arriving late.

I was angry and disappointed that this was happening now. In the past few days I'd been gathering bids for taking down an enormous cottonwood tree, and the average quote was $6,000–$7,000. The added expense of a ticket was the last thing I needed.

"What the heck is taking him so long," I said, glancing at the clock and noticing he'd already been gone seven or eight minutes. Wild thoughts began to run through my head. Could there be a warrant for my arrest? Is he calling for backup? . . . *Don't be ridiculous*, I thought.

Closing my eyes, for a brief moment, and breathing slowly began to center me. This simple act shifted my energy and my mood. I was immediately calm with a great sense of peace. Of course, I knew there wasn't a warrant for my arrest, so I was sure he wouldn't be calling for backup. And I also knew that ultimately, I was safe. I understood I'd been going too fast—although I had no idea that I was going as fast as I was, which in itself was kind of disturbing. I realized, in that moment, that I was kind of embarrassed that I had been caught so absentminded and unaware while driving down a residential side street.

Suddenly, there he was again at my window with the dreaded blue slip in his hand. Again, with the I-am-the-authority voice projecting forcibly at me, he gruffly said, "Going 45 in a 30 zone is $160 and four points on your license." I gasped. "But I gave you a bit of a break. Here's your ticket for going 39 in a 30, which is $95 and one point." I reached out my hand to him, and before he could leave, I said strongly, "I'd like to say something. First, I'd like to apologize." He giggled somewhat nervously. "You don't need to," he answered quickly. "Yes, I do," I said firmly. "I had no idea how fast I was going. But the fact is everyone goes fast on this road. I've been the front car with people on my tail because I wasn't going fast enough for them. But honestly, I had no idea how fast I was going today."

"We had a complaint, and that's why I'm here. This is a big problem on this road."

"I understand. And I'm relieved that I didn't endanger anyone this morning. I appreciate the wake-up call, even though it comes at a time when money is an issue for me, so it's a doubly good lesson to slow down!"

The gruffness was gone from this Jefferson County sheriff as his face softened. "You have a good day ma'am. Thank you."

My frustration, anger, and sense of hurry had turned to acceptance and appreciation. I was speeding and had, in fact, caught myself twice earlier that week doing that very thing on different streets and thought, "I need to slow down before I get a ticket." Third time and my number was up! It wasn't the cop's fault that I was speeding; yet, how often do we get angry and lash out at the messenger? It's a relief to assess the situation honestly and take responsibility for what is within our control. And that perspective not only shifts the energy of the situation but also opens the door of opportunity moving forward.

Probably my biggest stress is time—most specifically not feeling like I have enough of it. Life is rich and full, and I rush more times than I'd like. As I left the scene of the ticket that morning, I decided to leave extra early for appointments and tote a book along for those rare occasions when everything falls into place and I might arrive twenty to thirty minutes early. Meditation also fits nicely into that space of extra time. My spirit was lifted even further with the thought of consciously building in these luxuries, and I felt myself breathe a little easier. Turning a negative into a positive is an empowering action! So, a traffic ticket may seem a little mundane and unimportant to you, and yet, what I did with that situation changed the quality of my life. I have another story that demonstrates this technique of consciously shifting emotions . . . and hers is one that literally gets to the heart of the matter.

Mary Ann is a generous, considerate person seemingly with a big heart. But there's a lot of residual pain from a difficult childhood in a large family—one in which she stepped up to a responsibility when no one else would. Her fancy-free childhood ended when her beloved father died, and she took on his role as physical and emotional caretaker for her mother in so many ways for many years.

Mary Ann is learning to love herself. And learning how to be attentive to her own needs and nurture herself. For most of her life, she pushed her needs away in the line of duty. I've witnessed many layers of

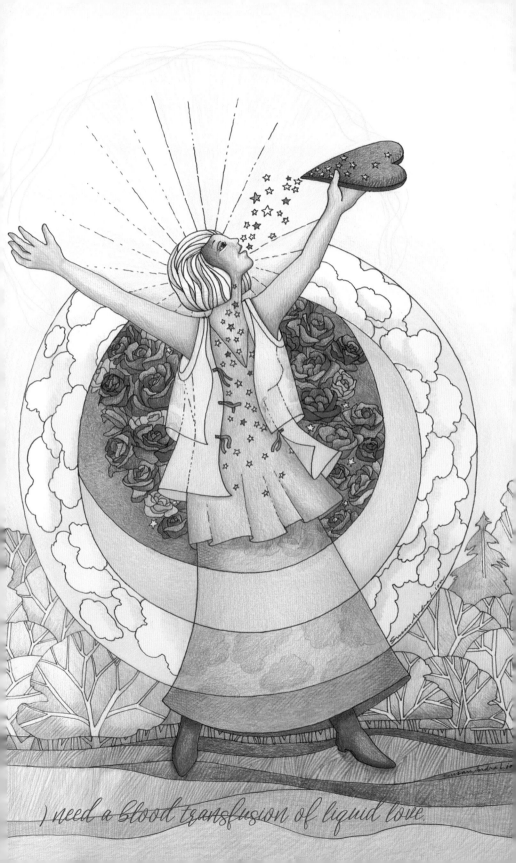

I need a blood transfusion of liquid love.

pain and resistance being shed as she uncovered and revealed her deepest heart. Her process has not been an easy one, and I often marvel at her courage, persistence, and deep insight.

Mary Ann reached a point in her healing where she said everything felt so raw. She became emotionally tender, crying easily, often without knowing why. She also became easily "pissed off," even though she hadn't felt much anger in years. My response was that even though these strong emotions arising without control were sometimes uncomfortable, they were also very good. Emotionally raw is several steps upward from "numb," which is what many of us experience when trauma or suffering is so great that we suppress our feelings in order to survive.

People are starved for love. They may have had limited attention or not been shown enough love as child, still leaving younger parts of themselves aching. Perhaps their family didn't know any better, or perhaps circumstances caused a wounding in some way. But it's never too late to go back and nurture, go back and love that child within. She's waiting for you! And if she's crying and doesn't know why or what she needs, just be there with her. She needs you most of all.

Even though Mary Ann already nurtured herself, buying roses to celebrate a new home and making a fine oyster dinner to treat herself, she recognized that she needed so much more. "It's an inside-out job," she wisely mused. "A cozy blanket won't do it, because the problem isn't feeling warm on the outside. It's my inside that needs it."

"I need a blood transfusion of liquid love!"

 Write of Passage: Fluid Emotions

Explore how your emotions are like Water:

➢ Is there a current raging fast and deep?

➢ Do you have a river of tears within you needing to flow?

➢ Are some of your emotions frozen like an ice cube?

➢ Is your happiness and joy like a gurgling mountain stream turning into a fast-moving river as it comes down to the foothills below?

What words could you put on your emotions right now? At other times in your life? How have they changed?

➢ Sit and imagine bodies of water: a clear, gentle mountain stream, a strong and powerful river; see rapids and compare them to the calmer eddies.

- Oceans large and mighty

- Warm Caribbean waters (one of my favorites!)

- Now consider how those bodies of water relate to your emotions and in what way.

- Engage in stream-of-consciousness writing to see what surfaces for you.

KEEP FROM DROWNING: LEARNING TO SWIM IN OUR FEAR

Wise elders have said that our greatest journey is moving from fear to love. But fear may have a strong hold that threatens to pull us down beneath the churning waters, literally choking off our life's breath. Fear can be debilitating. Chronic fear in the form of severe anxiety affects many; if your fears are paralyzing, please summon the strength to seek professional help.

For most of us, fear comes and goes relative to our outer and inner realities. Dangerous or threatening situations, perceived or real, may trigger fear. There are many forms of this emotion: a nervous quickening, difficulty in speaking through a dry mouth, shortness of breath, a feeling that you might faint, a desire to flee, a reactive defensiveness, or a need to fight to try to keep yourself safe, and sometimes all-out panic.

I've often heard the idea that FEAR is "false evidence appearing real," and in some cases that may be true, especially with a repetitive fear projected outward onto different situations. At other times, we might build things out of proportion because of an unresolved feeling that's triggered within us. A dear friend was afraid to ask her loving husband about something because she was trapped in a fear that was ungrounded within the reality of their longtime successful relationship. Once we broke the feelings down, looking at their innards, she was able to easily see that the fear was projected from within her and was not relevant to him or his possible reactions to her task at hand.

Avoiding fear or trying to avoid fear won't minimize it. If there's a genuine reason for fear to be felt, it will build in strength and power until it is seen. It's helpful to explore acceptable ways to manage or release our fears. In many cases we're called to meet them directly, walking into the fear and out the other side. I like to imagine offering my fear an outstretched hand, so we can walk hand in hand as we transcend the current "stuck place" and travel into the distant horizon.

Dealing with our fear is not simple or easy, but moving through our fears is often empowering. One morning as I went to water my plants, I found an unusual pattern in the dirt and after a quick minute realized there was a coiled snake in my jade plant pot! What!!! It was remarkable how much fear could be attached to picking up that pot and taking the snake outside—it was quite the ordeal.

> What I observed during my process was that thinking things through certainly helped quell the surge of fear. "First I'm going to place this bag over the top of the planter (which was odd shaped, just to complicate matters), then I'll pull the drawstring to contain him, then I'll carry it outside to the back fence by the field."

> Next, I found practice useful even if it was a common bed pillow that I practiced my moves on.

> Self-talk was important: "You've got this." "He's only a foot or so long." "He's sleeping and won't move very quickly if he wakes up." "You've GOT this!" Yikes!

> I don't know about you, but I sang a favorite tune to lift me up.

> *Viola!* Done deal. :)

> And yes, that was not as easy as it looked!

Awareness is key. By bringing awareness to it, your fear already shifts. Fear can be turned into something useful: Singers and speakers learn how to turn stage fright into powerful energy that catapults them into a successful presentation. Chronic fears that replay often may be soul imprints poking their heads out to get your attention and lead you in the direction of growth. There may be valuable keys within those kinds of fears.

Judgment is a major contributing factor. We label people or situations and assign them a meaning that colors our emotional state. Healing sometimes takes the form of transcending the attachments of our emotional judgments. How can you go from a limited, stuck, or stagnant perspective and see something for its hidden value? How can you break free of a limited state and move to a greater one? Changing or reframing your thoughts and beliefs can have valuable impact on all your emotions, especially fear. Are you working toward coping or are you reinforcing a fear's fierceness? Change the idea and you will reshape the experience even if you remain in the same spot.

Nancy hated her job. Every morning she woke with dread because of the trap she felt she was in, with no hope of escape. As the sole support of her family, she had to work . . . and the thought of leaving a job that provided for the family terrified her.

Through our exploration, Nancy was able to determine that her fear was responsible for holding her in what seemed like a long jail sentence—only to end when retirement came many years from now. I pointed out that she was in a position of choice. Even though she had to work, Nancy chose to get up in the morning and go to this particular job, and she did for good reason. It provided nicely for her

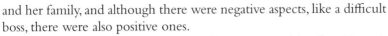

and her family, and although there were negative aspects, like a difficult boss, there were also positive ones.

Once she let go of the feeling of being trapped by fear, Nancy's attitude shifted, and she approached her days from a different perspective: She looked for what she liked about this company, appreciating how they did business; she savored her professional relationships; she immersed herself in a very challenging project and received a lot of recognition from the upper echelon, which resulted in a transfer to a more prestigious position with a raise in pay.

Nancy didn't run from her situation, but rather by meeting her inner resistance and fears and then redefining them, she was able to shift her outer circumstance.

FORGIVENESS: RAIN TO NOURISH YOUR SACRED GROUND

To err is human. To forgive, divine.

—Alexander Pope

Forgiveness is often essential to provide the freedom to explore our soul creativity. Bitterness and resentment take up such precious space when held within us, space better suited for worthwhile development and soul expression. Forgiveness is an incredibly powerful process, one that affects us far more than it does the one we forgive. Each piece of bitterness or resentment that we neutralize, and release, lightens our heavy burden and quickens our step.

There was a woman who had a woven basket—it was simple in its shape and form, and it was a very sturdy container. In this basket, the woman placed her disappointments, her resentments, and her bitterness. In the basket, the woman placed her wounds. She held the basket tightly to her, guarding its contents, unknowingly believing them special and unique. In spite of their weight, they were precious to her . . .

And so, the woman carried her basket with her everywhere, clinging to it as she cradled it in her arms. Her disappointments, her resentments, her wounds, and her bitterness were not shared or given to others. . . . Or so, the woman thought! When she spoke with her neighbor across the fence or bent down at the market to select her vegetables, some of the contents of the basket unwillingly spilled out, polluting those around her with their rotting stench. Still the woman clung to her basket, adding to it from time to time, until the woman grew very, very old. The weight of the basket became too much to bear.

The very old woman sat down under a tree with the basket huddled next to her, clinging to its rim. A young boy came down the path and saw the old woman under the tree. He also saw her basket, which was very odd, since for all these years no one had seen the basket even though it was with her always. The young boy peered into the basket, struck by the weight of all that was inside. "Grandmother, why do you keep all that rotting stuff?" he asked. "I don't know," the woman replied honestly.

Together, they hoisted the basket full of its heavy contents, carefully turning it over at the nearby river's edge—into the river tumbled her disappointments, her resentments, her wounds, and her bitterness, and the old woman watched as they moved away. She watched until they were out of sight, and she felt a little strange because they had been so much a part of her. The little boy smiled, since he knew more than he could say to this old woman. Together they took to the path homeward, the now-empty basket swinging between them.

—Donna DeNomme (2008)

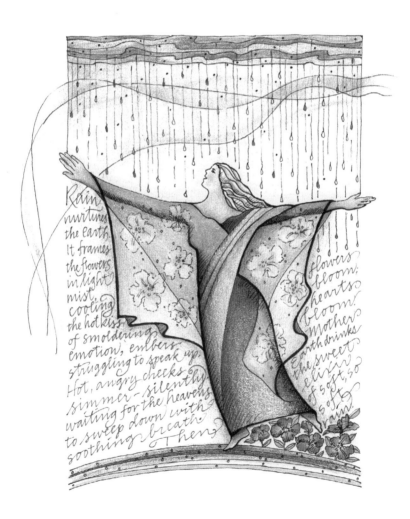

Rain nurtures the earth. It frames the flowers in light mist, cooling the hot kiss of smoldering emotion, embers struggling to speak up. Hot, angry cheeks simmer—silently waiting for the heavens to sweep down with soothing breath. Then... flowers bloom, hearts bloom. Mother earth drinks the sweet elixir of soft, so soft rain.

TRUSTING RIGHT TIMING

Lorraine told me about a memory of herself at age four: She was strong, feisty, and bold. She felt that, at the time, she was also kind of mean, and she recognized in the reflection of those around her that this quality was not seen favorably. She remembered pushing that piece of herself away and choosing instead to be a gentler, people-pleasing girl who could be better received.

Now in her thirties, Lorraine wanted that part of her back. Being quite perceptive, Lorraine realized that still within her was not just that four-year-old, but older pieces, also strong and bold, who had been held back and pushed down too. And they were very angry! Just acknowledging them and wanting to embrace them was not enough to heal the rift. And so, we did some deeper work to connect with these parts of her.

What struck me as so significant in listening to Lorraine's story is the clarity of what happens when we're at one of those crossroads, conscious or unconscious choice points, where we choose one emotional or behavioral aspect of ourselves over another and reject, banish, or bury the other. As Lorraine described the circumstances and her family dynamics, it was clear to me that, at the time, she needed to choose one way of being over the other. It was not yet possible to embrace and express both. Her development was not evolved enough to be able to move back and forth between the two very different, almost diametrically opposed ways of being. If she had not buried the more defiant bold one, she might have buried the gentle people-pleaser and had a very different childhood because of it. Her little self was not yet ready to integrate these two polar-opposite pieces.

That time was now.

With many of my clients who experienced some form of abuse in their childhood, which was the catalyst for lost or abandoned pieces, I don't typically see a conscious decision to choose one aspect of themselves over another. Because hers is not a story of physical or sexual abuse causing a fragmentation, Lorraine's story easily demonstrates why we might do this for better interpersonal relations or for our physical or emotional survival. As we grow and evolve, these hidden aspects arise in the perfect time and space for further healthy emotional development.

A situation occurred in Lorraine's marriage that precluded that stronger, bolder, opposite of the people-pleaser self to stretch into view. The specific content is unimportant. What's interesting to note is if Lorraine simply tapped back in and expressed from that feisty four-year-old self, it would most likely have been overreactive and inappropriate for her current reality. I doubt it would have been effective. Lorraine was wise in reaching out for help to take this beautiful, somewhat raw and undeveloped piece . . . and give it the opportunity to grow.

This is one of the most fascinating aspects of emotional healing—watching a younger emotional piece find its voice and expression and, consequently, begin to evolve. There may be many steps along the way, and patience serves us. As we continue to move forward with our newly reclaimed piece, we become lighter and lighter as the old, heavy, dense captive energy spins into a fine golden thread, a newly integrated piece of the wholeness of who we are and how we express in our world.

IT'S A PROCESS—WHAT PROGRESS ARE YOU MAKING?

Look closely at the present you are constructing. It should look like the future you are dreaming.

—Alice Walker

Our emotional healing and development is not a destination to arrive at, but rather an evolving process.

> Pause at various points along the way and reflect on the progress you're making.

> Observe and celebrate your maturity milestones.

> Let go of what you don't want, so you can open your arms to what you do want.

> Are you moving in that upward spiral? If something has you sliding along the downward spiral, reach out for help or act to shift into upward movement.

> Again affirm: "I am healing the past, being mindful in the present, and visioning the future."

MEETING FAILURE, TRUSTING SUCCESS

Out of the environment of what we could consider a failure, true genius may flourish, if we can entertain an openness, honest communication with all concerned, and a curiosity to understanding the inner and outer workings of what has occurred. Chase Jarvis says, "Allow yourself the freedom to step away from perfection because it is only then that you can find success." I like to entertain an "Isn't that fascinating!" philosophy when life throws me a curve.

It felt like a typical day. There'd been no warning . . . in fact, quite to the contrary. Sheila called me into her office and began our unscheduled meeting. With her sweet southern drawl, she was kind of blubbering without making much sense, but my mind finally rested on one key comment: "You have a son. You're a mother." I had an immediate vision in my mind's eye of a small window opening and puffy flowered drapes fluttering inward in response to a strong, cold wind.

"Are you *firing* me?" I asked.

"Yes . . . they're making me," Sheila blurted out as she laid her head in her hands and sobbed uncontrollably. I just sat there staring at her in disbelief . . . as an eerie calm and sense of peace washed over me.

I was getting fired from an apartment-leasing job in spite of being consistently in the top three nationwide with my sales, and often number one. A new company was buying the property I had helped build and fill with good residents. I loved helping people find their new home, and I was super good at it. Now I was being let go.

The incoming company promised we'd all keep our jobs, and now, two hours after the head honcho signed the paperwork, I was being fired (and within a month, the last of us was gone). Because I was the first and I'd been such a good employee, they gave me an excellent exit package. And during the only six months in my adult life that I was ever unemployed, I completed my teacher training as a conscious-energy teacher and began advanced spiritual-coaching training, which both catapulted my life in another direction and reshaped my career.

That fateful day, as I cleaned out my desk, my dear friend Gina arrived, picking me up to go to the newly released *Steel Magnolia* movie set in Louisiana, coincidentally the home of the company taking over our apartments. Gina jokingly said, "What'd you do, get fired?" and I nodded. She was stunned. Gina was the manager who originally brought me in as a leasing agent for this property, courting me from another one within our company because of my desirable skill set.

There's a couple fascinating pieces I feel I must share. I'd been getting the inner guidance to leave this job for close to a year . . . and I kept saying, "Give me an option. I'm not going to quit a perfectly good job that provides my income and our housing." And on top of that, as someone who didn't typically use grocery coupons before this, I caught the wave of the triple-couponing fad and set the alarm for the wee hours of the morning when they restocked the shelves, so I could buy shopping carts full of products for very little money. Now the decision to leave this job had been taken away from me, while at the same time I was being cared for in mysterious ways. When I unpacked my things after moving to a new place, I laughed until I cried as I stocked shelves with boxes and boxes and cans and cans of products. I didn't have to shop for core staples for well over a year. And the next six months of completing my advanced training while unemployed changed my life forever.

In the midst of great adversity, we may find an opportunity to reorganize or refine our personality, or to reach in and draw from the core of our character. And if there's a sense of failure, it's important to know that making mistakes—even big ones—is a part of living and learning . . . and sometimes "failure" leads to success. It's a trust walk to lean in, and sometimes to literally fall into the unknown, to draw on our resilience and rise above what presents itself. Edison says that the "most important ingredient for success is failure. Every time you fail, you eliminate one more way that won't work, being one way closer to the one that will," and Confucius says, "Our greatest glory is not in never failing, but in rising every time we fail."

When we let go of the shore of what is known and move into the emotional void, we may have a sense of being cut loose, floating aimlessly in a vast sea. What was useful no longer is, and we don't know what's next. We associate discomfort with danger, and uncomfortable emotions with something to be avoided, but we can reprogram that natural reaction with the understanding that there is value in traversing ominous terrain. And at times, what has been avoided and is actually waiting for our precious attention is our untapped potential, our creative genius. Condition yourself to hold your vulnerability, be courageous, and move into what might come next. By opening wider, you could awaken a possibility, moving beyond your present reality.

Sometimes we fear failure, but other times we may surprisingly fear success. Have you ever observed someone who worked for years toward a goal and then, just before achieving it, suddenly switched directions and missed the mark? In the field of physical and personal healing, this shows up when someone is not ready for the healing; perhaps there's still something needing to be experienced or learned to fully accept their resolution. Succeeding may sometimes cause us to be vulnerable or visible in a way we fear. If we can honor ourselves and our emotions through the process of healing and personal evolution, it can open us to the greater scheme of things.

Write of Passage: Microscope and Telescope

Remember to look up at the stars and not down at your feet. Try to make sense of what you see, and wonder about what makes the universe exist. Be curious.
—Stephen Hawking

Focus in and zoom out to observe yourself emotionally. Draw yourself inward and examine your emotions in detail, seeing their every fiber and dissecting their deepest meaning. It's as if you're looking at them through a powerful microscope:

➢ What am I feeling?

➢ What are the aspects and nuances of that feeling?

➢ Observe how the feeling is changing (if it is) simply by examining it.

Then zoom outward to see how those emotions interact with the broader picture. It's as if you're looking at the cosmos through a powerful telescope and marveling at the constellations. Examine the overall view:

> What was the context in which my emotions were felt?

> Who else was involved? How did their behavior affect my emotions? How did mine affect theirs?

> And what might be triggers tapping to another time, another place?

> When you let go of ideas of "right or wrong" and "true or false," what can you observe about the interrelations?

> Notice how the feeling is changing (if it is) simply by examining it in its greater relational constellation.

By focusing in, and then zooming out, you can escape the limited myopic perspective that comes from being overwhelmed by an all-encompassed feeling, and instead glean a fuller perspective.

A grandfather cottonwood held the boundary between my yard and my neighbor's yard: Year after year the tree stood beautiful and tall, blessing us with its sweet shade. But there was danger lurking in its three massive trunks ominously leaning in three different directions—the largest trunk being 103 inches in diameter, over eight and a half feet around. After twenty-seven years of good care, it became evident that it was time. I needed to take the tree down before it fell on something (or someone). Even the tree had let me know that it was time . . . and the day after it did so, the huge kindred cottonwood in the field behind me fell, shaking the ground with a penetrating "thud."

I settled on Forestry Tree Care, an arborist who was also a rock climber, to help me dismantle the huge tree. For days prior I did gratitude ceremonies for all the tree had provided. I shared my love and appreciation with the tree. Mark brought in his crew of six, and the guys did a phenomenal job. Navigating the tree with their climbing ropes, Kyle and Zach sawed sections off and lowered them down to safety; a ground crew scurried around feeding the branches into the chipper, and the larger pieces onto a trailer. Several loads left for disposals; unfortunately, cottonwoods are extraordinarily heavy and crack easily, making them unusable for recycling purposes.

On day two it became evident after a morning of grueling work that the guys had taken on more than they envisioned regarding this job. The cost was rising above the bid, and Mark was working very hard on a job that now was costing him money. What I found exceptional was that when he presented that information to me, he said things like, "I made a mistake when I calculated the cost of this one. And I take full responsibility for my bid. I just want to keep you informed on what I'm planning. I'm going to bring in a crane, which will up my cost $1,500." He was noticeably distraught, but in no way did he try to make me wrong or pressure me. I was very appreciative of the good work they had all done with my tree, and the care they'd taken with my yard while doing it, and sad for Mark's difficult predicament. In addition, I was impressed with the way he was handling this.

I also knew it wasn't my responsibility to rescue him, yet how we treat others makes a mark, not only on our character but on the overall collective too. We're all in this life together, and I didn't want the full burden to be on this small-business owner. I went to my checkbook to see what I could juggle and was able to come up with an extra $500. Perhaps it could help. When I offered it to him, Mark was ecstatic. He said he could bargain with the crane guy, and this would make all the difference to him; it'd be a bonus if they could finish sooner and get on to other jobs this week. Mark's way of dealing with the problem and my response to it left good juju in place of the old cottonwood, and the remnants of that lives on well beyond the time frame it was shared in.

Write of Passage: Balance of Giving and Receiving

In our Transformation segment, we touched on who supported you and whom you support, and the idea of giving and receiving. One of my Native American teachers, years ago, spoke about the "sacred hoop of giving and receiving" and there being an essential need for finding balance between the two aspects. Just like it isn't healthy to be taking all the time, we can't just give and give and give.

> ➤ Are you the rescuer? Do you attract people to you who are in constant crisis, so you can be the one to help?

> ➤ Do you feel emotionally exhausted from meeting other people's needs?

> ➤ Is there an "emotional vampire" who sucks the life force right out of you?

> ➤ Are you an emotional trash can for others to unload their worries and dump their emotional garbage?

> ➤ Are you driven to help?

In *How Can I Help* (1985), Ram Dass and Paul Gorman pose important questions such as "What really helps?" and "How much is enough?" They also urge us to explore our own motivation for helping and to look at what we might be avoiding in our own life when our time is immersed in helping other people.

- Is an unattended part of you crying for attention?

- Is there something you might be emotionally avoiding?

- Could helping others be an outer projection of a need to help yourself?

- Can you stop . . . and be with your own pain?

- What makes you uncomfortable emotionally?

- What is the most difficult to deal with emotionally? Why?

- Do you have any emotional karma—what did you bring in as your emotional nature? In what way?

- What would you need to feel safe emotionally?

- Explore ways to nurture self and receive support and care from others.

Whatever has been your pattern up until now, strive for a healthy balance in giving and receiving: be there for others, be there for yourself, and open your heart to receive from others. Look for ways you can support another in finding their own solutions. Be conscious in your choices regarding how you help and how you receive help.

Write of Passage: Your Heart's Desire

If you follow your heart, you're gonna feel better than if you hold back because of fear.

—Pema Chodren

One way to move in the direction of your greater story is to look into your heart of hearts and ask: "What is my heart's desire? My soul's craving? What do I hope for? What direction do I want to take, and what experiences do I wish to have? What brings me joy?" You owe it to yourself to explore and pursue these longings. You owe it to those you love, your family, your community, and the world at large to do so too. When one realizes their soul potential, we all benefit from the repercussion, delightfully releasing energetic glitter in celebration!

- Make a list, write in a journal, or speak aloud what you are grateful for in your life. Remember to include the qualities about your personality or your accomplishments that you are grateful for in yourself. You literally create an atmosphere of appreciation, which builds on its own vibrational momentum, creating even more to be thankful for.

➤ Now what is your heart's desire? Write with abandon, noting everything that comes to mind. Keep returning to the question of "What is my heart's desire?," noting what surfaces until nothing else arises. Then write about each idea further, developing and exploring your initial thoughts.

➤ Finally, create a collage of pictures as a visual reminder to embrace the things you love every day.

Integrate these interests and pursuits into your life, balancing them with your obligations. When you're fulfilled, you are a well overflowing, who has much more to offer. As you replenish your own vitality by doing the things you love simply because you love to do them, your joy has an impact on those around you.

★ We explore and deepen with these activities in the "Coming Home to Yourself: 30-Day Invitation" online program.

 ## Write of Passage: The Pondering Pool

Begin by focusing on your breath . . . and being with the awareness of your beautiful spirit . . . and your strong and healthy body (even if it has shortcomings, see it as strong and healthy). . . . Let go into that inner sanctum that always exists within you as you open to receive whatever is here for you in this centering process . . . call up in your own mind's eye a beautiful body of water, whether it's a pond or a lake, its calm water with strong boundaries just like you. Gaze upon this body of water and appreciate it for all its natural beauty, all of its natural essence. See it in as much detail as possible.

Search for a spot on the water's edge where you're able to bend over and look into that beautiful pool of water . . . and you see your own reflection looking right back with wise eyes greeting you there. Beautifully knowing eyes look up at you, and you move into the depth of wisdom held in those insightful eyes.

Listen as you open to receive the understanding of your enlightened self—exactly right and perfect for where you are right now in your life. Perhaps you have a specific question you ask of those wise eyes as the reflective, crystal pool shows you your own inner strength and sage insight.

This pool shows you the magnificence of who you are. . . . You are in a receptive space of seeing and hearing, even what's said without words—as you hear your own heart communicate to you in a language that speaks of knowing what's right for you.

And in this moment, you honor your heart. You honor your character. You honor your brilliance and your deep wisdom. And you feel, with absolute appreciation, the gratitude of having been

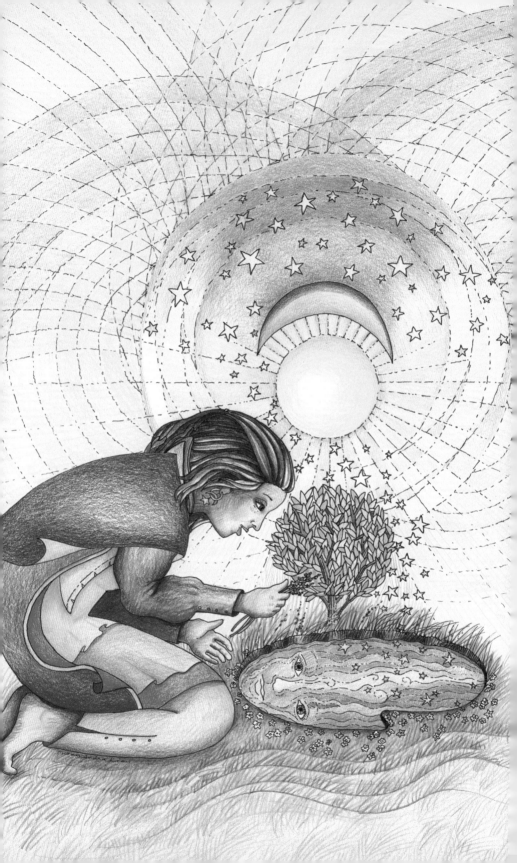

born . . . and gratitude for being the unique soul that you are . . . for without you there'd be a space in creation; a lack in the overall fiber of life. So, in this moment, fall into your heart of hearts, as you receive an even-deeper acceptance and trust of who you are and what you are at core essence. . . .

Draw into your mind's awareness the intentions you've had for your Writes of Passage. Draw into your awareness your heart's desires and soul's longings. Right now, in this blessed moment, imagine a magnetic field around you that is attracting toward you what you desire, what is for your good, what is for the best and the highest, that which is your greater-yet-to-be and the truth of who you are, the truth of your innermost core being. And you feel it coming closer and closer . . . closer and closer. You feel it coming closer and closer. You feel it coming closer and closer and you open your arms wide to accept and receive. And you embrace all that is yours, as you stretch into the capacity of your human self, expressing your soul essence. And life is very, very good! And you give great thanks! And life gives great thanks right back!

Taking a nice, slow, gentle breath to feel all that you've placed here . . . knowing you can return again and again and again to the sacred space of this reflective gazing pool to meet those wise eyes in whatever form they appear as they look back at you. Take your time with this. And when you're ready, come back to our page.

★ Access my extended guided meditation at WriteofPassage4me.com.

I believe your greatest potential is reaching, is stretching toward you. So, it's a good practice magnetizing it to you as you imagine yourself as a receiving port that's accepting your good. Recognize the gift you are and unwrap the many layers of that gift, as you transform into your beautifully self-realized butterfly self.

It is better to believe than to disbelieve; in so doing you bring everything to the realm of possibility.

—Albert Einstein

 ## Write of Passage: Give Yourself Permission to Be Happy

One birthday present I give myself is to write "birthday wishes." I list intentions, recording as many as the number of years I've been on the planet. It's a sweet gift because I receive more wishes each year! The eve before my next birthday, I review, celebrate how many wishes have come true, and decide which wishes or intentions I'll draw forward to the next year.

For my birthday this year, I crafted a personal mala. malas are strings of 108 beads that can be used to focus on, one bead at a time, as you say an affirmation or mantra. My personal mala is constructed with

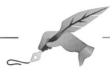

Have you given yourself permission to be happy?

crazy lace agate beads, sometimes called the laughter stone, symbolic of providing a nurturing, accepting, and playful nature. One of my spiritual practices is to meditate with this mala, while focusing on affirmations about laughter, joy, and happiness for twenty-one-day periods of time. I've found it delightfully uplifting.

There have been so many books written on happiness, and I think Barry Neil Kaufman said it first: Happiness is a Choice (1991). Happiness is not something that happens to you; it's something you choose to create. What surprises me is the prevalence of an attitude or belief that for some reason we aren't supposed to be happy. That suffering is our lot in life. Perhaps this is an old generational or cultural belief from times past . . . or one that conveys that in order to "get ahead," we need to struggle. Regardless of where it came from, it is alive and well among us. Yikes!

So, you may need to give yourself *permission* to be happy. It sounds silly, but I've found it to be true. Have *you* officially given yourself permission to be happy? Assume a positive attitude about your life and commit to enjoy it as much as possible. Be a fun instigator! Albert Einstein claimed: "The most important decision we make is whether we believe we live in a friendly or hostile universe." This brilliant man knew that our attitude and approach to life colored our experiences.

> Check in with yourself: What are your thoughts, your attitudes, and your beliefs about happiness? Record these in your journal.

> How did family, early conditioning, and societal norms shape those beliefs?

> What do you think now?

> Who or what impedes your happiness?

> What is within your power to change?

> How do you respond to the words "happy," "happiness," "joy," and "bliss"?

- Are those states of being within your reach? Or do they seem unattainable?

- Do you even know when you're happy? Do you know when you feel joy? Are feelings of joy and happiness the same for you? Or what is the difference?

- Do you laugh out loud? How often?

- How can you shift your thoughts or attitudes about happiness to open the door to more of it?

- Choose a day this week and observe each and every moment of joy or happiness. Record it. Describe it in detail. Savor its sweet nectar.

- When you focus on the good, it expands and grows!

In *Solve for Happy* (2018), Mo Gawdat says: "Happiness shouldn't be something you wait for and work for as if it needs to be earned. Furthermore, it shouldn't depend on external conditions, much less circumstances as fickle and potentially fleeting as career success and rising net worth." He makes the point that we'll never be happy if we hinge that happiness on something we wish to acquire or a certain benchmark of success. The greatest attainment is your happiness; the greatest adventure, seeking and finding your joy. Practice being keenly aware of what makes you happy, and express wholehearted gratitude for what you receive.

affirm:

I am worthy of joy and happiness. I open to accept my happiness.
I am happy!

THE ADVENTURE OF SOUL CREATIVITY

Through sacred initiation, we come from the awakening of our self-discovery phase, crossing the threshold into our transformational phase, and the trials of our sacred-path phase, to enter the personal reflection and illumination found by going into our inner cave and drawing forth our soul creativity. We express our unique soul essence coming into form through the fluidity of our thoughts and actions, in what Carl Jung referred to as individuation. Our precious life expression becomes our uniquely blessed contribution: our abilities and talents are our gift from life, and how we express them is our gift right back. Further explore the area of your soul creativity by pursuing one or more of the following ideas:

1. "ME TIME"

Use your soul creativity to live a life of your own design. Monitor yourself to avoid the "forced march" kind of existence, where you stumble through your days numbly checking off your to-do list. Contemplate and cultivate activities that bring you joy and happiness, and seed them throughout your busy schedule. Like a kid in a candy store, you can choose what you'd like, but you don't have to eat one from every jar!

2. CARETAKING THE BABY (THAT'S YOU!)

Would you let a baby's bum get raw from lack of lotion and powder? What do YOU need today? This week? This month? Attend to your own needs as if you were a little one in your loving care. And just like a baby, there'll be times of yucky caca and proverbial dirty diapers. As any parent or caregiver knows, there's nothing you can do to escape it. It's inevitable; you simply must deal with it. If you ignore them, they won't go away. If you turn the other way, well, that smell is still there. And if you leave it there too long, the baby's bottom will become raw and inflamed. The same is true for us. No matter what terrible caca presents itself, take care of it. And then take out the trash!

3. SENSORY FOCUS: IT'S GOOD TO BE ALIVE

Visit or meditate on things with a strong sensual experience and f-e-e-l the richness they offer. Some of my favorites are a warm, sandy beach; the texture of an intricate weaving; the smells of a farmer's market at high noon; or the richness of cobalt blue. What are yours?

4. YOU ARE LISTENING (SO WATCH WHAT YOU SAY)

Have you ever shared something with a friend—a story, a fact, or some snippet of information—and then a couple of days later have them recount to you, word for word, what you said as if they are sharing the most fascinating news with you! And when you mention that you spoke about that the other day, they still look at you cluelessly as to who mothered this information? They honestly don't remember you talking about it because it's become an integral part of them.

This is another reason why our Writes of Passage are so powerful. Everything you do is creative, and your words hold great power. As you shape and reshape your emotional understanding through the words you write, that creative action has its way with you. When you focus on the negative or the difficult and process it through, the act leads to healing. When you focus on the positive and draw that thread forward, it will replicate through many blessings. The Writes of Passage enable you to hear your own words and learn from your own wisdom, accepting your innate power to put into action your ideas or desires through your soul creativity.

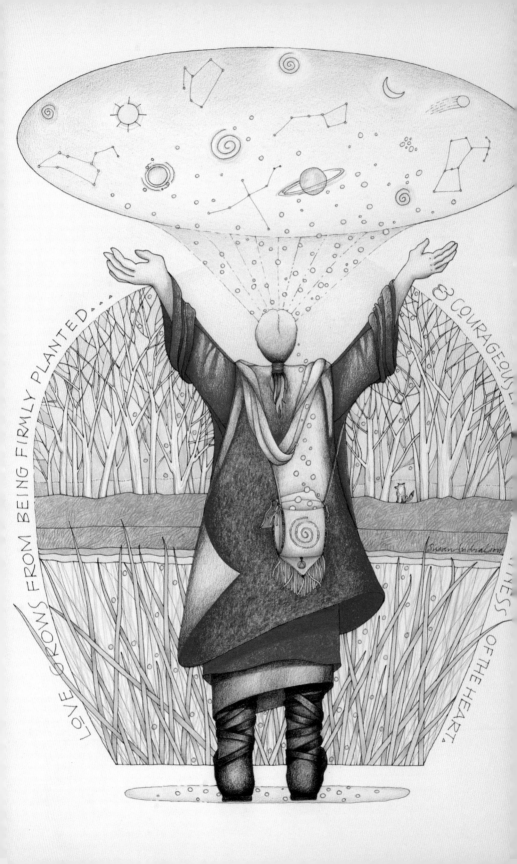

LOVE GROWS FROM BEING FIRMLY PLANTED... & COURAGEOUSLY WITNESS OF THE HEART.

Chapter 5

THE GREAT MYSTERY OF LIFE

Our job is to hold fast to the conviction that there is a power, to discover that power, and to use it.

—Ernest Holmes

Ancient peoples recognized the natural world as being created from the four elements of Earth, Fire, Air, and Water. But there is a fifth element that is more elusive and not necessarily seen with the naked eye. It is the intelligence or the consciousness that is the basis for our very life essence. Although the ancients intuitively sensed and grew to intimately know this fifth element, it has only been in our lifetime that modern science has substantiated it. Ether is the "stuff" that supports all of us, holding up the sun, the moon, and the stars and cradling our planet within the solar system. Remarkably vast and somewhat intangible, ether is what holy people and shamans call "the Great Mystery." Within this Great Mystery, there is a divine intelligence and an infinite space, or void, that holds the potential for all of creation. Ether is great possibility, inspiration, receptivity, and manifestation; the fifth element is the spark of life itself.

You can illuminate your emotions with the fire of your heart, transmuting what is difficult or painful into something useful. You can ground your intentions into the earth, blessing them with the sound of your breath and the gentle rain of your tears; yet, within the element of ether, you truly open and access the greater yet-to-be, moving beyond what you know and believe is possible to the greater spiritual potential. This is a land beyond your wildest dreams!

EXPLORING THE VOID

Within the element of ether, there is a great void; much can be discovered in this place of emptiness. Buddhists speak about a transcendent state where there is no suffering and no desire. Deep meditation is an example of accessing this infinite potential. Have you felt even a brief moment when you transcended the density of the physical world and existed in the purity of your spiritual essence? Or perhaps you've glimpsed your mystical connection with the cosmos and all of creation? Have you sensed Oneness? Many people struggle to attain this, which in a way is missing a bit of the point. In our struggle we remain locked inside our bodies, trapped in the human condition. If you haven't felt complete emptiness, no worries; you can still dip your toes in this Center Space of Spirit where all things are possible.

Practice discovering your own spiritual nature and living in integrity with your soul essence. Discover greater inspiration and truth, that luminous insight helps you access the vast potential held within ether. You can create more than what you're now experiencing when you draw on the remarkable gifts of this ethereal well. Infinite potential is available to us in every moment; it's not reserved for monks and shamans. Ether is a place you and I can visit daily . . . and we, too, provide a significant value for this Great Mystery because, ultimately, we are the vessels that contain its spaciousness and ground it into form.

> ➢ Did you ever go to sleep with a problem, only to awaken with the answer? That's going into the void, drawing from the fifth element.

> ➢ Did you ever see a sign in the rocks, in the trees, in the clouds? That's recognizing ether's subtle messages.

> ➢ Did you ever see a symbol in your dream that led you to a solution or a resolution to something troubling you? Your subconscious, which often communicates in symbols, has a clearer channel to the Great Mystery and can act as a bridge from there to here through your dreams. You can find valuable insight if you pay close attention to yourself.

> ➢ Another way this might happen is in those moments when things just spill out of your mouth, unexpectedly, and you hear yourself and think, "Oh, yes. That's what I've been trying to say." Or, "That's exactly what I want to do." We often call those "aha moments" of truth and realization.

> ➢ And if you're open to it, the Universe may call "plot twist" and send you in an expansive new direction. Step into the void and see what arises!

Dancing in the vast field of the fifth element brings forth the requested, sometimes the unexpected, and other times the downright "never thought it could be." We learn to follow the threads down the open trail that leads to our destined path. Or perhaps, a possibility we've never considered presents itself and becomes our newfangled chosen path.

As an author, I check in on Amazon from time to time. One day I noticed an ad at the bottom of one of my book pages that said, "People who like *Turtle Wisdom* love Pacifica Graduate Institute." What! I clicked over to see what this university was about, and found it intriguing. I signed up for Pacifica's snail mail and email newsletters.

Several months later, I received an official email offering a small number of scholarships for their spring session. "Well, I'm not going back to school," the words audibly escaped my mouth. But an odd thing happened: I soon filled out the application, including an essay, and submitted it with a $50 application fee. It was as if I was on autopilot.

They graciously accepted me, offering the maximum scholarship amount available, and to my complete surprise, I returned to school after a twenty-nine-year hiatus. Wow! Honestly, this had not been on my personal radar.

And that master's degree literally changed my life, as I wrote about my story of childhood wounding partnered with in-depth trauma research for my master's thesis. What eventually followed was the award-winning, internationally published *8 Keys to Wholeness* book and the online transformational journey "8 Essential Keys: Tools for Hope-Filled Healing and Expansive Evolutionary Growth." These are significant pieces of my life's work, the culmination of my personal and professional experience. It was truly meant to be, and it was the direct result of a "coincidental" Google ad!

Drawing from infinite possibility is often like having many pieces already present but needing that one exactly right piece to bring the entire puzzle together. The Spiritual Source knows where that piece is. If we release control and open to greater guidance, it may manifest as better than what we imagined it could be.

There was a time when I was teaching classes in Connecticut and needed to find a suitable meeting space. After writing a list of my needs and desires, I spoke words of acceptance for the highest and best for all concerned. And then I opened to possibilities, as well as letting go of the way my needs could be fulfilled. And it came to pass. I stumbled upon a lovely Catholic retreat center that was a sweet connection for me, having been raised Catholic. The cozy library where I gathered my groups had floor-to-ceiling bookshelves packed with priceless volumes. There were soft, rolling hills with gorgeous flower beds and plush grass for picnicking on our lunch breaks. Comfy benches and a contemplative labyrinth invited us to pause a while in this peaceful garden.

The one piece I couldn't possibly have scripted, because I didn't think to include this idea on my wish list, was that this spiritual center had small rooms with single beds and a desk that could be rented for $12 a night, including breakfast. Because of that unforeseen opportunity, people came from far and wide to attend my events. This experience taught me never to limit what is asked of the Universe because Her vision is so much greater than my own.

The thing about this element of ether, the Great Mystery, is that we can sense it, we can describe it, the ancients believed in it and used its power, and now science has substantiated it, but it's still difficult to comprehensively define or measure. *The Power of Eight* (2018) by scientist Lynne McTaggart documents the expansive possibilities found when groups send energy to the collective without any strings attached, offering support unconditionally. What I love about this material is it demonstrates our value to the Great Mystery. In many traditions, this same idea is echoed: when we selflessly ask for something for another, it holds great merit. A group of us formed a circle of eight (well, it ended up being six) and found that letting go of our own requests or expectations while going into collaborative meditation was remarkably powerful. We saw comforting, expanded visions and, despite putting aside our personal desires, had many of them manifest. It's difficult to say how we had an impact on the collective, but the microversion reflected in our own lives was quite impressive.

Monday, April 26: Weird. I went in . . . and then felt nothing. I had a thought: "I've got too much to do today. Maybe I'm too amped up. I'm going to end early." Got up and went to turn off the music, only to discover that I was five minutes into another CD. I had been in the zone for over twenty minutes. Where was I? In the void!

 Your Write of Passage: Open Space of Uncertainty

I begin with an idea and then it becomes something else.

—Pablo Picasso

There's an enormous space that opens when we let go of the idea that there's one perfect answer or one specific path. How often have you searched for that "right" piece instead of exploring possibilities? When we see with our intuitive insight, we can move beyond human limitations, letting go of the musts and the shoulds and moving into the realm of what might be. By being brave enough to remain in a state of "not knowing" instead of pushing a particular agenda, we make friends with uncertainty and many of our reactive emotions relax, as this attitude and perspective of "let me see what is possible" helps us discover which way we'd like to choose. This approach enables us to appreciate not only the destination, but every step of the journey.

Focus on what's truly important to you, and let extraneous points of control relax. This practice will bring positivity, a belief in your ability to navigate through life, a centeredness, and a comforting peace. Jon Kabat-Zinn, well known for his stress-reduction and meditation work, says: "Mindfulness is about love and loving life. When you cultivate this love, it gives you clarity and compassion for life, and your actions happen in accordance with that." Marianne Williamson adds that "Ego says, 'Once everything falls into place, I'll be at peace.' Spirit says, 'Find your peace, and everything will fall into place.'"

So instead of trying to force a specific agenda into fruition, can you sit and watch the proverbial fruit tree grow? And play in the shade of its growing? And lie down in the grass and watch the leaves twinkle in the wind?

Don't get me wrong, I like getting things done as much as the next person, but I've found it's all too easy to become one of those hamsters on the wheel of life . . . putting forth great effort to run aimlessly round and round. Best to slow it down a bit and open to what might be missed in the haste of life's demands.

> Find a special spot. It may be in your home or your garden or at a park. Focus on where you are at this very moment. Be completely present and mindful of the surroundings outside you.

> Now feel your physical body. Take a soft, gentle breath. Be present in this space and time. Feel your spirit in and through your physical form. Be aware of your body and the distinct personality within that body.

> Become acutely aware of your thoughts.

> Now draw your attention inward. Be fully present to yourself. Notice the richness of your feelings in this moment. Observe what you know to be true . . . and then, move beyond.

> Let your thoughts and your feelings move in and move out, gently, without effort. Focus on your breath: breathe in, breathe out. Now let the breath breathe you. Just be.

GOING NOWHERE

Acclaimed travel journalist and TED talk sensation Pico Iyer says: "In an age of speed, nothing could be more invigorating than going slow. In an age of distraction, nothing could feel more luxurious than paying attention. And in an age of constant movement, nothing is more urgent than sitting still." Although he's logged over 1.5 million air miles, Pico promotes "going nowhere"—by going within. He says the idea of going nowhere is "as universal as the law of gravity;

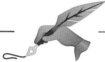

Whoever you are and wherever you are, the most incredible adventure you'll ever have is when you journey within.

that's why wise souls from every tradition have spoken of it." Going nowhere opens us to the space between the thoughts and the potential of the center space where all things meet in the Great Mystery. When we escape the clutter of our everyday world and find a safe haven in the stillness of just "being," we can experience the great mystery firsthand: We become immersed in the inner landscape, learning the contours of who we truly are and the vast potential of what we can experience while in our human suits, and we learn about what's possible long after we leave this Earth plane. Whoever you are and wherever you are, the most incredible adventure you'll ever have is when you journey within. That's been our focus with *As You Feel, So You Heal: A Write of Passage*. In *The Art of Stillness: Adventures of Going Nowhere* (2014), Pico Iyer instructs: "Travel can give you sights, but silence gives you insights. I sit still to find out what moves me the most and what brings me joy, and that is where, for me, true happiness lies."

 ## Write of Passage: Your Sacred Promise (to Yourself)

Just write it down. There's power in that action.

—Donna DeNomme

This is a good time to pause again and take a personal assessment and to look at what this Write of Passage has been like for you and where you'll go from here.

> ➢ What have you learned during our time together? What have you discovered about yourself emotionally? Did your curiosity serve you?

> ➢ How has your emotional process changed? What has been healed? What has been transformed?

> ➢ Have you cultivated a greater acceptance of yourself and life as your sacred path? In what ways have you grown?

➤ Have any avenues of expression opened to you? And do you know and appreciate everything you do as your unique soul creativity?

➤ What needs further refinement?

- -

➤ Do you feel complete? Or is there more to discover? Will you place this inquiry aside or continue with your written exploration of your emotions?

➤ This is a good time to make note of what exactly is your commitment to yourself moving forward. The energy of conscious commitment is a catalyst for healing, change, and growth.

ANCIENT ONES

The Great Mystery includes interdimensional and interspecies communication bringing forth enlightening information. If you're open to the signs and symbols around you, you can learn to speak the language of the soul . . . and the more you open to its musings, the more it will communicate with you in the most fascinating ways:

Many years ago, several of us trekked up the mountain to scatter the ashes of our beloved brother, Bill John. With a ceremonial drum strapped to my back, I climbed over large boulders on the last part of the trail as we hiked up above the mountain tree line. We made a ceremonial circle in a natural basin, anchoring a tall shaman's staff with sacred feathers barely fluttering in the sparse wind of this desolate tundra. We set the intentional altar by speaking words of gratitude for this ceremony of blessing and release for our dear friend. Once preparations were complete, we settled in to begin our honoring ceremony. A lone gray wolf made his way down the short distance of the south wall that cradled the saddle of the basin we were sitting in. . . . I watched as he approached us, and although I'd been crouched on the Earth, intent on the sacred space we were blessing, I slowly rose to my feet as this beautiful animal circled our group, looking intently at each one of us. He looked right in my eyes, which was thrilling, and at the same time, quite intimidating. I felt my heart race. What does he want with us?

Time seemed to stand still. After what seemed like an eternity, and what was most likely a few minutes, he walked away from our small circle, climbing slowly up the steep rise. He looked back at us a time or two and then he called to his pack, and they immediately answered—with beautifully eerie howls echoing toward the lake below, the sound reverberating down the mountain. Mesmerizing! Wolf looked upon our group huddled in prayer, once more, before he crested the peak and disappeared on the other side.

When we returned to base camp, we asked our neighbors if they heard the wolves, and no one had. According to the Department of Wildlife, there were no wolves at that time in Colorado. But the seven of us know what we saw watching our ceremony on the top of the mountain that day. He was most certainly *not* a coyote but a *gray wolf* . . . and I'll never forget the wonder of that sound, the wolf calling to his clan and the pack answering with a harmonious symphony of wilderness sound. A compelling "coincidence" is that Bill John's strongest alliance was the wolf—and we most certainly saw and heard wolf that day. Goodbye, dear brother. Until we meet again.

Even if you aren't aware of this ethereal realm and if you aren't keen to its subtle messages, it will get your attention when need be:

Dazed. I'm physically and emotionally exhausted from a grueling schedule of double shifts at the all-night diner, while caring by day for an active nine-month-old wonder child with an almost insatiable curiosity. It's five forty-five in the morning, and I'm walking the few short blocks to pick up my young son from the sitter. I worked through the night, desperately trying to make enough tip money to pay a few daunting bills.

My husband is no help. Bill's focus is wholehearted partying while flirting with young women in an effort to prove his manhood. Last week, I had to wrap my baby in a kitchen towel and leave him with the next-door neighbor while looking for my wandering husband, whom I'd sent to buy Pampers. I found the undelivered diaper box in the Better Days Pub, sitting next to his almost-empty beer. Bill was nowhere in sight until I heard him playfully calling out to another woman when he emerged from the toilet. He had no idea his wife was in the room.

Bill's in jail. He got in a fight several nights back and broke a man's leg, so he was charged with aggravated assault. That was the same night my "prince" rode down the main street of our small town with a shotgun between the handlebars of his motorcycle. Bill's a gem. I struck it rich when I fell for this one. Well, young and foolish, as they say. At least we have Michael. My boy is beautiful and smart beyond his meager months, already way ahead of the developmental curve. I delight in watching him grow and change as every day brings a new discovery. Life is a thrilling adventure as I see it reflected in my young son's eyes.

Still, in this moment, I'm physically and emotionally wrung out. Life's one big challenge, and I'm weary from the weight of it all as I shuffle zombielike through the deserted street with its abandoned stores darkened for the night's rest. It'll be hours before they reopen for business. Shoppers are snug in their comfy homes, soon to awaken to a warm, family breakfast; my heart aches for the normalcy of such simple things. Turning left, I head down 8th to continue the two short blocks to the sitter's house. I'm grateful that I have someone willing to watch my baby through the night.

I shuffle along, mesmerized by the movement and sound of my feet hitting the pavement, deep in thought about nothing in particular. I'm moving in a mindless trance. I appear to be there, but my mind has gone asleep days ago—tired of the constant struggle to understand how I ended up in this little hick town with a womanizing, alcoholic husband and a small child. I've always been a smart girl. What happened to my common sense?

Lifting my right foot a little higher to clear a thick black rod, I notice the contrast of wood beneath me as I pull my left foot to join its sister. In front is another black rod. Perched atop a small incline with an elevated view of what's ahead, I glance over at the solitary white cottage tucked in the "V" of Summer and Vine. I'll be there in minutes, and then I can take my Michael home.

A loud noise summons me from my waking sleep, causing a natural reflex to automatically jerk my head to the right in the direction of the sound. A magnificent black form looms close by, radiantly glowing in the reflective light of the just-rising sun, still soft and low in the sky. "Hoonnnkk, Hoonnnkk!" the sound comes from the black form. I have no idea what is happening, no sense of where I am or what is heading right for me. All I can think about is how strikingly beautiful the image is—it looks like something right out of a picture book! I stand mindlessly still, just watching the form move closer . . . and closer.

A strong, firm hand presses against the middle of my back, between my shoulder blades and right behind my heart. "Honk, Honk! . . . Honk, Honk!" The sound is closer and more frequent, urgently pleading. I feel the hand push stronger, sinking into my flesh as it pushes me forward and my feet mindlessly follow suit. "Honk, Honk! Honk, Honk! HOOOOOOOOOOOOOOOOOOONK, HOOOOOOOOOOOOOONK!"

I clear the thick black rod and the rush of the close-at-hand train flattens me on the gray gravel next to the track when I fall to the ground, knocked over by the substantial force of that huge form moving past me at great speed. I lie still for a moment, as the delayed reality of what just happened mixes with the rough gravel beneath me. "Oh, my God, that was a TRAIN! I almost got hit by a train!" I look around but see no one. When the train completely passes, I look on the other side of the tracks, and no one's there either, and I wonder, who could push me over the tracks with such a steady hand behind me, yet not be hit by the train themselves? The close-by train literally took me to the ground with its fierce force.

Then reality hit me with as much impact as that big black engine. With all my family troubles and the state of my messed-up life, common knowledge in this small town, if I had been taken out by that train, people would say I threw myself on those tracks. The conductor would confirm that he repeatedly sounded the horn and I just stared at him, refusing to move. I would have abandoned my young son with a missed opportunity to change our life course. He would never have known that he was enough to encourage me to keep going no matter how rough things got, to keep moving so I could get us out of this caustic place. "Oh, no, there has to be more than this," I thought, tears running down my flushed cheeks.

My mind now fully functional, I realized the only explanation was that a guardian angel was watching over me that early morning and saved my life by pushing me to the other side of those tracks. That jarring experience woke me up in more ways than one. I soon found a program that helped me enroll in community college, graduated first in my class, received a scholarship to Cornell University, and years later went on for my master's degree in psychology. My chosen field enabled me to work with underprivileged and emotionally challenged kids, displaced homemakers, and female felons, as well as many people challenged by their seemingly typical lives. Because of what happened on those tracks that day, I know appearances can be deceiving, and never settle for what's at face value. And I've learned not to judge. What might look horrible from the outside is not necessarily the truth of what's going on inside. Sometimes in the darkest room, you discover the brightest light.

We can trust it'll be all right, even if we're presented with something that seems unbearable or insurmountable. Your support goes far beyond what you can see, so even when you aren't aware of it, there may be an angel or a guide with a strong hand on the back of your heart, encouraging and guiding you forward. Your angels, guides, and helper beings are there for you. The teaching I received as a child said that everyone has one guardian angel watching over us. In my lifetime, I've been blessed to see and feel many of them, my guardian council or the "head office" as I like to call them. Their guidance is priceless to me. They were the saving grace keeping my inner psyche intact while I was being sexually and ritually abused; they literally saved my life when I put myself in physical danger as a rebellious teen, and they've been the consistent motivation that has encouraged and driven my professional mission, illuminating my life's path. I know and believe wholeheartedly that I'm not special in this regard. Having sat with many beautiful souls over decades of service, I know that we all have angels, guides, and helper beings. Some of us just listen more intently or open to receive their inspiration through spiritual practices such as meditation and, yes, sacred journaling.

This is another reason why your Write of Passage is so important—it can open the channel for your helpers to speak to you. We may receive guidance in words, in pictures, or in feelings presenting a powerful vibe, "Like whoa, there may be something here for me." Be hypervigilant for the signs and symbols when they present themselves. Angels and guides are calling you. Will you pick up the line?

TRUSTING SELF, TRUSTING LIFE

My years of study with Native American teachers were particularly precious to me. Their teaching validated ideas I'd always held true, and they introduced me to new kindred perspectives too. One of the most impactful lessons had to do with insecurity. Humans have a tendency toward having feelings of insecurity, and my teacher's response was "Of course, you do! The wingeds fly above with keen sight, mountain lion can move at great speed with fine precision; all the animals carry coats that adapt to the changing seasons, and even the ants know more about cooperation than humans do. No wonder people feel insecure." They taught me it was better to accept my weaknesses, my foibles, and the parts of me still in development, rather than focus on how these parts aren't good enough in the moment.

We learn to trust ourselves. And we learn to trust life. We find ways to let go of any false security that causes us to cling to the shore or hug the ground of what's known, and instead recognize that nothing external can provide that kind of safety for us. At any time, a wave can come by pulling us away from the shore, or the ground can shake with a great tremor, throwing us off-balance. Safety—true safety—only lies within us in our ability to move through the changes of our lives, whatever they may be. When we have confidence in our own ability to adapt, then we can gain security in every step because even the shaky ones have a purpose. You may not have exactly what you need in any given moment, but you can trust in your ability to acquire it. You know it is there. Like looking at the dark side of the moon, you see the potential and know the fullness of light is only hidden from view. You soothe any negative self-talk, replacing it with comforting and encouraging stories. Aligned choices born of your belief and trust in yourself bring forward a life that is healthy, expansive, and abundant.

HONOR YOUR EMOTIONS, HONOR YOURSELF

Cracking the emotional code is really very simple: Reject no part of your emotional self. This simple approach develops emotional intelligence. As I've suggested, draw your emotions to you, look them in the eyes, give them a voice, dialogue with them, and learn from them. When necessary, fashion changes by sculpting and resculpting yourself: wiring and rewiring your emotions. Ultimately, embrace them and integrate them into the wholeness of your being. That is the richness of spiritual alchemy.

Your unique self in all its beautiful nuances is not something to "figure out" and "fix." You are never broken. You are unfolding and evolving into your greater soul self. I call this expanding into your soul creativity. As you've explored your outer expression and your inner landscape, you've learned more about who you truly are . . . and there is still so much more! I encourage you to continue working with the prompts and the processes outlined in *As You Feel, So You Heal*, since they will serve you for many years to come.

 ## Ritual Write of Passage: Marry Your Emotions

I cheated on my fears, broke up with my doubts, got engaged to my faith, and now I'm marrying my Dreams. Soon I will be holding hands with Destiny!
—Eddie A. Rios

In my first book, *Turtle Wisdom: Coming Home to Yourself* (2007), we look at how the most important relationship in your life is the relationship you have with yourself. No matter where you go or what you experience, you are the constant. So, you might as well love the one whose skin you're in! Commit to accept yourself with no excuses and no regrets as you know that you are a masterpiece in the process of being created. If ethereal Great Mystery holds the potential for everything and you are made of that essential "stuff," then you hold great potential too. Spirit is called by many names too numerous to share; regardless of the name you speak with reverence, know that you are born of that Sacred Source. Never lose sight of the wonder of life itself and bring forth the integrity of your highest self. Remember who you are; claim your divine inheritance. Joy N. Hensley says: "You are not a drop in the ocean. You are an ocean in a drop."

Every part of you longs to evolve into who you were meant to be, and as we've seen, emotions can be helpful guideposts. The call of *As You Feel, So You Heal* is to truly see and fully claim yourself. Learn your own love language and nurture true intimacy between all your emotions, so you can embody lasting peace and happiness. In *Solve for Happy: Engineer Your Path to Joy* (2018), Mo Gawdat says: "A device fresh from the factory, set up the way its creators think best, is said to be in its 'default state.' For human beings, simply put, the default state is happiness."

Design a Marriage Ceremony:

> Make an official and sacred commitment with your emotions.

> Choose the setting.

> Decide what things will help set a sacred space; create an altar.

> Whom would you like to witness this event?

> Write your vows.

> If you choose, perform this wedding privately or with one or more guests.

Your vision will become clear only when you can look into your own heart. Who looks outside, dreams. Who looks inside, awakes.

—Carl Jung

SHAPE-SHIFTING: POWERFUL PERSONAL TRANSFORMATION

I danced with my shadows until they became part of my light.

—Jodi Livon

We are being called to transform our icky sludge into something useful—to use our wounding, our suffering, and our pain as new potential. Healing is recognizing the part of us that is always well, realizing the truth of our core nature or our soul essence. Within the ethereal realm of infinite potential, we can also ask "What's missing?" and grab ahold of untapped fibers of our being. It isn't as simple as speaking it into existence; yet, I've seen miracles come to those who are able to imagine the possibility of what may seem impossible. A basic shamanic principle focuses on creating the desired container, so the Divine Creative Force can fill it in. "If you build it, [they] will come" is a message that can season the space for your own field of dreams.

We are at a pivotal point in our human evolution, one in which we can expand our ability to shape and reshape who we are and to maturely sculpt our future from a place of conscious choice. We can no longer be at the mercy of what life gives us. We cannot allow ourselves to feel trapped within our own skin, prisoners to the human condition. Rather, we must be empowered to create the life we envision and to manifest our dreams. We possess the potential for shifting into a dynamic way of being, if we can recognize our personal responsibility for how we are living and our ability to successfully affect change in our own life and beyond.

There is inherent good that seeks a path of expression through you. Explore the great unknown and live in a way which brings forth a planet that we have never seen, a reality we have only glimpsed, and a future bright with potential. If you want to experience what you have always experienced, keep doing what you have been doing. If you can envision a grander scheme, shapeshift! (*Turtle Wisdom: Coming Home to Yourself*, 2007)

It is an honor to connect with you through these pages, and I feel your presence as you read my words. We live in an exciting and pivotal time. What we each do in our individual lives affects not only those around us, but our entire planet. Our personal process serves as an energetic purifier for the collective energy. As we heal ourselves, that healing energy spills over and affects our world. And as we face our emotions, and our emotional pain, we can better notice the sorrow all around us; our emotional and spiritual maturity enables us to be brave as we gaze into the face of what's happening in our world.

Will you step up to the call? As you feel, so you heal—and then your healing ripples forth as you, too, become the healer who is a light unto others. Know your worthiness, know your ability, know the power of your actions, and believe that the time has come.

EXPANSIVE EVOLUTION

We cannot solve our problems with the same thinking we used when we created them.

—Albert Einstein

When you actively engage with life in a manner that is co-creative, you will never be hopeless or helpless, because there will always be something you can do to make a positive difference—you can hold the idea that healing and growth are possible even when you don't know the "how." Furthermore, your individual consciousness contributes to the collective consciousness and has the power to help make positive shifts as we collectively evolve. We have a personal responsibility to tend to the soul of the world in whatever way we can; acknowledging the suffering of others and reaching out to help is a sacred and holy act. There's a collective chaos and heaviness in our world and toxic energy rampant in our culture. When I began this book, we had just endured a rapid succession of severe weather tragedies and cataclysmic natural disasters, and on top of that, we had a racially charged shooting, a shooting that turned a concert into a war zone, and number of school shootings. When these devastating events occur, we are often at a loss, but the one thing we can contribute is to hold the high consciousness that things can be different; we can imagine and work toward a better world. We can support each other through the pain and hold the faith that healing will come.

You make a difference. The world can be brighter and more beautiful because of you. Regardless of whether your actions are small or grand, there is a powerful ripple effect. I'm sure you've heard of the Butterfly Principle, where small actions like a butterfly's wings flapping can be shown to have an impact a great distance away. You make a difference. You matter.

THE ADVENTURE OF LIFE'S GREAT MYSTERY

Life reflects our inner state: The key to experiencing a better life is in mastering your thoughts, your beliefs, and your emotions. If we keep trying to fix it "out there," we'll keep spinning in the patterns we've created. James Redfield called it our "control dramas." Be grateful for the growth cycles you have already gone through (think about where you were five or ten years ago), be grateful for where you are now and all that you're doing to grow into a better way of being, and be grateful for what lies ahead.

In this final stage of our initiation, we open to the greater-yet-to-be within the Great Mystery of Life, and at the same time we draw forth the lessons we've learned from our sacred trek within, as we integrate those insights into our wholeness of self and share them with others as our contribution to the collective whole. Our journey has included a focus on the elements that we've observed in relation to the shapes and forms of our emotions. The Earth may appear as a lush green meadow with wildflowers speckling its belly, or a vast, dry dessert with prickly cactus stretching toward brilliant stars shining in a dark night sky. Fire can be a warm candle's glow or a raging wildfire out of control. In the gurgling of a crisp mountain stream or the reflection of a still lake, we find Water; the warm Caribbean salt water holds our body as we float lazily on a delightful vacation day. The Air all around us wisps in a gentle breeze or gusts of hurricane force or tornado speed. The elements can be gentle or strong, welcomed or a challenge, just like our emotions. They are precious allies for helping us understand and come to peace with our natural and necessary emotional expressions.

You can draw further strength and support from your spiritual helpers, mentors, and guides from every direction and every kingdom, and most certainly you can draw sustenance from the Spiritual Source Itself. Life is created through the intangible Great Mystery, and yet, like that drop that never ceases to be ocean water no matter how far it's taken away from the shore, we are spiritual beings at our core. And that spiritual essence expresses in and through all we are and all we do. Each human being makes an impact, each one significant. As we observe the richness of life all around us, perhaps it becomes easier to see the value of our changing emotional terrain too. When we cultivate acceptance of our precious emotional selves and open to the understanding of those emotions, we truly embrace a significant part of our humanity. And by being more present to what it is to be human, we remember what it is to be divine.

1. RELEASE TO THE ETHER

Sometimes letting go means deciding not to struggle to be understood or to understand. When it's futile to process or negotiate any further, you may want to release the challenge or the relationship to the element of ether. By realizing and accepting that any further change is beyond your control, surrendering to the unknown or untapped potential can be an empowering act. When you've already done everything you can possibly do, let go of the struggle . . . and just let it be.

affirm again:
I heal the past, am mindful in the present, and envision my bright future.

2. COMING HOME TO YOURSELF: THE POWER OF SELF-REFLECTION

Taking time each day to witness our own feelings—whatever they are—is the foundation of self-love. And we can only connect with others to the depth that we are willing to connect with ourselves.

—Jessica Moore

Continue to deepen your understanding of yourself through writing and creative imaging to vision what more is possible. Where could you go from here?

3. CREATING THE STORY OF YOUR LIFE: FALL MORE IN LOVE EACH DAY

If you imagine that through your thoughts and actions you are creating life, and that with all your experiences you are writing the story of your life, why would you let someone else dictate the lines, choose the paper, or move your pen? Take full personal responsibility; be mindfully engaged and attentively present. Write on the line, above or below it, or decide to use paper without any lines. Choose white paper, black paper, or paper of every color of the rainbow. Would it be better for you to write in pencil, with the luxury of being able to erase, or are you brave enough to "write" your life in permanent ink—recognizing you can always shape and reshape your words, your thoughts, and your actions to be in clearer alignment with your highest self.

Awaken with appreciation for each day as you imagine what's possible. The ancient Greek philosopher Pythagoras was the first to profess the idea that we ought to guard the initial moments of our day, because the ideas we hold and the company we keep at that receptive time of the morning seeds the creation of the rest of that day. Wake up grouchy and resistant and you'll have an uphill climb; rise with the promise of today and magnetize hopeful success. We can be better served by being purposefully positive and believing in the potential of all our days. Live life with emotional zest and mindful participation, choosing your focus consciously and knowing that whatever the outcome, your life is your own. Do it your way!

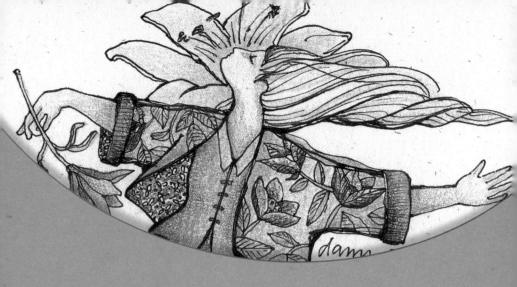

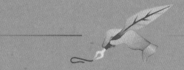

BECOMING AND EXPRESSING
WHO YOU'RE MEANT TO BE
IS LIFE'S PROMISE!

BE MORE,
HAVE MORE,
SHARE MORE OF YOUR TRUEST SELF.
WHY? BECAUSE YOU CAN.

FINAL BLESSING

ACCEPTANCE FOR THE HUMAN SELF

You could call it a glass half empty or a glass half full; if you focus on what you don't have, you'll be unhappy with what you've missed, but if you focus on what you do have, you'll fill your cup to overflowing with appreciation and gratitude.

—Donna DeNomme

We aren't born with nasty inner voices telling us we're unworthy or incapable. A baby doesn't question her cry because she doesn't like the sound of it; nor does she resist her smile because she's comparing it to the one next to her. In our youngest state, we accept who we are . . . until the world reflects something else or we're taught differently. We had a beautifully pure emotional openness and sincerity. We cried when we needed something and smiled when we were happy. Negative self-talk is learned behavior, internalized with a destructive time bomb just ticking away.

I walked past the nursery on my way to Weston's room to put away an armful of toys we'd just finished playing with—in my nanny position, I'm paid to play. This job was the perfect solution to my inner urgings to be around young ones again: I found a loving family who needed help with their children instead of having another one of my own.

The new baby was brought home this week, and I glance in on her as I'm passing by. Grandma cradles the little pink bundle in her arms, rocking gently back and forth in the strong wooden chair. I hear the tracks moving along the carpet with a subtle, "whoosh, whoosh," a comforting and somewhat timeless sound of a grandma rocking; the perfect accompaniment to her cooing voice: "We waited for you for so long. Do you know how precious you are? You are the most special girl in the whole wide world . . . and we are so happy you are finally here." Grandma nuzzles the little one's cheek with a soft "I love you" and a sweet kiss.

What a dear sight I witnessed that day. Not all of us are lucky enough to be born into a loving and attentive family; not all of us had emotionally available parents and grandparents. If you did not experience that kind of childhood, I want to say that you are a blessing to this world . . . and without you, our world would not be complete. "We waited for you for so long" is true even if it was never spoken to you.

Your life is an opportunity to get to know and love your uniquely precious self and to come to believe in the healing power and potential of the Great Mystery. Accept yourself, in this moment, as the one who has conscious choice and dominion over your own destiny, and choose a path of tenderness, compassion, acceptance, understanding, and love. Believe you can manifest those qualities in and through you and you can also attract those qualities through others. Allow the divine flow of spirit to move positively through the creation of your life.

affirm

I am a worthwhile person. I am blossoming every day into more of who I truly am . . . all I do is significant for my growth. I am lovable. And I am uniquely precious.

YOUR SACRED WRITE OF PASSAGE

Buckminster Fuller, during a pivotal heart-to-heart talk with himself when he was on the edge of despair and self-destruction, said, "You do not have the right to eliminate yourself. You do not belong to you. You belong to the Universe." Then he made a bargain to search and "discover the principles operative in the universe and turn them over to my fellow man." He recognized the responsibility to show up as fully as he could in pursuit of a life that would benefit not only himself but the greater good.

There is so much more to us human beings than what we are now portraying— and there is so much more to you too. Through the Heroine's journey, you can move past seeming limitations and venture out into the world (and inside yourself) to bring back priceless treasure.

Like a mountaineer, you meander through open fields with your eye on the mountain ahead; you traverse steep trails, picking your way over rocky overhangs and stepping mindfully across narrow passages so you can summit the peak for a clear view. Like a miner, you sift through the dark earth, excavating priceless gems, and like a gardener, you cultivate a beautiful bed of roses and a back field of wildflowers, appreciating the tenderness and the resilience of both.

Your most important trek is the one within your own inner wilderness to face the trials and tribulations of the dragons and the demons hiding there, to cross the most-treacherous moats stocked with snapping alligators, being brave enough to push through anything that stands in your way, as you clutch the keys to the darkest dungeons where you'll release weary prisoners who've given up hope of ever again dancing in the light. Along the way, you discover archetypal patterns that have been repeated over and over, and you break the magic spell that has held you captive to their control dramas. You choose new, healthier patterns of being and banish all darkness from the past to the land of transformation and healing; defense modes thereby released, for their time has expired and their duties fulfilled. And along the way, you discover the greatest treasure—precious gold held within you. Some of it is the result of the alchemical process of healing your wounds and spinning its heavy, dense material into something of great and lasting value.

Be grateful and bless your path, all of it, and know that no matter what, you are held in the loving arms of your guardians, guides, and helper beings and that you are protected. Fill your inner reserves of peace, love, and happiness . . . and know that to feel whole, you must be at peace with your emotions. Finding that peace comes from embracing rather than denying them and coming to terms with them even on your messiest day, when your eyes are leaking and your nose is running, even when you're feeling such anger that there's steam escaping from your ears! Being emotionally healthy means being okay with your human feelings, no matter what, and finding ways of support, guidance, and management so you can navigate the sometimes-treacherous pathway through to the other side. It's about knowing that your inner core is so strong and resilient that your center is unbreakable.

Praise what is right now in your life and also imagine what else is possible. Envision your wildest success and sweetest happiness built on the foundation of where you are, right here, right now. Set yourself free from any remaining chains of the past, while letting go of your victim self and accepting the role of healer who can tend and heal your own wounds. See the evolving potential of the seed, plant it within the void, and water it with trust and faith. Step up to the truth of your being the one that can contain and be the place of manifestation for the Great Mystery; your emotions are one way you help shape spirit into form. Right now, regardless of what is or is not happening in your life, where could you go from here?

As You Feel, So You Heal celebrates what makes you delightful human and, also, essentially divine. What is your true purpose? Maya Angelou says: "Nothing can dim the light which shines from within." You are here to radiate the beauty of your evolving soul essence through your human experiences and to create Heaven here on Earth. Call in the Light . . . and know it's waiting to shine through you. Right now, in this moment, know you are blessed. And know you are the blessing.

Though we travel the world over to find the beautiful, we must carry it with us or we find it not.

—Ralph Waldo Emerson

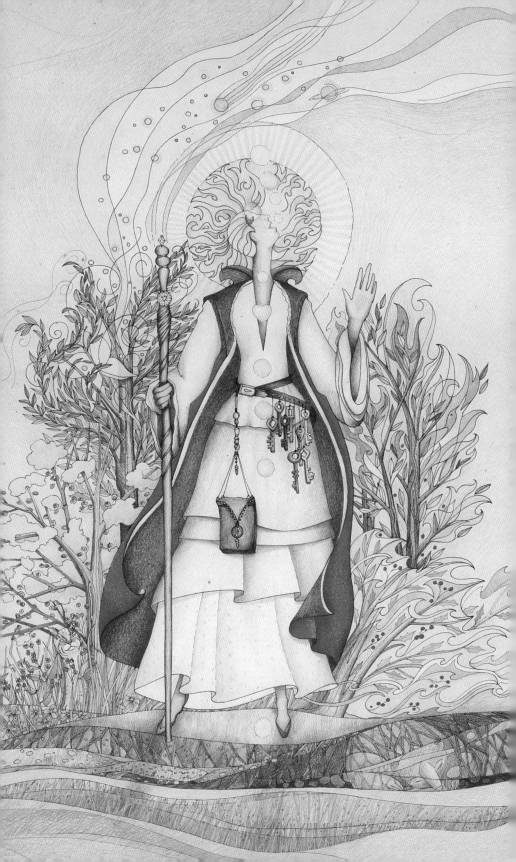

ACKNOWLEDGMENTS

The inspiration for a "Write of Passage" series has been present within me for a very long time. *As You Feel, So You Heal* is the culmination of many incarnations, refined through interactions with clients and students in sessions, classes, workshops, and retreats. Its contents are "tried and true." Some ideas originated in my earlier works and have found further maturity here. I am grateful to all who've contributed—both teachers and students—as all of life is our eternal classroom.

The Hero's Journey (Joseph Campbell) and the Heroine's Journey (Maureen Murdock), as well as studies on initiation (both formal and experiential), are so finely woven into my being that they are truly an integral part of me after many years as a ceremonial creator and facilitator. I bow with humble respect to the great teachers of these timeless sacred practices.

Thank you to Kent Rautenstraus who first introduced me to Pico Iyer through his article "Your Next Exclusive Destination: Nowhere" in the February 2018 *Science of Mind Magazine.*

Dianne Fresquez, you are so dear to me, and I love how you have an uncanny knack for seeing what I've somehow missed and broadening my perspective. And to Coleen Hampf, Tina Proctor, and Hollie McIntire—my besties—thanks for reading earlier versions of this manuscript. Sherry Ray, my confidant. Sweet ones, I am honored to share so many adventures with you!

With sincere appreciation to Christopher McClure for your belief in this project, all the wonderful folks at Schiffer Red Feather for your support, and especially to Dinah Roseberry, my editor, whose patient guidance has been invaluable.

Thank you to those who willingly shared their personal stories to highlight and deepen our understanding of this Write of Passage. Some are clients, or compilations of clients; others are friends. Many of the names have been changed to protect their privacy.

This work is heavily influenced by my background in traditional and depth psychology, and I am grateful for the exceptional training I received from Cornell University and Pacifica Graduate Institute.

I acknowledge, with deep appreciation and great respect, many years of conscious energy practice and shamanic wisdom study through several Native American, Peruvian, and Mayan lineages, most especially the Moonwalker Lineage. Special thanks to Tu Moonwalker and Lané Saan Moonwalker. And to my Guardian Council of Light and the natural world that supports me from every direction and every kingdom on this dear planet—you bring meaning and purpose to everything I experience. I am truly blessed with such a strong and supportive team. You are my precious North Star.

And heartfelt thanks to

Susan Andra Lion, the illustrator of this (and most) of my books.

Sue is a fine artist and inspired illustrator whose work has been displayed in many galleries and exclusive shows. Her visual images collaborate with my words in a way that reflects a connection only a soul sister can know. Sue believes imagination and creativity are keys to opening a peaceful and personally productive space inside of us—a space that brings light to a sometimes difficult and dark, yet receptive world. She is the author and illustrator of her own books, most recently *Night Threads: A Weaving of Soul Stories from the Dreamtime.* Sue lives with her cat, Tucker, and an abundance of wild life around her home in the foothills of the Colorado mountains.

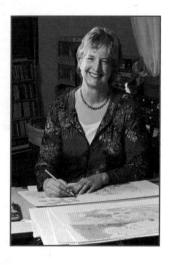

www.suelion.com

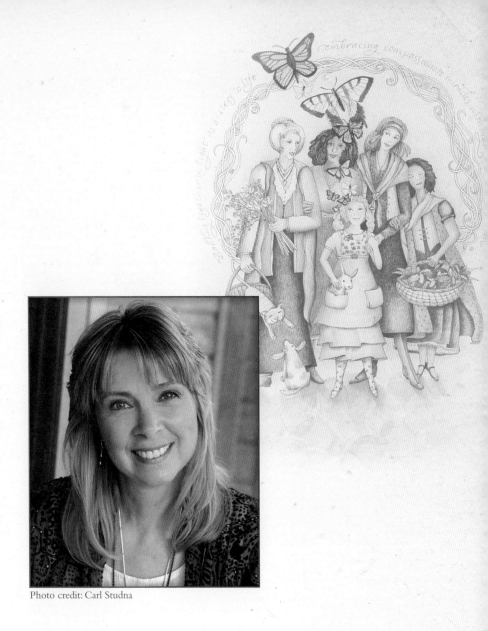

Photo credit: Carl Studna

DONNA DENOMME, MA, is an award-winning, internationally published author of self-help and motivational books. With a background in traditional and depth psychology, rites of passage, and ceremonial traditions, she recognizes that ceremonies give us a deeper understanding of self, as well as a sense of security, belonging, and purpose. Donna was voted Colorado's "Spiritual Health Guru" by the prestigious *5280 Magazine* for her unique combination of innovative therapeutic and self-realization techniques. She has been a Master Success Coach in private practice since 1987.

"How often we try to control feelings we don't like, yet they have a life of their own. In *As You Feel So You Heal*, author Donna DeNomme takes you on a powerful journey through hidden, sabotaging feelings to uncover your sweet spot of deeply knowing you are more than enough! If you are ready to have what you want, this book is for you. I highly recommend."

—Deborah Sandella PhD, RN, #1 International Bestselling author of *Goodbye Hurt & Pain, 7 Simple Steps to Health, Love and Success*

"Accessing a new cycle or setting out on a new adventure? Check out this book of timeless wisdom! Intuitive empath, life coach, and spiritual sherpa, Donna DeNomme, offers a compassionate insider's guide to self-discovery. *As You Feel, So You Heal* poses probing questions that ask you to explore the deep and varied terrain of human emotions, enabling you to access your inner compass, in order for you to achieve a life of success, joy, and bounty."

—Renee Baribeau, Hay House author *Winds of Spirit: Ancient Wisdom Tools for Navigating Relationships, Health, and the Divine*